Functional Anatomy and Physiology for Emergency Care in the Streets

Functional Anatomy and Physiology for Emergency Care in the Streets

JOSHUA S. YAMAMOTO, M.D., EMT-P

Fellow, Department of Medicine,
Johns Hopkins University School of Medicine;
House Officer, Osler Medical Service,
Johns Hopkins Hospital, Baltimore

STEPHEN A. BRADA, M.D.

Resident Physician, Department of Anesthesiology,
University of Utah Medical Center,
Salt Lake City

Little, Brown and Company
Boston New York Toronto London

Library of Congress Cataloging-in-Publication Data

Yamamoto, Joshua S.
    Functional anatomy and physiology for emergency care in the
streets / Joshua S. Yamamoto, Stephen A. Brada.
        p.   cm.
    Includes bibliographical references and index.
    ISBN 0-316-96726-2
    1. Human anatomy. 2. Human physiology. 3. Wounds and injuries.
4. Physiology, Pathological. 5. Emergency medical technicians.
I. Brada, Stephen A.
    [DNLM: 1. Anatomy—handbooks. 2. Anatomy—terminology.
3. Physiology—handbooks. 4. Emergency Medical Services—methods.
QS 39 Y19d]
QM23.2.Y36 1995
612—dc20
DNLM/DLC
for Library of Congress   95-22329
                                                       CIP

Printed in the United States of America
MV-NY

Editorial: Evan R. Schnittman, Robert J. Stuart
Editorial and Production Services: Silverchair Science + Communications
Designer: Thane Kerner
Cover Designer: Linda D. Willis

To Morag

And isn't it a terrible thing to find yourself in the presence of a serious accident, to see blood flowing in large streams from a gaping wound, death approaching with each shower that spurts up, and not to know how to behave in order to prevent the imminent danger?

—Dr. Frédéric von Esmarch
*First Aid to Be Given in Case
of Accidents Suffered*, 1897

All bleeding stops . . . eventually.

—Anonymous

Contents

To the Instructor

The goal of this textbook is to provide emergency medicine students with a useful framework for learning and understanding anatomy and physiology. Every act that an emergency medical technician (EMT) or paramedic performs is based on human form and function and, more specifically, how that form and function can be damaged or diseased. The more the EMT or paramedic understands about the human body and its functions, the better prepared he or she will be to treat the prehospital patient. Any experienced EMT knows that a "cookbook recipe" is not always a sufficient guide for treatment. The rules for emergency care in the streets are different from those that apply in well-lit, warm, dry, hospital wards; however, in both cases, the need to know and understand anatomy and physiology is constant.

However, anatomists do not necessarily make good EMTs or paramedics. Anatomy and physiology are important to an EMT or paramedic only in terms of what he or she will be confronted with in the field. The emphasis of this book, therefore, is *functional* anatomy and physiology. All information presented is done so in terms of what EMTs and paramedics need to know to work most effectively.

A conscious effort was made to omit minute details that are not clinically important. For example, no paramedic ever needed to identify the origin and insertion of the flexor digiti minimi muscle, but paramedics should *understand* the circulatory pathway of blood through the heart, why left-sided heart failure leads to pulmonary edema, and how to treat it, without mindlessly memorizing lists of information.

Each chapter presents anatomy, normal function, and abnormal function or injury in that basic order. The diagrams are related specifically to the text and emphasize only the most important details so that students are not lost in a sea of labels; specific anatomical terms are important to the EMT or paramedic only insofar as they are used to communicate information. An effort was also made to keep the medical vocabulary as simple and practical as possible. Anyone should be able to read this book without relying on a medical dictionary. When a name or term is important enough to remember, it appears in **bold** type. All bold terms are redefined in the vocabulary list at the end of each chapter, and again in the glossary, which appears at the end of the book. Terms in *italics* are of conceptual importance but are less important to memorize.

The clinical correlations are perhaps the most important part of the text. Whenever something has a clinical correlation, it is worth knowing and makes anatomy and physiology easier to remember. This entire text is designed to support clinical correlations. They are clearly marked and can be read by themselves, with the text, or not at all.

This book will be most beneficial to EMTs on their way to becoming paramedics. Essentially, this book is everything I wished I had known as an EMT student, a paramedic student, a working paramedic, and an EMT/paramedic instructor. It can be used either in a formal course on anatomy and physiology or in any EMT or paramedic course. It will make an ideal companion to Nancy Caroline's *Emergency Care in the Streets*, Fifth Edition, also published by Little, Brown, and other EMT and paramedic textbooks. The book also will be a valuable reference for experienced providers and would be an appropriate addition to a station house library.

Any errors or oversights in this text hopefully are intentional omissions I made for the sake of simplicity. I welcome all comments and criticisms.

J.S.Y.

To the Student

This book is designed to meet the needs of the prehospital worker at each level of training but is probably best used by those studying to become paramedics. A few general principles hold throughout the text. Any term in **bold** is a term you should probably know. Every bold word is defined both in the vocabulary section at the end of each chapter and in the glossary at the end of the book. A term in *italics* is not something you must memorize, but the concept presented is important. Clinical correlations are set off from the text and emphasize how the material discussed directly affects your work. This book is not intended to be an exhaustive discussion of anatomy and physiology; rather, it addresses only the essential information emergency medical service (EMS) personnel must know and understand.

FOR THE BEGINNING PARAMEDIC OR ADVANCED LIFE SUPPORT STUDENT

Try to read the section of this book that pertains to the material you are covering in class; do this before your lectures if possible. This will give you time to digest material before you have a chance to discuss it with your instructor. Don't try to read the book from cover to cover, unless you're good at that sort of thing. When you first begin your training, you are not expected to know everything, but the more you understand about how things work, the easier your training will be. Another key is vocabulary. Learning medicine is a lot like learning a foreign language. Make sure you *understand* all of the bold terms. Don't just memorize them—dictionaries make poor paramedics.

FOR THE EXPERIENCED PROVIDER

Whether you are certified for advanced life support (ALS) or basic life support (BLS), this book will be a valuable reference—it is not just a textbook for new students. Review a subject in the book that interests you or a subject you always wanted to know more about. On your next call, see how many things you can ask "why" about. Even the most routine calls elicit many questions. Look up the answers. Better yet, if you have a rookie working with you, have him or her look up the answers and explain them to you.

FOR PEOPLE WITH LIMITED READING TIME

Go through the book reading only the clinical correlations and figures. If there is something that strikes you as odd or new, try reviewing that section for more details.

Acknowledgments

There is an old adage that states, "If you want to get something done, ask a busy person." Well, a great many busy people helped in the creation of this book. Thanks to:

Dr. Heinz Valtin, without whose guidance this book would never have been written or published;

Tom Manning, for making it happen;

Rob Stuart and the Medical Books Department at Little, Brown, for putting it all together;

Dr. Jim Bell, personal mentor and friend, who not only did a lion's share of review work but also helped us define our careers;

Drs. William Boyle, Nicholas Ferrintino, Katherine Little, Harold Manning, David Schloesser, and William Young, all of Dartmouth-Hitchcock Medical Center, who graciously gave their time and talent to the preparation of this text;

Denny Kurogi, EMT-P, and Ray Wright, EMT-P, of Johnson County Community College in Shawnee Mission, Kansas, for their review of the manuscript;

Margaret Satchell, M.D., who could always give up medicine to be a full-time photographer;

Scott Brown, Susan Chi, Tisha Gallanter, M.D., Timothy Horita, Charles King, M.D., Anne-Marie Lemal, Travis Marl, Charles Owyang, Lucille Vega, and Michael and Zachary Yamamoto, for modeling for the text.

J.S.Y.
S.A.B.

I would also like to thank the following:

Dartmouth Medical School and its faculty and staff, to whom we will always be in debt (in more ways than one);

The Alexandria, Virginia, Fire Department, for the opportunity to work, serve, and learn;

xvi

Nancy Caroline, whose work inspired me to
   pursue medicine in the first place; and
Chip and B.J., my old partners, and two of
   the best paramedics I have ever known.

J.S.Y.

Functional Anatomy and Physiology for Emergency Care in the Streets

1

Terminology

Comedian Steve Martin once joked about his recent trip to Paris, "*Chapeau* means hat. *Oeuf* means egg. It's like those French have a different word for everything!" So it is true for medicine as well. It often is said that learning medicine is like learning a foreign language. There is nothing about the body that cannot be expressed by a fancy "medicalese" term. At first, the use of a long Greek-sounding word for an otherwise simple-sounding term seems outrageous, but there are reasons to do it. The most important reason is that the use of appropriate medical terminology allows you to communicate clearly, concisely, and unambiguously to other medical professionals. Terminology also provides a common reference point, or framework, for learning medicine.

For example, terms like *up* and *down* seem clear and simple. But imagine a patient lying facedown in a ditch. If you tell someone to "go up" on the patient, what do you mean? Up out

of the ditch? Up toward the patient's head? Up toward the patient's feet? Suddenly, common sense terms become cloudy, and you risk horribly miscommunicating. The right words at the right times will make your meaning clear to everyone.

This chapter sets the framework for communication about anatomy and physiology. Again, medical terms are not used for the sake of sounding important. Medical terms are used for clarity. Throughout this book, any word in **bold** is a term that you should be familiar with.

PLANES OF THE BODY

The first order of business is to establish a starting point or posture for describing relations between body parts—the **anatomical position**. The body in anatomical position is just as Leonardo da Vinci drew it hundreds of years ago: standing upright, arms comfortably

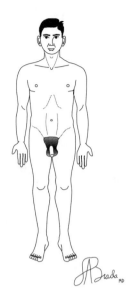

Fig. 1-1. Anatomical position.

at the sides, palms open and facing forward (Fig. 1-1). Now that we have a starting point, we can begin to divide the body into parts by passing three imaginary planes through it.

Transverse Plane

Imagine that the first plane, the **transverse plane** (Fig. 1-2), passes through the body parallel to the ground, dividing the body into top and bottom segments. The upper portion of the body, above the plane, is referred to as **superior** and the lower portion, below the plane, as **inferior**. *Superior* always means "toward the head" and *inferior* means "toward the feet," regardless of how the patient is lying. Superior and inferior can replace the terms *above* and *below*, which are confusing if the patient is not standing.

A commonly used transverse plane is the so-called nipple line passing through both nipples. For example:

The shoulders are *superior* to the nipple line.
The navel is *inferior* to the nipple line.
The shoulders are *superior* to the navel.
The navel is *inferior* to the shoulders.

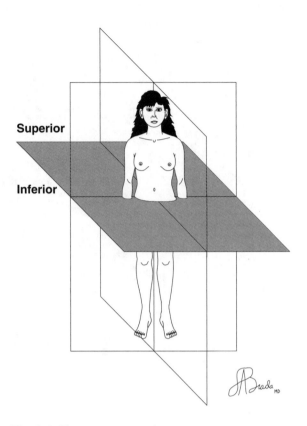

Fig. 1-2. The transverse plane.

Frontal Plane

The second plane, called the **frontal plane**, extends vertically from floor to ceiling and from side to side. It is the plane you pass through every time you walk through a doorway, and it divides you into front and back portions (Fig. 1-3). Again, parts of the body can be described in reference to this frontal plane. You can call the front portion of the body **anterior** (or **ventral**) and the back part of the body **posterior** (or **dorsal**, like the *dorsal fin* on a shark's back). One example of a frontal plane is the midaxillary line, which divides the patient into ventral and dorsal by passing through the middle of the axilla (armpit). For example:

The breasts are *anterior/ventral* to the midaxillary line.
The back is *posterior/dorsal* to the midaxillary line.

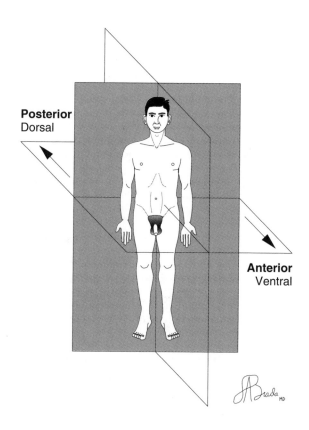

Fig. 1-3. The frontal plane.

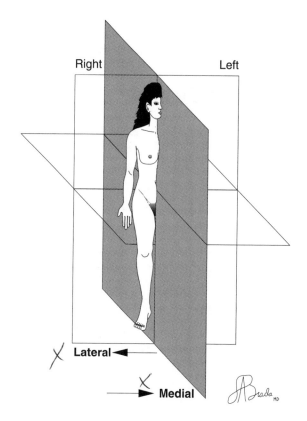

Fig. 1-4. The sagittal plane.

The breasts are *anterior/ventral* to the back. The back is *posterior/dorsal* to the breasts.

Sagittal Plane

The final plane, called the sagittal plane, divides the body into left and right parts (Fig. 1-4). Also, because the human body is symmetric on either side of the sagittal plane (at least on the outside), one special plane, the **midsagittal**, divides the body exactly in half from the top of the head to the crotch. This makes an excellent landmark for describing locations, as in "5 cm left of the midsagittal line." It is also a break for us, because there are no words more specific than **left** and **right**. Just remember to refer to the *patient's* left or right rather than your own. It takes some practice when you are facing patients. **"Left" and "right"** *always* **refer to the patient's left and right, not yours!**

Locations around a sagittal plane other than the midsagittal are described as either **lateral** or **medial**. Things that are medial (sounds almost like middle) are closer to the **midline** of the body (the midsagittal line) than the point of reference. Things that are lateral are toward the side of the body (as a *lateral* in football is a sideways pass). Just be careful not to confuse medial with the word **median**, which means actually lying *on* the midline rather than just close to it (like the *median strip* down the middle of a highway).

Emergency medical technicians and paramedics frequently refer to the midclavicular line. It is a sagittal plane that passes through the midpoint of either clavicle (thus, left or right midclavicular line). For example:

The axilla (armpit) is *lateral* to the midclavicular line.
The navel is *medial* to the midclavicular line. It is a *median* structure.

The inner side of the knee is the *medial* side.
The outer side of the knee is the *lateral* side.

POSITION AND MOTION

Extremities

The next set of relations between body parts deals with locations along the length of the arms or legs. When we say something is **proximal**, we mean that it is closer to the point where the extremity attaches to the rest of the body (something in *proximity* means it is close by). That is, something is proximal if it is toward the trunk. Meanwhile, if something is **distal**, it is farther away from the point of attachment, or farther away from the trunk. That is, it is more *distant*. For example:

The elbow is *proximal* to the wrist.
The wrist is *distal* to the elbow.
The knee is *proximal* to the ankle.
The ankle is *distal* to the knee.

Joints

Not all of your patients (that is, probably none) will be in anatomical position when you find them. Short of trying to reposition them (not always in your best interest or theirs), you need terms to describe the position of the joints in the body. People tend to bend at their joints, unless they have suffered major trauma and have bent in other unnatural places. Each of the terms below can have three forms—for example: flex, flex*ed*, and flex*ion*. "To flex" is the act of bending a joint. *Flexed* describes the position of the joint once it is bent, and *flexion* describes the motion of the joint to put it there.

Flexion and Extension

When you **flex** a joint you bend it out of the straight position, as when you flex your elbow. Notice that in anatomical position there are no flexed joints. In a few special cases (the neck, the spine, the wrist, and the hip) the joint can bend in two directions; it can be flexed or extended. Now consider the fetal position. Flexion of all your joints puts you into fetal position, including chin to chest (neck flexion), trunk rolled forward (spinal flexion), knees to chest (hip flexion), and wrists bent bringing the palms toward the arms.

Extension of a joint means that it is straightened out to make the body as long as possible, as when you extend your fingers. Notice that in anatomical position, almost all the joints are extended except the neck, spine, wrist, and hip, which are all in **neutral position**. Extension of the neck and spine tilts the head back and bends you over backward. Extending your hip places your thigh behind you, while extending the wrist brings the back of your hand toward your arm, as when a traffic cop gives you the signal to stop.

Keep in mind that you flex joints by *contracting* muscles. Even though you may be used to saying that you are "flexing" your muscles, you are actually contracting (shortening) them (see Chap. 6). By contracting your biceps you flex your elbow. People commonly say you "flex" your biceps, but they're technically wrong, which can lead to confusion.

Abduction and Adduction

Movement of the limbs laterally away from the midline of the body is called *abduction*. The opposite motion, bringing the limb back toward the midline, is called *adduction* (Fig. 1-5). Remember these by thinking that to *abduct* a person is to take him or her *away*, whereas when you *add* things you bring them *together*. The only joints that can be abducted or adducted are the shoulder, hip, fingers, and, if you are really talented, the toes. Motion at the shoulder or hip moves the entire limb, as shown in Fig. 1-5. When referring to the fin-

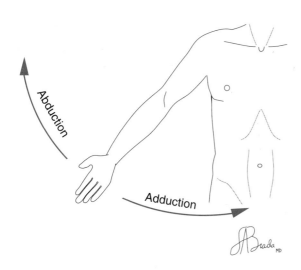

Fig. 1-5. Abduction and adduction at the shoulder.

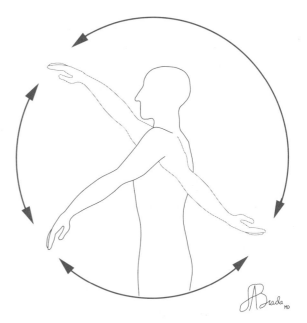

Fig. 1-6. Circumduction at the shoulder.

gers or toes, rather than thinking about the midline of the body, we think about the midline of the hand or foot (the middle finger or toe). Abduction spreads the digits apart. Adduction brings them back together.

Circumduction

The shoulder is the most mobile joint in the body. Not only can it be abducted and adducted, it can also be moved forward and backward in a complete circle. This is called *circumduction* (Fig. 1-6).

Pronation and Supination

The two bones of the forearm (see Chap. 6) rotate about each other at the elbow so that the palm of the hand can face either up or down. Turning the palm up is called *supination*. When the palm faces up it is said to be **supine**. This is also a way to describe the posture of your patient. A patient lying faceup (which would place the palms up in anatomical position) is said to be supine as well. You might want to remember this by thinking of the word *supplication*, another word for begging, which you do by holding your hand out with the palm up. Or you might want to think

of the famous scene from *Oliver Twist* when Oliver holds up his bowl in the soup line and says, "Please, sir, may I have some more?" He is *supinating* in order to *supplicate*. (Soup line...supine. Get it? Sure, it's corny, but you'll never forget it.)

The opposite of supination is *pronation*. When either the palms are turned down or the patient is lying facedown they are **prone**. You can think of firing a rifle from the prone position. You are lying facedown to shoot; no one fires a rifle lying faceup.

Internal and External Rotation

The last six motions deal specifically with the lower leg and foot. *Internal rotation* is rotation of the two bones of the lower leg to turn the toes inward toward the midline of the body. *External rotation* turns them back out.

Plantar Flexion and Dorsiflexion

These two may be confusing. *Plantar flexion* bends the ankle so that the toes point down toward the sole of the foot, which is the part you *plant* on the ground. *Dorsiflexion* is the opposite; it flexes the ankle so the foot and toes point up toward the *dorsum* of the foot. Just to be confusing, the dorsum of the foot is the "top" of the foot (even though this is not really on the dorsal surface of the body). The sole, or "bottom" of the foot, is also known as the *plantar* surface.

Inversion and Eversion

Inversion is motion at the ankle to roll the sole of the foot inward so that it faces the midline of the body. *Eversion* turns the sole outward. Inversion and eversion are what sprain ankles.

MEDICAL VOCABULARY

The practice of medicine has a foreign language with its own vocabulary. There *is* a method to the madness of medical vocabulary. Medical terms tend to be divided into three parts: prefixes (which come first), root words, and suffixes (which come last). The combination of prefix-root word-suffix creates a medical term. The idea is that it is quicker to use one long word than a sentence to describe something. The only problem is that the prefixes, root words, and suffixes are all Greek or Latin.

Tables 1-1, 1-2, and 1-3 list some of the more common prefixes, root words, and suffixes. There are many more, but only the ones emphasized in this book are listed. They may seem cumbersome at first, but once learned allow you to use fewer words. For example, rather than saying "inflammation of the liver," you can say "hepatitis." Or, rather than saying "too little fluid in the body causing a decrease in the body's circulating volume of fluid and/or blood," you can simply say "hypovolemic."

Historical note: There is a story behind almost every anatomical name. About 2,000 years ago, the Romans built on the knowledge

Table 1-1. Medical prefixes

Prefix	Meaning
a-, an-	absence of
ante-	before
anti-	against, in opposition to
brady-	slow
e-, ec-, ex-	away from
epi-	outside of, near to
extra-	outside of, not a part of
hypo-	low, too little
hyper-	high, too much
intra-	within
inter-	between
peri-	surrounding
post-	after
sub-	below
super-	above
tachy-	fast

Table 1-2. Medical root words

Root word	Meaning
cardia	heart
cerebro	brain
cutaneo	skin
entero	intestines
gastro	stomach
heme, hemato	blood
hepato	liver
myo	muscle
nephro/reno	kidney
neuro	nervous system
oxia	oxygen
pnea	breathing
pneumo	air
pulmo	lungs
thorax, thoraco	chest
vaso	blood vessels

Table 1-3. Medical suffixes

Suffix	Meaning
-genic	caused by or causing
-itis	inflammation of
-ectomy	surgical removal of
-oma	mass, collection of something
-ostomy	make a hole in
-otomy	to cut into

of the Greeks to assign anatomical names. For example, the temporal bone (which makes up the temples on the head) is derived from the word for *time*. We tend to get gray hair in our temples first—thus showing the effects of age and time. The sacrum, found at the base of the spine, comes from the root word for *sacred*. Because the sacrum is the densest bone in the body, it is the last to decay. Since it is the last to decay, ancient farmers often plowed up old sacrums. Because all of the other bones were gone, the ancients thought that the soul must be kept in it, so they called it the "sacred bone."

Also, Greek soldiers going into battle lined up in rows to form a *phalanx*. Our fingers and toes are called *phalanges* (the plural of phalanx) because they make little rows just like the Greek soldiers. *Tibia,* the shin bone, is Latin for "flute." Romans made flutes out of shinbones (presumably, *horse* shinbones).

VOCABULARY LIST

anatomical position	the common reference point in describing anatomy: standing upright, with the palms facing forward
anterior	the front, or toward the front with respect to a frontal plane
distal	away from the trunk (along an extremity)
dorsal	posterior
extend/extension	straightening out a joint
flex/flexion	bending a joint
frontal plane	a vertical plane separating the front from the back
inferior	toward the feet, referring to the transverse plane
lateral	away from the midline, toward the side
left	the patient's left
medial	toward the midline
median	in the midline
midline	the centerline of the body, defined by the midsagittal plane, separating the body's left from right
midsagittal plane	a sagittal plane down the center of the body, separating the body's left from right
neutral position	neither flexed nor extended (with regard to the neck and back, hips, and wrist)
posterior	the back, or toward the back with respect to a frontal plane
prone	facedown or pronated (palm down)
proximal	toward the trunk (along an extremity)
right	the patient's right
sagittal plane	a vertical plane separating left from right
superior	toward the head, referring to the transverse plane
supine	face up (on your back), or supinated (palm up)
transverse plane	any horizontal plane across the body
ventral	anterior

2

Head, Neck, Spine, and Nervous System

BONES OF THE HEAD

It is useful to think of the bony structure of the head as having two parts: the **cranium** (the case for the brain) and the face. Although the two obviously are connected, it is possible to damage one and not the other. For example, gunshot wounds to the face can be grotesquely disfiguring but leave the cranium and the brain intact. Always remember that the patient's airway is your highest concern.

The adult **cranium** is a fixed, rigid box consisting of the **frontal** bone, paired **parietal** bones, **temporal** bone, and **occipital** bone in the back (Fig. 2-1). Connecting these bones are *suture lines*. By providing a firm shield, the cranium protects the brain. The rigid nature of the bones, however, can be a problem when the brain is injured. When any tissue is injured, it swells. When the brain swells, it is trapped inside the skull and has little place to go. When

this happens we often see a rise in **intracranial pressure,** or pressure inside the cranium, from the swelling brain pressing against it from the inside. An increase in intracranial pressure can cause severe brain dysfunction.

Because the skull is a box, it is important to remember that it has a bottom surface as well. The bottom, or base of the skull, cannot be seen directly from the outside.

CLINICAL CORRELATION *A basilar skull fracture, or fracture of the bottom of the skull, classically will show pooling of blood, or ecchymosis, which looks like bruising, about the mastoid process—known as Battle's sign—or around the orbits—known as "raccoon eyes" (Fig. 2-2).*

In the face, the bony **orbits** protect the eyes. The weak spot of the orbit is the floor, which may be fractured by blunt trauma (getting hit in the face, for instance). In this case, the eye will drop down and the patient's face will appear asymmetric. It has been suggested that

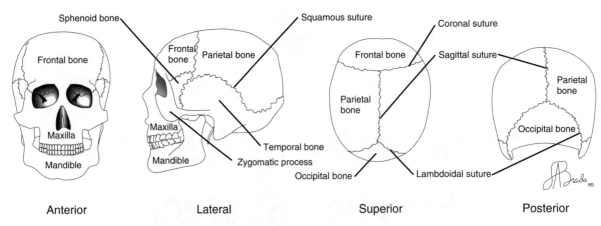

Fig. 2-1. The bones of the adult cranium.

patients with orbital fractures should be kept from sneezing, as this may cause the eye to "pop out."

The **maxilla** is the region below the nose. *Maxillofacial trauma* is a commonly used term to broadly refer to trauma of the face. These fractures are known as *Le Fort fractures*. They can be subclassified depending on the extent of injury.

CLINICAL CORRELATION   *In all head trauma, the greatest problem for the emergency medical technician is airway maintenance. Head trauma is a relative contraindication for the use of nasal airways, either nasopharyngeal or nasotracheal, due to the potential for a basilar skull fracture and inadvertent intubation of the brain.*

The **mandible** is more commonly known as the jaw. Obviously, mandible fracture (a broken jaw) can lead to serious airway problems. Below the mandible, deep in the neck, is the small and obscure *hyoid* bone, which is not attached to any other bone. It helps anchor some of the muscles of the front of the neck and is found above the thyroid cartilage (see below).

AIRWAY ANATOMY

The term airway refers to the entire path air must travel between the outside world and the lungs. *Airway maintenance is the single most*

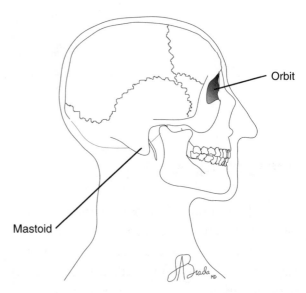

Fig. 2-2. In a basilar skull fracture, blood classically pools about the mastoid and orbits.

important responsibility a prehospital provider has, so know your anatomy.

Air travels through the **nares** or nostrils of the nose, across the nasal **turbinates,** which warm and crudely filter the air back into the **nasopharynx.** Alternately, air may pass through the mouth into the **oropharynx.** The oropharynx and the nasopharynx meet in the back of the throat, or **pharynx.** (Yes, it is possible to send a tube into the nose and out the mouth.) The pharynx then becomes the **larynx,** which houses the vocal cords and is protected on top by the **epiglottis** at the base of the tongue. It is protected in front by the **thyroid cartilage,** or "Adam's apple." Below the larynx is the **trachea,** which bifurcates (forks) into the right and left **mainstem bronchi** (singular = bronchus) (Fig. 2-3).

Nose and Nasopharynx

The nose is divided by the **nasal septum,** which is mostly cartilage. A large number of adults have what is known as a deviated septum; that is, their septums do not sit in the midline but are offset to one side. This is important only in that one of the nasal passages is larger than the other and thus airways will be more easily passed on that side.

CLINICAL CORRELATION *If your patient's nose is obviously crooked, pass nasal airways on the side that the septum is bent away from, as the nasal passage is more likely to be wider. If you have difficulty passing a nasal airway through the nose, try using the other side, as a deviated septum is not always obvious.*

In the nose, the turbinates are on the lateral side. The medial side is normally smooth and flat. Nasal airways thus should be guided down the medial side, not the lateral side, of the nose. Furthermore, notice the path of airway through the nose—it goes straight back. It does not follow the contour of the nose itself (Fig. 2-4).

CLINICAL CORRELATION *When inserting a nasal airway, it often is helpful to turn the tip of the patient's nose up, like a pig snout, to facilitate sliding the airway straight back into the nasopharynx, and not up into the body of the nose.*

Mouth and Oropharynx

Notice the size of the tongue; it is much larger than it appears when you stick it out of your mouth. Also notice that it is firmly attached to the front of your mandible. Unless you cut it off, you cannot swallow it.

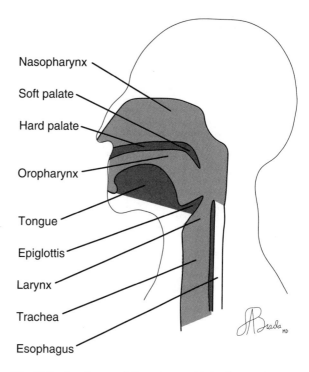

Nasopharynx
Soft palate
Hard palate
Oropharynx
Tongue
Epiglottis
Larynx
Trachea
Esophagus

Fig. 2-3. Anatomy of the airway. Note the pathway air must travel to the lungs: through the mouth or nose, into the pharynx, past the epiglottis, into the larynx, and to the trachea. Notice also the size and attachment of the tongue. In the supine position, the tongue can fall back and occlude the airway.

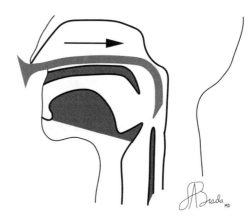

Fig. 2-4. Proper passage of the nasal airway. Notice that the airway travels straight back through the nose along the surface of the palate. When inserting nasal airways, avoid the temptation to follow the exterior contour of the nose. Also, when using nasal cannulas, point the prongs down rather than up so that air can follow its natural course.

When a patient is supine, however, the tongue will slip back into the pharynx and may block the airway. Any unconscious patient may lose muscle tone in the tongue and be at risk for airway obstruction. (Loss of muscle tone in a sleeping person is a common cause of snoring.)

Pharynx

The nasopharynx and oropharynx meet in the throat, or pharynx proper. The pharynx then divides into the larynx in front and the **esophagus** (food tube) in back, which leads into the stomach. The epiglottis acts as a "flapper valve" to close off the top of the larynx and protect the airway whenever we swallow food.

Larynx

The larynx is at the top of the trachea. When orally intubating a patient, you will directly visualize the larynx with a laryngoscope. It is imperative that you recognize all of the anatomy. First, you will see the **epiglottis** at the base of the tongue. The region between the epiglottis and the tongue is known as the **vallecula,** which is where the tip of curved laryngoscope blades are placed. The **vocal cords** themselves are normally white and lie in an inverted V. They define the **glottis,** the opening that leads to the **trachea.** Posteriorly lies the **arytenoid cartilage,** which marks the lower border of the glottis (when the patient is supine) (Fig. 2-5).

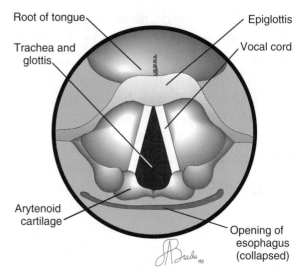

Root of tongue

Trachea and glottis

Arytenoid cartilage

Epiglottis

Vocal cord

Opening of esophagus (collapsed)

Fig. 2-5. The larynx as seen through a laryngoscope. It is absolutely critical to see the vocal cords and the open glottis between them when attempting to intubate a patient. If you cannot see the cords, a blindly inserted endotracheal tube likely will end up in the esophagus. If the cords are closed, do not force the tube past them, as you may cause trauma deep in the airway.

The larynx is protected in front by the **thyroid cartilage.** Just inferior to the thyroid cartilage is the **cricoid cartilage.** The cricoid and thyroid cartilage are *not* visible with the laryngoscope but are easily palpable on the front of the patient's neck.

Connecting the gap between the cricoid and thyroid cartilages is the **cricothyroid membrane.** This space is usually easier to locate on men and is the best site for gaining emergency access to the trachea when intubation is not possible. Puncture of this membrane with either a needle or scalpel is normally safe, as there are no major vessels or nerves running anterior to it (Fig. 2-6).

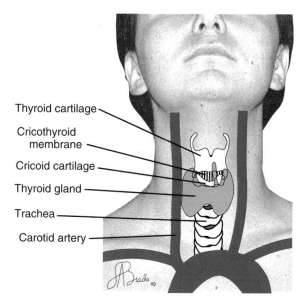

Fig. 2-6. Surface projections of the thyroid cartilage, cricoid cartilage, and thyroid gland. The thyroid cartilage is the "Adam's apple," more easily palpated and seen in men. It is an important landmark for emergency airway access through the cricothyroid membrane.

Trachea

The trachea continues below the larynx. It is a hollow tube approximately 2 cm across, protected only by C-shaped cartilage rings. It is important to remember that the trachea sits in the front of the neck and thus is susceptible to trauma.

The trachea descends into the chest until it reaches the level of the sternal angle (see Chap. 3), where it bifurcates (forks) at a point called the **carina**. At this point, the **right** and **left mainstem bronchi** branch off. The left bronchus branches at a much sharper angle than the right side.

CLINICAL CORRELATION *The end of endotracheal tubes ideally should be placed just above the carina. If a tube is advanced too far, it almost always will go down the right mainstem bronchus because it is the straighter route. If you hear nothing over the left lung when checking lung sounds for proper tube placement, back the endotracheal tube out, as it is most likely in the right bronchus.*

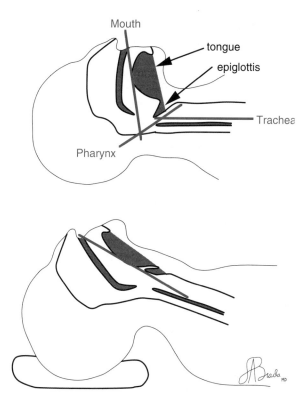

Fig. 2-7. Planes of the airway. Notice that in the supine position, the planes of the mouth, pharynx, and trachea are all askew, but when the patient is placed in the "sniffing position," the airway is much more in line.

Notice that the airway, from the outside world to the lungs, has essentially three different planes: the mouth, the pharynx, and the trachea. In a natural position, these planes each are pointing in different directions. Therefore, to establish an airway on a patient, it is necessary to bring the planes in line, which is accomplished by placing the patient in the "sniffing position." With the patient supine, the patient's head should be elevated (anteriorly) and the neck slightly extended (Fig. 2-7).

CLINICAL CORRELATION *To intubate a patient in the field, it is best to place a folded towel behind the patient's head to raise it off the floor approximately 2 inches. Anterior displacement with the laryngoscope and not hyperextension of the neck is the best way to line up the planes of the airway and bring the cords into view.*

VASCULAR ANATOMY

There are two types of blood vessels in the body: **arteries** and **veins.** Arteries carry blood away from the heart. They are firmer structures (that is, they tend to have thicker muscular walls) and are under pressure. Pulses are felt over arteries.

Veins carry blood back to the heart. They are usually not under much pressure and tend to be more superficially visible (see Chap. 3). (Ever seen those muscle-men who have veins sticking out everywhere?)

Arteries

Common and Internal Carotid

The **carotid arteries** are the major supply of blood to the head and brain, providing 80% of the blood to the brain. (The other 20% comes from the *vertebral arteries*, which travel up the cervical spine.) The common carotid arteries travel up the neck and can be palpated in the groove lateral to the trachea and just medial to the **sternocleidomastoid muscle.** The sternocleidomastoid is the big, strap-like muscle in the front of your neck connecting the mastoid process to the clavicle and sternum. It stands out when you try to turn your head against resistance (Fig. 2-8).

CLINICAL CORRELATION *The easiest way to palpate a carotid pulse is to place your fingertips on the thyroid cartilage and gently slide them laterally into the groove in front of the sternocleidomastoid muscle.*

Just below the **angle of the mandible** (the point where the jaw is bent), the common carotid artery divides into the internal and external carotid arteries. Just distal to the bifurcation in the internal carotid lies the **carotid sinus,** or the **carotid body.** (Some authors use the two terms interchangeably; distinction is not important.) Within the carotid body are pressure receptors, or *baroreceptors*, which are

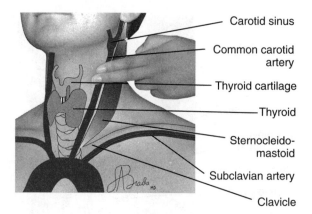

Fig. 2-8. Palpation of the carotid artery. This pulse is readily palpable in the groove between the trachea and the anterior border of the sternocleidomastoid muscle. The carotid sinus lies just caudal to the angle of the mandible.

sensitive to the blood pressure in the internal carotid artery that feeds the brain. If the pressure drops, a *sympathetic* response is triggered (see section below on The Nervous System). If the pressure is high, the opposite will occur (a parasympathetic response).

CLINICAL CORRELATION *Supraventricular tachycardias may be treated by a number of vagal maneuvers, including carotid sinus massage. To perform this procedure, palpate the carotid pulse in the groove between the sternocleidomastoid and the trachea—just inferior to the angle of the mandible—and briskly massage. This will increase vagal, or parasympathetic, tone and may slow the heart rate back to a normal sinus rhythm.*

The internal carotid artery at the bifurcation is also the most common site for the development of atherosclerotic plaques. Atherosclerotic plaques are formed from the deposition of fat and cholesterol in the walls of arteries. Plaques tend to form at the bifurcation due to the turbulent flow of blood past this area. A blood clot or thrombus may form on the plaque, which may totally block blood flow downstream. Clots, or pieces of the plaque itself, can break free, and form an *embolus.* An embolus is any free-floating particle in the bloodstream. An embolus from the internal carotid artery will travel into the brain and get stuck. This will block blood flow distal to the embolus, causing a stroke.

CLINICAL CORRELATION *Because of the risk of a stroke, a carotid sinus massage should not be performed on elderly patients or patients with a history of atherosclerotic vascular disease (previous strokes or heart attacks). A massage may break free pieces of plaque or blood clots. It also is prudent to listen with a stethoscope over the carotid sinus. If a significant plaque is present, you may hear a bruit (pronounced "brew-ee"). A bruit is a swishing sound made by turbulent blood flow. This sign, however, is not foolproof. When in doubt, do not use a carotid sinus massage.*

Strokes

A stroke, or **cerebrovascular accident** (CVA), is defined as a neurological deficit or a dysfunction of the brain caused by an area of the brain not receiving enough blood or oxygen. There are four major causes of CVAs: (1) free-floating particles or clots becoming stuck in blood vessels (*embolic*), (2) blood clots forming in the vessels and blocking the flow of blood (*thrombotic*), (3) bleeding (*hemorrhagic*), or (4) a global decrease in blood or oxygen supply (*hypoxic*).

When an embolus lodges in the brain it causes an *embolic stroke* because no blood is able to flow downstream from where the embolus is stuck. A major source of emboli, as mentioned above, is the carotid artery, which tends to form plaques that are prone to embolize. Another major source of free-floating blood clots is the heart, especially in patients with chronic atrial fibrillation (see Chap. 3). Atrial fibrillation is a condition in which the heart beats abnormally and blood pools within the atrium, becoming stagnant. When this happens, clots form in the heart that may then be pumped out into the brain and become stuck.

The second major cause of strokes occurs when a blood vessel inside the brain or feeding the brain clots up, closing off the blood vessel. The medical term for clot is *thrombus*, so this type of stroke is called a *thrombotic stroke*. The area of the brain downstream from the clotted-off blood vessel will not get the blood it needs.

Additionally, a person can literally burst a blood vessel inside of his or her head. It may be a small blood vessel deep inside the brain or a major artery. When a patient bleeds inside the head, it is known as a *hemorrhagic stroke*.

CLINICAL CORRELATION *Bleeding in the brain may be precipitated by rapid increases in blood pressure called a hypertensive crisis. They are characteristically preceded by severe headaches, nausea, and vomiting. Patients in hypertensive crisis are best treated with careful blood pressure control, usually with agents such as sodium nitroprusside, nitroglycerin, beta-blockers, or calcium channel blockers.*

The last major type of stroke occurs in the setting of decreased oxygen delivery to the brain. Not having enough oxygen is known as hypoxia, so this type of stroke is a *hypoxic stroke*. Situations that might cause a hypoxic stroke include airway obstruction, drowning, respiratory or cardiac arrest, or profound hypotension (very low blood pressure).

The symptoms of CVAs depend entirely on the location of the stroke. Absolutely any area of the brain can be affected, so *any* normal function of the brain may be disrupted. Commonly, only one side of the body will be affected, so that differences in the patient from left to right—for example, one-sided weakness—are a sign of a stroke. The signs or symptoms may not be permanent. In fact, many will disappear completely in minutes to hours. Such cases are called **transient ischemic attacks** (TIAs), as opposed to CVAs, which have lasting effects.

CLINICAL CORRELATION *The clinical manifestations of strokes are extremely variable and too numerous to list here. The most important thing to* *remember for patients with either a CVA or TIA is airway maintenance. Even conscious patients may have difficulty protecting their airways due to problems with swallowing their own saliva or an inability to control the tongue.*

CLINICAL CORRELATION *The ability to speak often is lost with a stroke. Patients, however, often can hear and understand you despite their inability to respond. Remember: Always watch what you say to or around your patients, even unconscious ones.*

External Carotid and Scalp

The external carotid artery, the other branch of the common carotid artery, supplies blood to the face, the meninges (discussed in the next section), and the **scalp**. The scalp is under tension from front to back (less so from side to side). Problems arise when the scalp is lacerated *coronally* because the muscles of the forehead (the *frontalis*) and the muscles of the back of the head (the *occipitalis*) pull the scalp apart, preventing the superficial arteries from collapsing and clotting off.

CLINICAL CORRELATION *Even superficial scalp wounds can be rapidly life-threatening due to hemorrhage. Direct pressure and appropriate volume support are necessary, but you must be wary of underlying skull injury. Clotted blood in hair and the darkness of night easily can hide injuries. You must make a special effort to find the exact injury as best as possible to control the bleeding. But be careful not to put pressure on fractured bones in the skull!*

The external carotid artery also branches into the middle meningeal artery, which travels along the inside of the **temporal bone** (Fig. 2-9).

CLINICAL CORRELATION *Because the temporal bone is so thin, blows to the side of the head are likely to cause temporal bone fractures, which tend to tear the middle meningeal artery. Temporal bone fractures are the most common cause of epidural hematomas (see next section).*

Veins

The **external jugular vein**, a superficial vein, drains the scalp and face. As with all superfi-

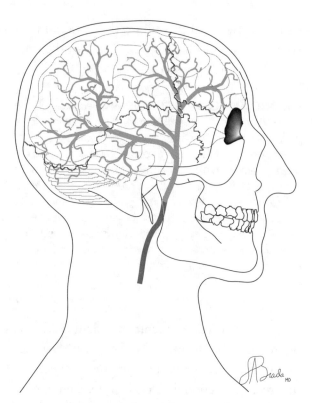

Fig. 2-9. Middle meningeal artery. This branch of the external carotid artery lies just beneath the skull and external to the dura mater. Notice how it passes behind the intersection of the coronal and parietal sutures at the pterion (temple), making it vulnerable to injury in skull fractures that can result in epidural hematomas.

cial veins, the anatomy varies from one person to the next, but the external jugular vein tends to run vertically across the top of the sternocleidomastoid muscle in the neck (Fig. 2-10).

CLINICAL CORRELATION *An intravenous line can be started in the external jugular vein just as in any other peripheral vein. This can be advantageous when only one advanced life support provider is available for both airway maintenance and intravenous access. To make the vein stand out, apply mild pressure to the downstream end of the vein, which is closer to the heart and chest. This pressure acts the same way a tourniquet does and helps distend the vein.*

The **internal jugular vein** drains blood from the brain and the inside of the skull. Much larger than the external jugular, it lies deep to the

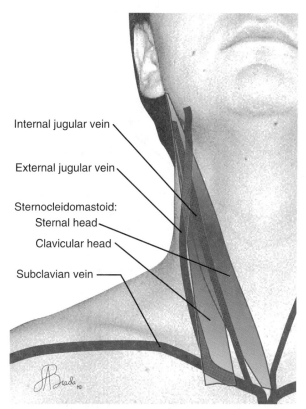

Internal jugular vein

External jugular vein

Sternocleidomastoid:
 Sternal head
 Clavicular head

Subclavian vein

Fig. 2-10. Jugular veins. The external jugular vein is normally a readily accessible peripheral vein. The internal jugular vein is the best place to look for jugular venous distension (JVD), which is best appreciated in the neck between the heads of the sternocleidomastoid muscle.

sternocleidomastoid. The internal jugular vein is considered a *central vein*, or one of the major vessels leading back to the heart. The internal jugular drains into the *superior vena cava*, which then empties into the right atrium of the heart. The right side of the heart normally is under very low pressure, but in cases of *right-sided* **heart failure**, pressure will rise and blood will back up into the internal jugular vein causing it to become engorged (see Chap. 3), a condition known as **jugular venous distention (JVD)**.

CLINICAL CORRELATION *The best place to check for JVD is in the notch between the two parts of the sternocleidomastoid muscle in the neck. One part connects to the sternum, the other to the clavicle. Between them is a gap where the internal jugular vein is nearest to*

the surface. If you look closely, pulsations can be seen that represent back pressure from the beating of the right atrium and right ventricle. This point between the two parts (or heads) of the sternocleidomastoid is also the point for placing a central venous line into the internal jugular.

Some authors suggest that the external jugular veins can be used for checking JVD. The problem is that the external jugular veins are highly *valved*; like all superficial veins, they contain one-way valves to prevent backflow of blood. Central veins, like the internal jugular, have fewer, if any, working valves. Therefore, the internal jugular vein better reflects the pressure in the right side of the heart. Almost anyone can tense up the neck muscles to make the veins stick out, but this does not mean that he or she is in right-sided heart failure. In a relaxed patient, however, obvious distention of the external jugular veins is significant for possible right-heart failure.

INTRACRANIAL ANATOMY

The Brain

The **central nervous system** (CNS) consists of the **brain** and the **spinal cord**. The human brain can be anatomically and functionally divided into several three major parts: the **cerebrum**, the **cerebellum**, and the **brain stem** (Figs. 2-11 and 2-12).

Brain tissue includes both *white matter* and *gray matter*. Gray matter is on the surface and consists of the billions of cells, called *neurons*, that make up the functional parts of the brain. White matter consists of all of the connections and pathways between different brain cells. Cells of the central nervous system are unlike most other cells of the body in that once they are destroyed, they can never regenerate. Acute processes such as ischemia (lack of blood, as from strokes or very low blood pressure), hypoxia (lack of oxygen, as from drowning or

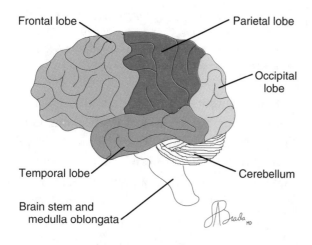

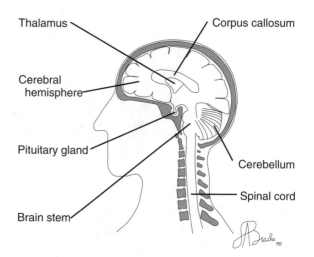

Fig. 2-11. Lobes of the brain. The different lobes of the cerebrum each have specific functions that can either be turned off by strokes or turned on by seizures.

Fig. 2-12. The central nervous system.

respiratory failure), or direct trauma can cause death of brain cells. In addition, chronic processes such as aging, alcohol, and drug use can cause widespread death of brain cells.

If a brain function is lost, it does not mean that the function is lost forever. Remaining brain cells often can "relearn" tasks other parts of the brain used to carry out.

The *blood-brain barrier* is another unique feature of the brain. The blood vessels in the brain, especially the capillaries, are different from those in the rest of the body in that they are impermeable to most substances. This keeps most toxins, poisons, and drugs out of the brain while allowing oxygen, glucose, and other important molecules to pass through. Although largely effective, the blood-brain barrier is not perfect.

Anatomy

The **cerebrum**, also known as the cerebral hemispheres, is the major part of the brain in which all higher brain functions (such as thinking) are carried out. The cerebrum is divided into right and left hemispheres, connected by the *corpus callosum*. There are four *lobes* in each hemisphere, corresponding to the region of the skull where the lobe lies: *frontal, pari-*

etal, temporal, and *occipital* (see Fig. 2-11). Although the precise workings of the brain are still largely a mystery, there are many functions that are well localized. For example, the frontal lobe controls movement, the parietal lobe controls sensation, the temporal lobe receives odor and sound, and the occipital lobe receives visual input (which is why you may see stars if hit on the back of the head).

It also is true that the right side of the brain controls the left side of the body, and vice versa. The reason for this is unknown. Midline body structures, such as the muscles that move the spine and face, often get input from both sides of the brain. When a region of the brain is damaged or stressed, it may not function properly or may not function at all.

The **cerebellum** is located posteriorly and inferiorly to the cerebrum. Its primary function is coordination of movement. (The movement is initiated in the frontal lobe.) The cerebellum is what allows us to move smoothly and never forget how to ride a bicycle. It is commonly damaged by chronic alcohol use, which is why alcoholics often stagger when they walk, even when sober. The *inner ear,* or *vestibular appa-ratus,* works in close proximity with the cere-

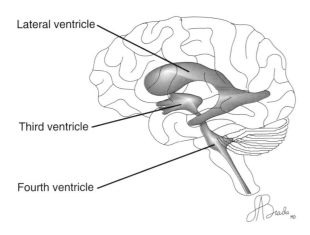

Fig. 2-13. Ventricles of the brain. Cerebrospinal fluid (CSF) is made in the ventricles and circulates within the confines of the arachnoid, surrounding the entire central nervous system (CNS).

Lateral ventricle

Third ventricle

Fourth ventricle

bellum to maintain balance. Infections of the inner ear, known as *labryinthitis*, will cause dizziness, balance problems, nausea, and vertigo (the subjective sensation of movement—"the room spinning").

The **brain stem** is the stalk on which the brain sits and leads continuously into the spinal cord. The brain stem is our primitive brain, sometimes referred to as a "reptile brain" because it is the human equivalent of the brain of a lizard. The brain stem controls our most primitive functions: arousal (whether we are awake and how awake we are), breathing, and autonomic function.

The brain starts in the early fetus as a tube. At the center of the brain are hollow spaces, or *ventricles* (Fig. 2-13). There are four ventricles in the brain, which have absolutely nothing in common with the four ventricles of the heart. The *choroid plexus* is a vascular structure within the lateral ventricles that produces **cerebrospinal fluid** (CSF). CSF fills the ventricles and flows through channels to the outside surface of the brain. The entire nervous system thus floats in a cushioning sea of fluid. Head trauma that causes a fracture in the cranium may cause CSF to leak.

CLINICAL CORRELATION *Check for CSF leakage from the ears and nose in all patients with suspected head trauma. CSF is a clear, colorless fluid thinner than blood and often tinged with or mixed with blood in trauma. If bloody fluid is coming from a patient's ears, place a little on a gauze pad. If CSF is present, a clear ring will form around the central dark area of blood. More practically, while you are holding the patient's head stable with your gloved hands, watch to see if CSF separates from the blood as it runs down your fingers. The presence of CSF is a bad sign; the patient needs to go to a trauma center with neurosurgical capability.*

At the base of the front of the brain in the midline, the *pituitary gland* is suspended from a short stalk, surrounded by a bony cradle. The pituitary gland is the master gland of the body. It receives nerve signals from the brain and secretes hormones into the bloodstream that control most of the other glands in the body. It also secretes *oxytocin*, a natural form of the drug *Pitocin*, which stimulates labor contractions in pregnant women.

Seizures

The brain functions by sending small electrical impulses from neuron to neuron. When normal electrical activity of the brain is interrupted, a seizure results. Seizures can be either *primary generalized*, affecting the entire brain all at once, or, more commonly, they can be *partial*, initially affecting only part of the brain (Fig. 2-14).

There are four types of generalized seizures: **grand mal, absence** (or *petit mal*), myoclonic, and atonic. Grand mal seizures are the classic "generalized motor seizure" usually characterized by a period of muscle rigidity (*tonus*) throughout the body followed by spastic movement of the extremities (*clonus*). The term *tonic-clonic seizures* also has been used. Grand mal seizures always are followed by a **postictal** period during which seizure activity has stopped but the patient's brain has not returned to normal function. Patients often will be confused or unconscious.

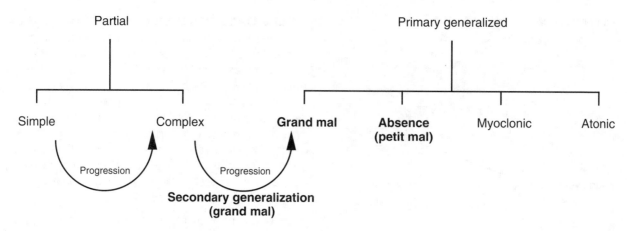

Fig. 2-14. Types of seizures.

Absence, or petit mal, seizures are primary generalized seizures seen almost exclusively in children. They are characterized as "staring spells" during which the patient literally stares off at nothing, totally unaware of his or her surroundings. Absence seizures may last only a few seconds but may occur hundreds of times a day. These spells often are brought on by hyperventilation.

Myoclonic seizures are more unusual. They are characterized by very brief, random muscle jerks associated with an alteration of consciousness—not the prolonged contractions and spasms of grand mal seizures. Atonic seizures also are not as common. *Atonic,* meaning the absence of muscle tone, describes these seizures exactly. These seizures are "drop spells" during which the patient instantaneously loses all muscle tone and drops to the ground. These patients sometimes are referred to as "crash helmet kids," usually going through life wearing helmets because their seizures are not well controlled.

A *partial seizure* can begin in any part of the brain. Just as a stroke can turn off any part of the brain, a partial seizure can turn on any discrete part of the brain. Partial seizures may begin with muscle twitching, for example, as with the so-called focal motor seizure. The seizing area of the brain may spread, a phenomenon known as the *Jacksonian march*. For example, a seizure may begin in the area of the brain controlling the hand, causing uncontrolled hand movements, and then spread to involve the rest of the arm.

A partial seizure that does not cause any alteration of consciousness is known as a *simple partial seizure*; a seizure that does cause an alteration of consciousness is known as a **complex partial seizure.** A common type of complex partial seizure is **temporal lobe epilepsy** (a seizure that starts in the temporal lobe). Patients with temporal lobe epilepsy often display bizarre, repetitive behavior, staring, lip smacking, and possibly strange noises but may not show any sign of tonic-clonic posturing or motion. As with generalized seizures, a postictal period, which likewise can be very bizarre, usually follows the seizure. Any postictal patient may display a lot of confusion and paranoia. Unfortunately, this is when most EMS personnel first encounter seizure patients.

CLINICAL CORRELATION *Postictal patients must be observed carefully and restrained if necessary. Patients may run into traffic, climb out of windows, or try to leave the ambulance while you are driving to the hospital.*

Any partial seizure may go on to generalize into a grand mal seizure. This is the most common cause of generalized seizures. A generalized seizure that persists is known as **status**

epilepticus, which is defined as a recurrence of a seizure before the effects of the initial seizure have been alleviated, or a seizure lasting more than 30 minutes. More practically, it is a seizure that just won't stop.

CLINICAL CORRELATION *Status epilepticus is an extremely life-threatening emergency that must be treated rapidly. Currently, the drug of choice to stop a seizure before arriving at the hospital is a benzodiazepine such as lorazepam (Ativan) or diazepam (Valium).*

Some seizures are preceded by an **aura,** or vague feeling, indicating a seizure is coming. Some patients, knowing a seizure is coming, will call for an ambulance. Seizures have many causes, some of which are correctable (Table 2-1), but it is important to remember that seizures are just a sign and not a disease in and of themselves. *Recurrent idiopathic seizures* (seizures of unknown origin) are termed **epilepsy;** however, not everyone who has a seizure is epileptic. It is important to rule out treatable reasons for seizures as much as possible.

CLINICAL CORRELATION *Although a clear airway is our highest concern, never forcefully manipulate the airway of a patient having a grand mal seizure; you will cause trauma. Instead, lay the patient on his or her side, allowing secretions to better drain out of the mouth.*

CLINICAL CORRELATION *There is a standard "cocktail" used to treat suspected seizure patients in the generic category of "unconscious/unknown": oxygen, glucose, naloxone (Narcan), and thiamine. This combination corrects most of the easily reversible causes of altered mental status, and most of it can be administered by non–advanced life support providers. Furthermore, none of these drugs is dangerous. However, thiamine should be administered prior to glucose. Glucose given to someone who is thiamine-deficient (as many alcoholics are) can cause metabolic brain damage (known as Wernike's encephalopathy).*

CLINICAL CORRELATION *A good intravenous solution to administer to seizure patients is normal saline. Phenytoin (Dilantin) often is given intravenously at the hospital but cannot be mixed with D5W because the mixture precipitates in the intravenous tubing.*

Table 2-1. Causes of seizures

Epilepsy (idiopathic)

Hypoxia

Hypoglycemia

Hyperglycemia (less common)

Alcohol and drug overdose

Alcohol and drug withdrawal

Poisoning

Trauma (head injuries)

Fever (hyperthermia)

Infections: meningitis

Metabolic: electrolyte disorders

Brain tumors

Cerebrovascular accidents and transient ischemic attacks (rarely)

Psychological disorders and pseudoseizures

Meninges

The brain has three membranes, or **meninges,** covering it: the *pia mater, arachnoid*, and **dura mater** (Fig. 2-15). Stuck to the brain's surface is the thin, filmy pia mater ("gentle mother"). Above the pia is the arachnoid, so named because of its spider-like connections to the pia. Between the pia and the arachnoid is the *subarachnoid space. Subarachnoid hemorrhages*, bleeding from abnormal or weakened blood vessels in the subarachnoid space, are characterized by a severe headache and stiff neck (patients will call it "the worst headache of my life") and can be life-threatening. They are seen more often in women, smokers, and users of oral contraceptive pills. The best course of action when a person has suffered a subarachnoid hemorrhage is to keep the patient's head elevated (if he or she can tolerate it) to help venous drainage of blood from the head and rapid transport to a hospital with neurosurgical capability.

The outermost covering of the brain is the dura mater ("tough mother"), or the dura.

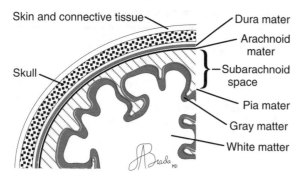

Fig. 2-15. The meninges. The outermost layer, the dura, is a thick, waterproof layer that holds the CSF and surrounds the entire CNS. In the head, it is applied closely to the skull; thus, the epidural space is only a potential space. Bleeding into the epidural space (epidural hematoma) requires rupture of an artery. Bleeding beneath the dura (subdural hematoma) is venous and occurs between the dura and the closely applied arachnoid. CSF circulates in the subarachnoid space between the arachnoid and the pia mater, which follows the contours of the brain.

Held more closely to the skull than to the brain, it is a waterproof barrier containing CSF. The space between the dura and the arachnoid is the **subdural space** ("below the dura"); the space between the dura and the skull is the **epidural space** ("outside the dura").

Injuries

Bleeding into the subdural space, known as a **subdural hematoma**, results from head trauma, causing venous tearing, with or without skull fractures (Fig. 2-16). Subdural hematomas can be minor and associated with minimal trauma. Subdural hemotomas are common in alcoholics, who are prone to falling.

Bleeding in the epidural space, or an **epidural hematoma**, is caused by arterial bleeding and is a much more serious matter (see Fig. 2-16). Most commonly, the middle meningeal artery is torn as a result of a temporal or parietal bone fracture on the side of the head. Classically, the patients with epidural hematomas temporarily lose consciousness. They then regain consciousness and may be asymptomatic during a period called a **lucid interval.** Unfortunately, later that day they may lose consciousness again and go into a coma. If not operated on, epidural hematomas can be fatal.

CLINICAL CORRELATION *The nursery rhyme about the old man who "bumped his head, went to bed, and couldn't get up in the morning," actually describes a man with an epidural hematoma. Any patient who has suffered enough trauma to lose consciousness needs to go to the hospital.*

Bleeding inside the head, whether epidural, subdural, subarachnoid, or *intraparenchymal* (within the brain tissue itself), causes a rise in **intracranial pressure** (ICP). Increased ICP makes it more difficult for the heart to push blood into the brain because of the pressure inside the head it has to overcome. The brain is the most important organ in the body and will do everything possible to get blood to it. The brain sends out a signal that causes systolic blood pressure to go *up*. Higher blood pressure, however, often makes the bleeding worse, which in turn causes ICP to rise even higher. Thus, a vicious cycle is started.

As blood accumulates in the skull, it begins to act like a solid mass, causing a *"mass effect."* A solid mass inside the skull will push on the brain. The only place for the brain to go is out the bottom of the skull through the *foramen magnum* (Latin for "big hole"), where the spinal cord normally leaves the brain through the skull. As the brain is pushed from the mass effect, the brain stem is squeezed into the foramen magnum (a *herniated brain stem*). The squeezed brain stem will not function properly, inhibiting proper function of the patient's cardiorespiratory control.

CLINICAL CORRELATION *The characteristic vital signs for a patient with bleeding inside the head and ICP are (1) rise in blood pressure, (2) slow pulse, and (3) irregular respirations. (The latter two effects usually are due to dysfunction of the brain stem from compression as the brain swells.) In some cases, the difference between*

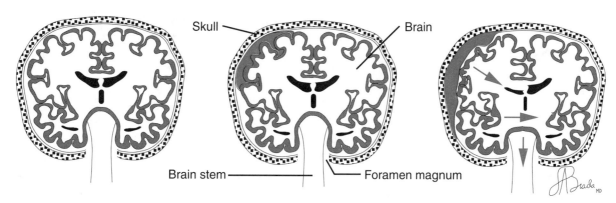

Skull   Brain

Brain stem —   — Foramen magnum

Fig. 2-16. Intracranial hemorrhages. The diagram on the left shows the normal relation of the dura to the inner surface of the skull. In the middle diagram there is free venous blood in the subdural space with minimal mass effect on the brain. The epidural hematoma (right) shows blood under arterial pressure separating the dura from the skull and creating a mass effect that compresses brain tissue and ventricles, shifts midline structures to the contralateral side, and depresses the brain stem down toward the foramen magnum.

systolic and diastolic pressure also increases, called a widened pulse pressure (see Chap. 3).

CLINICAL CORRELATION *Isolated closed-head injuries (bleeding inside—not outside—the head) do not cause shock. If you see signs of shock (see Chap. 3), look for other injuries.*

The blood vessels in the brain are controlled in part by the autonomic nervous system (see section on The Autonomic Nervous System) but also respond locally to concentrations of gasses in the blood (see Chaps. 3 and 4). A high level of CO_2 in the blood causes the brain's blood vessels to dilate. This is a natural response. CO_2 is normally a waste product that needs to be cleared, which is why an increased CO_2 level causes an increased blood flow. An increase in blood flow to the brain when it is swelling, however, makes swelling worse and further increases ICP.

CLINICAL CORRELATION *Patients with head injuries should be hyperventilated to lower the body's CO_2 level and cause vasoconstriction in the brain, thereby reducing swelling and ICP.*

Meningitis

All of the layers of meninges cover the brain and the entire spinal cord. **Meningitis,** or spinal meningitis, has several causes and occurs when the meninges become infected or inflamed. It is most common in infants and young children but also occurs in teenagers and the elderly. Most commonly, meningitis is caused by a viral or bacterial infection. Most viral meningitis is benign—that is, people rarely die from it. Bacterial meningitis, however, can be fatal if not quickly treated in the hospital.

Meningitis is characterized by a stiff neck, headache, fever, and general flulike symptoms and also can be associated with a rash. It may be highly contagious and is spread via the respiratory system.

CLINICAL CORRELATION *Little can be done for a patient with meningitis before arriving at the hospital except for the standard ABCs in severe cases. It is important to protect yourself from exposure to this disease by putting a surgical mask on patients first to avoid their breathing germs on you; then put a mask on yourself.*

THE SPINE

Bony Structure

The **spine,** or spinal column, is the bony structure that makes up the backbone, supports the head, and provides a protective case for the **spinal cord,** the part of the central nervous sys-

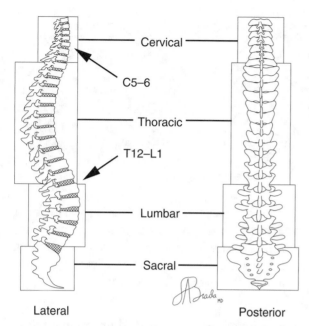

Lateral   Posterior

Fig. 2-17. The spinal column. Notice that the spine changes curvature at C5–6 and again at T12–L1. These are the most commonly fractured sites because of their mechanical instability.

tem carrying nerve fibers from the brain to the rest of the body (Fig. 2-17).

The spine consists of individual bones known as a **vertebra** (plural: vertebrae) and is divided into three sections (Table 2-2): **cervical spine, thoracic spine,** and **lumbar spine.** The neck, or cervical spine (C-spine for short), is made up of seven vertebrae. The chest, or thorax, covers the thoracic spine, which consists of 12 vertebrae. A rib is attached to each thoracic vertebra (see Chap. 3). The lower back is the lumbar spine and is made up of five vertebrae. These lumbar vertebrae are the largest in the spinal column. Below the lumbar spine are the fused **sacrum** and **coccyx,** or "tail bone."

Notice the curvature of the spine when viewed laterally. The neck curves backward, the upper back curves forward (hunches), and the lower back curves backward again. Thus, the curvature of the spine naturally changes twice.

CLINICAL CORRELATION *The most common places for a fracture are C5–C6 (the fifth and sixth*

Table 2-2. Segments of the spine

Segment	Common name	Number of vertebrae
Cervical	Neck	7
Thoracic	Chest	12
Lumbar	Lower back	5
Sacrum	Tail bone	5 fused
Coccyx	Tail bone	3–5 fused

cervical vertebrae) and T12–L1 (the last thoracic and first lumbar vertebrae) because these are the points where the spine changes curvature and are therefore the most structurally unstable.

Spinal Cord

The spinal cord carries nearly all information to and from the brain. *The terms spinal cord and spinal column are not interchangeable.* The spinal column is the bone; the spinal cord is the nerve pathway.

CLINICAL CORRELATION *The spinal column can be fractured or otherwise damaged without damaging the spinal cord. In these cases, prehospital spinal precautions are critical to prevent cord injury.*

Spinal fractures endanger the spinal cord when the bones are moved transversely, or side to side. Transverse movement creates a shearing effect that can cut the cord. A twisting motion is likewise dangerous. The only safe way to move the spine is *axially*, along the long axis of the spine (up or down).

CLINICAL CORRELATION *The log roll, which moves the spine and body as a single unit, is the best way to turn a patient with spinal injuries to avoid dangerous side-to-side or twisting motions of the spine.*

With the exception of 12 pairs of *cranial nerves* coming from the base of the brain and the brain stem, essentially all other nerves in the body lead to or from the spinal cord. A spinal nerve leaves the spinal cord and emerges from the spinal column between each pair of vertebrae

(Fig. 2-18). *Notice, however, that the spinal cord extends only to the level of L1–L2.* It sends a tail of nerves down the spinal column that exit between the vertebrae lower down. The entire spinal cord is less than 18 inches long.

CLINICAL CORRELATION *Because the spinal cord itself reaches only the level of L1–L2, movement below this level does not threaten the spinal cord. This is why patients can sit forward when being extricated from vehicles without risk to the spinal cord, as long as proper cervical precautions are maintained.*

Another key landmark in the spinal cord is the point where the **phrenic nerve** comes out. The phrenic nerve innervates the **diaphragm,** the muscle separating the chest cavity from the abdomen and the major muscle that allows breathing (see Chap. 3). The phrenic nerve comes from roots that emerge above C3, C4, and C5.

CLINICAL CORRELATION *A person whose spinal cord is cut above the level of C3-4-5 cannot breathe because of damage to the phrenic nerve. If the phrenic nerve is damaged, the diaphragm won't work. If the diaphragm won't work, the patient can't breathe. This is why broken necks can be fatal. (Remember: "C3-4-5 keeps the diaphragm alive" or "Above C4 you'll breathe no more.")*

If the spinal cord is completely cut, all function below it is lost. The spinal cord can be partially damaged, or swelling from nearby bone injury can cause compression and dysfunction of the cord. Such injuries may be reversible.

CLINICAL CORRELATION *It is imperative to eliminate movement of the bones of the spinal column to prevent any further spinal cord damage in patients suspected to have spinal trauma. Remember that a loss of function below the level of the injury may not be permanent, including that caused by neck fractures. A patient with damage above C 3-4-5 may not be able to breathe but otherwise may be intact. A patient with this kind of injury needs artificial respiration, preferably with intubation and 100% oxygen.*

CLINICAL CORRELATION *Intubation in a trauma patient or a patient with suspected neck injury*

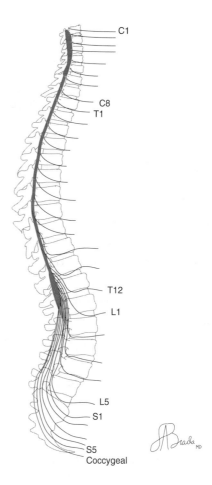

Fig. 2-18. The spinal cord. Notice that the cord itself (shown in red) ends at the level of L2–3, even though spinal nerves exit at each vertebral level of the spinal column. Lumbar punctures are performed below the L2–3 level, as there is no risk of piercing the spinal cord and the smaller roots move out of the way of the advancing needle.

must be accomplished without moving the patient's neck. This is known as "in-line" intubation because the neck is kept "in-line" by a rescuer holding the patient's head immobile. It can be performed orally or nasally, with or without a lighted stylette. Whatever technique used should be well practiced before a field situation arises.

THE NERVOUS SYSTEM

The human nervous system is divided into the *somatic* and **autonomic** systems (Fig. 2-19). The somatic system includes voluntary motor movement and sensation of the outer world

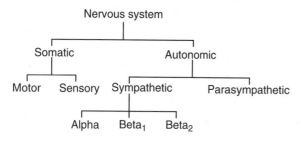

Fig. 2-19. Divisions of the nervous system.

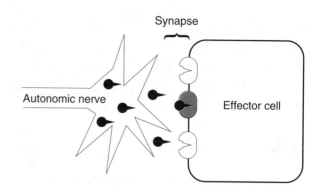

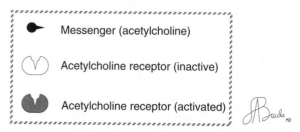

Fig. 2-20. Autonomic nerve terminal. When the nerve receives a stimulus either from the brain or a reflex arc, chemical mediators are released from the end of its axon. These mediators float across the small synaptic space where they bind to and activate receptors on the next cell. The net result depends on the type of nerve, the mediator it releases, and the type of responding cell.

(touch, pain, temperature, etc.). All of the somatic nerves carrying these impulses either to or from the brain come out of the spinal cord. The autonomic nervous system affects everything in the body, taking care of bodily functions we do not think actively about and cannot control voluntarily such as digestion of food, sweating, control of heart rate, and so forth. Many drugs administered by paramedics work by directly affecting the body's autonomic function.

The Autonomic Nervous System

The autonomic nervous system has two major divisions that differ both anatomically and functionally: the **parasympathetic** and the **sympathetic** systems. Generally, they work in opposition to each other; one produces the opposite effect of the other. Both parasympathetic nerves and sympathetic nerves work similarly, however. When a signal travels down the nerve, the end of the nerve releases a chemical messenger. This chemical then moves to the next cell (for example, a heart cell) and binds to a specific receptor, much like a key fitting into a lock (Fig. 2-20). When the messenger (the key) binds to the receptor (the lock), the cell is stimulated to do something. What the cell does depends on what type of cell it is and whether it was the parasympathetic or the sympathetic key that turned it on.

Acetylcholine is the messenger for the parasympathetic system; thus, the parasympa-

thetic nervous system often is called the **cholinergic** system. The messenger for the sympathetic system is *noradrenalin* (also called norepinephrine); thus, the sympathetic nervous system also is called the **adrenergic** system (Fig. 2-21). Freely circulating drugs or hormones (like **adrenaline**, also called **epinephrine**) that mimic the messengers also fit into the receptors and turn cells on.

Sympathetic Nervous System

The sympathetic nervous system is the "gas pedal" for the body; that is, its general effect is to speed up everything. It stimulates the body's natural, primitive "fight or flight" response. Imagine your reaction if you encountered a hungry saber-toothed tiger. Your heart would race, you'd breathe faster, you'd turn pale and

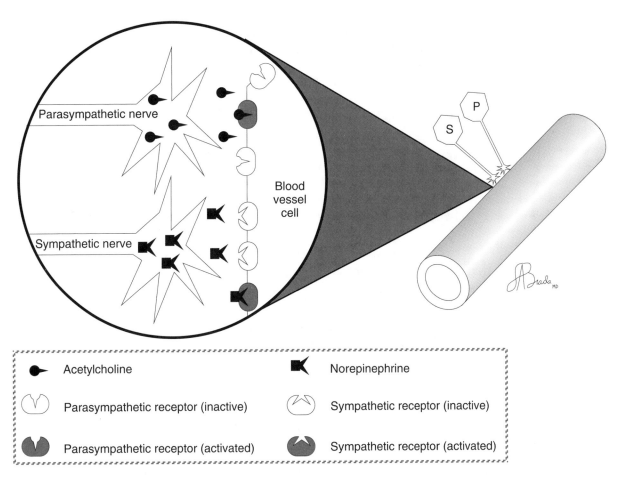

Fig. 2-21. Parasympathetic and sympathetic nerve endings. The parasympathetic nerve's mediator is acetylcholine; the sympathetic nerve releases norepinephrine. At a blood vessel, parasympathetic stimulation signals it to dilate, while the sympathetic stimulation sends a signal to constrict. Thus, the blood vessel remains balanced.

break out into a cold sweat, your eyes would widen, your blood pressure would rise, and you'd run like mad. I think we would all feel pretty *sympathetic* for you.

Anatomically, the nerves that carry sympathetic fibers come out of the spinal cord between T1 and L2. They travel in a chain that lies alongside the spinal cord, spreading diffusely throughout the body (Fig. 2-22). These nerves go everywhere, but the organs of principle interest are the heart, the bronchi and lungs, the blood vessels, the skin, and the adrenal glands.

In the sympathetic nervous system, there are several different receptors, or locks. The same key (noradrenalin) fits into all of them but fits into some receptors better than others (Fig. 2-23). The major receptors are **alpha**, **beta$_1$**, and **beta$_2$**. The location and function of each of these receptors are outlined in Table 2-3. In simplest terms, beta$_1$-receptors are found in the heart; stimulation of beta$_1$-receptors increases heart rate and the force of contraction. Beta$_2$-receptors are found in the lungs and *bronchi*, airways leading into the lungs; stimulation of beta$_2$-receptors causes relaxation of the muscles surrounding the bronchi. Relaxation of these muscles causes dilation, or opening, of the bronchi, resulting in easier breathing. One way to remember the location

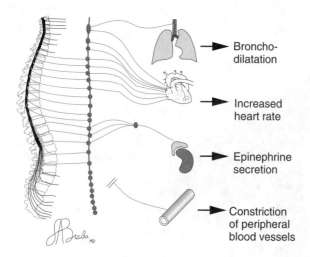

Fig. 2-22. Schematic diagram of the sympathetic nervous system. Sympathetic nerves arise between T1 and L2 in the spinal cord but reach all levels of the body by traveling up and down the sympathetic chain (shown in red). They have significant effects on the lungs, heart, adrenal glands, and blood vessels. The overall effect is to speed everything up in the "fight or flight" response.

of beta-receptors is that you have *one* heart (beta$_1$), and *two* lungs (beta$_2$).

Alpha-receptors are located primarily in the blood vessels. Stimulation of alpha-receptors constricts, or narrows, blood vessels, resulting in increased blood pressure. This effect causes the skin to become white as the blood vessels in the skin clamp down.

The sympathetic nervous system also innervates the *adrenal gland* (see Chap. 4), which secretes adrenaline (also called epinephrine). The effects of having "adrenaline pumping" in a stressful or exciting situation are fairly well known. Epinephrine, like the transmitter norepinephrine, binds to sympathetic receptors and activates cells. Because epinephrine is released into the blood from the adrenal gland, it acts all over the body.

All of these responses can be predicted by the tiger scenario. We need to increase our breathing and heart pumping capability to run from the tiger. Also, by shunting blood away from the skin, we save it for more important organs, such as the brain.

The body's natural response to any stress such as an injury, trauma, or blood loss is to increase the sympathetic output, or **sympathetic tone**. If you think someone who suddenly finds a tiger appears to be "in shock," you are mostly correct. Most of the visible signs of shock are caused by increased sympathetic tone.

Table 2-3. Sympathetic receptors

Type	Location	Effect
Alpha	Blood vessels	Constricts (raises pressure)
	Pupils	Dilates
	Hair cells	Erection (goose bumps)
	Heart muscle	Increase force of contraction
	Penis	Ejaculation
Beta$_1$	Heart muscle	Increase force of contraction
	SA, AV nodes	Increase heart rate
Beta$_2$	Smooth muscle	Relaxation
	Bronchi	Relaxation (bronchodilation)
	Blood vessels	Relaxation (vasodilation)
	Uterus	Relaxation (stops contractions)

SA = sinoatrial; AV = atrioventricular.

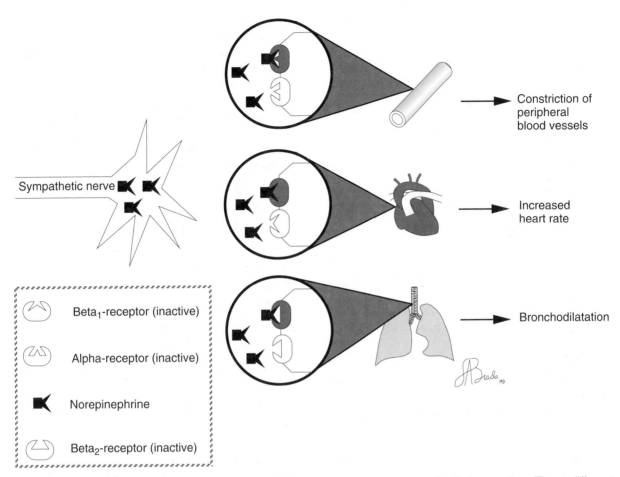

Fig. 2-23. Sympathetic nerve endings. Many different organs receive sympathetic innervation. Three different receptor types, each on characteristic organs, help differentiate the effects. Certain medications bind to one type of receptor more strongly than others, thus exerting influence only at specific organs. For example, isoproterenol binds beta-receptors (both 1 and 2) but not alpha, so it does not affect blood vessels. No drug or receptor is entirely exclusive, so there is always some overlap between effects.

CLINICAL CORRELATION *Because the body uses the sympathetic nervous system to combat any trauma or stress, the signs and symptoms of someone who has been shot are similar to those of someone having a heart attack. The symptoms result from the sympathetic nervous system's "kicking in" to keep the patient alive: rapid heart rate, rapid respirations, pale skin, sweating, and an increase, or at least a maintenance of, blood pressure.*

Epinephrine is very similar to norepinephrine, but the two are not identical. Norepinephrine, released from sympathetic nerve endings, stimulates alpha receptors more than it does beta-receptors. On the other hand, epinephrine, released from the adrenal glands and a commonly used prehospital drug, stimu-lates beta receptors more than it does alpha-receptors (Fig. 2-24).

CLINICAL CORRELATION *Injected epinephrine (or "epi") produces the same effect as the body's natural adrenaline, which is turned on by the sympathetic nervous system.*

Sympathomimetic, or **adrenergic,** drugs mimic the effects of the sympathetic nervous system (Table 2-4). Each drug is characterized by how much it stimulates alpha and beta receptors.

A certain baseline sympathetic tone always is maintained in the body; that is, the body always is using the sympathetic system to

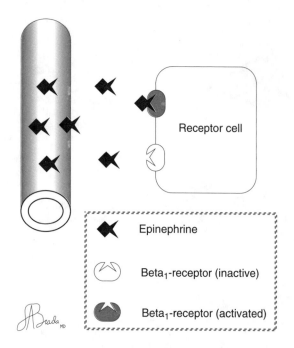

Fig. 2-24. Circulating epinephrine. Free epinephrine in the blood diffuses out of vessels and binds to sympathetic receptors. Epinephrine is primarily a beta-agonist but has some alpha activity as well.

"keep the foot on the gas pedal" just a little bit. Without sympathetic tone, the heart would slow down and the blood vessels would dilate, causing blood pressure to fall.

CLINICAL CORRELATION *If the spinal cord is severed above T1 in the neck, the body loses all sympa-*

thetic tone. Heart rate drops to 40–50 beats per minute, and blood pressure falls because the blood vessels dilate all over the body. The blood vessels in the skin also dilate, causing a red, flushed appearance below the point where the spinal cord has been cut. This is neurogenic shock, also called "spinal shock" or "hot shock," but is not the classic picture of shock (see Chap. 3), which depends on the response of the sympathetic nervous system. In addition to immediate fluid support, these patients often require an agent such as dopamine to maintain blood pressure.

Just as there are a wide variety of agents that stimulate alpha- and beta-receptors, there are drugs that *block* them, the most common of which are **beta-blockers**. The prototypical beta-blocker is propranolol (Inderal). Beta-blockers work by simply blocking the beta-receptors, preventing beta agents from working (Fig. 2-25). They are very often used by patients to treat high blood pressure. Beta-blockers affect the body's own natural sympathetic responses and block the effects of any beta drugs you might administer to patients.

CLINICAL CORRELATION *Find out if your patient takes a beta-blocker. There are many on the market and are so common that most patients know they are taking a beta-blocker even if they don't know which one.*

A trauma patient taking beta-blockers does not show the normal rise in heart rate you might expect to see in patients going into shock

Table 2-4. Sympathomimetic drugs

Drug	Receptor	Clinical use
Epinephrine	Beta$_1$, beta$_2$, alpha	Cardiac arrest, anyphalaxis
Isoproterenol	Beta$_1$, beta$_2$	Bradycardia
Terbutaline	Beta$_2$	Asthma, COPD
		Stop premature labor contractions
Albuterol	Beta$_2$	Asthma, COPD
Dobutamine	Beta$_1$	Cardiogenic shock
Dopamine	Alpha, beta$_1$, dopaminergic receptors*	Raise blood pressure
		Cardiogenic and neurogenic shock

COPD = chronic obstructive pulmonary disease.
*At low doses, dopamine activates a special dopamine receptor, also a sympathetic receptor, which increases blood flow to the kidneys and gastrointestinal tract (mesentery).

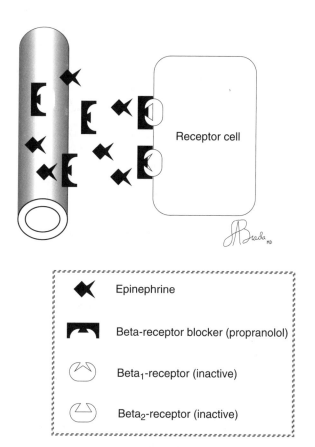

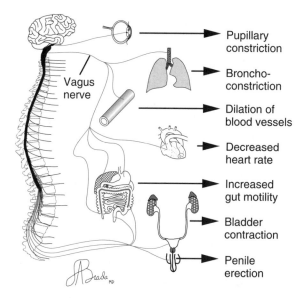

Fig. 2-26. The parasympathetic nervous system. Most parasympathetic activity arises from the vagus nerve, a nerve coming from the brain stem. Sacral spinal nerves also contribute to parasympathetic activity. The parasympathetic system stimulates most of the body's baseline functions (e.g., digestion).

Fig. 2-25. Beta blockade. Drugs such as propranolol are called beta-blockers because they bind to beta-receptors without activating them. By not allowing epinephrine to reach the receptor, propranolol prevents the sympathetic beta response.

because the patient's sympathetic response is blocked. Patients taking beta-blockers may be more prone to syncope (faints) or decreased levels of consciousness due to low blood pressure and not enough blood reaching the brain, which results when the heart is not pumping hard enough because of decreased sympathetic tone. These patients should be laid down with their feet elevated, and intravenous fluids should be administered if necessary.

If a patient taking a beta-blocker has an allergic reaction, do not indiscriminately treat him or her with epinephrine as you normally would (see Chap. 3). There is a normal balance between alpha- and beta-tone on blood vessels. With the beta effect blocked, however, blood vessels can constrict from unopposed alpha-tone, and the patient may go into a *hypertensive crisis* if epinephrine is administered. The patient's blood pressure may rise to dangerous levels, and the patient could die of a stroke. Use an antihistamine (such as diphenhydramine or Benadryl), contact your medical control, and use epinephrine only if the patient is dangerously hypotensive.

The Parasympathetic Nervous System

The parasympathetic system is much simpler from a paramedic's point of view. If the sympathetic system is the body's gas pedal, the parasympathetic system is the body's brakes, with the general effect of slowing everything down.

Anatomically, almost all of the body's parasympathetics arise from the **vagus nerve**, a cranial nerve arising from the brain stem (Fig. 2-26). Parasympathetic effects often are referred to as **vagal responses** because they are mediated by the vagus nerve. Because the vagus nerve does not arise from the spinal cord, it is not affected by spinal trauma. Parasympathetic fibers that innervate the pelvis also arise from the sacrum.

As mentioned, parasympathetic responses are mediated by acetylcholine and cholinergic receptors, found throughout the body as illustrated in Table 2-5. The most important parasympathetic effects for the paramedic to consider are those on the heart, lungs, and blood vessels. The vagus nerve innervates the *sinus node* and the *atrioventricular node* of the heart (see Chap. 3) with the net effect of slowing it down. Vagal tone causes bronchoconstriction, making it more difficult to breath, and vasodilation, which can cause a sudden drop in blood pressure.

CLINICAL CORRELATION *A classic swooning faint, or syncope, usually is caused by a vasovagal event. A sudden increase in vagal tone triggered by some stressful event (the sight of blood, for example) causes the blood vessels to dilate and blood pressure to fall. The problem self-corrects when the patient collapses to the ground and blood then returns to the head.*

The vagus nerve also can be used to our advantage to slow the heart and lower blood pressure by being stimulated in a variety of ways, the most common being the **Valsalva maneuver** and the carotid sinus massage. These methods trick the body into thinking blood pressure is too high so that the brain increases vagal output.

CLINICAL CORRELATION *The Valsalva maneuver is performed by "bearing down" as if one is having a bowel movement and can be an effective way to stop a supraventricular tachycardia (see Chap. 3).*

Many older patients who are constipated inadvertently perform their own Valsalva maneuvers when having a bowel movement. It is not uncommon to find unconscious people in the bathroom. Again, the problem usually self-corrects once the patient lies flat.

Table 2-5. Parasympathetic receptors

Location	Effect
Pupils	Constriction
AV, SA node (in heart)	Decrease heart rate
Blood vessels	Dilation (lowers blood pressure)
Bronchi	Constriction
Gastrointestinal tract	Contraction (increased motility)
Anal sphincter	Relaxation (defecation)
Bladder	Contraction
Urinary sphincter	Relaxation (urination)
Penis	Erection

AV = atrioventricular; SA = sinoatrial.

Just as the sympathetic system has beta-blockers that block beta-receptors, there are blockers for the parasympathetic cholinergic receptors. The prototype *vagolytic* drug is **atropine**, a **parasympathetic blocker** or an **anticholinergic** drug, which works by simply blocking the parasympathetic receptor (Fig. 2-27).

Simply put, atropine acts by "taking your foot off of the brake." In contrast, epinephrine, the sympathetic drug, works by "putting your foot on the gas." In either case, the "car" should go faster.

CLINICAL CORRELATION *The first choice of drugs for symptomatic bradycardias (heart rates that are too slow) is atropine. As a parasympathetic blocker, atropine prevents the vagus nerve from slowing down the heart.*

Another physiologic point should be mentioned. Normally, the vagus nerve releases acetylcholine, which moves to the receptor of the next cell. The acetylcholine is removed from the receptor by an *enzyme* known as *acetylcholinesterase*. This is the crane that removes the key from the lock that stops the response started by the vagus nerve (Fig. 2-28). (It takes a crane to remove the key because it's a very big key.)

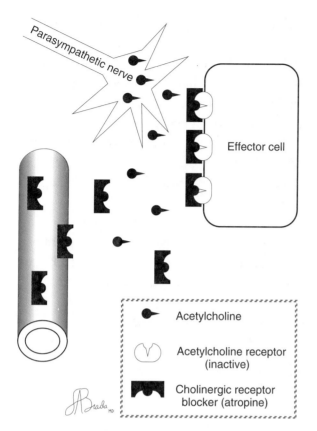

Fig. 2-27. Anticholinergics. Parasympathetic receptor blockers such as atropine prevent acetylcholine from reaching its receptors and prevent a parasympathetic response. Because much of the body's parasympathetic activity arises from the vagus nerve, these drugs also are referred to as vagolytics.

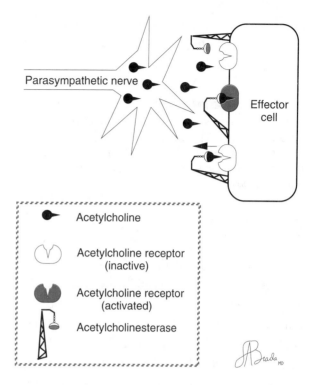

Fig. 2-28. Acetylcholinesterase function. In normal cells, acetylcholinesterase (the crane) removes acetylcholine from its receptor shortly after it binds. This limits the duration of the parasympathetic stimulus. Organophosphate insecticides short-circuit the crane, leaving the acetylcholine bound to the receptor. The net result is that the parasympathetics remain turned on and the patient may suffer a cholinergic crisis. Atropine (an anticholinergic) is the treatment of choice.

Organophosphates are chemicals found in most pesticides—both household bug killers and large-scale farm products—and in poison gas used by various armed forces as weapons of mass destruction ("nerve gas"). Organophosphates work by inhibiting acetylcholinesterase. They prevent the crane from removing the key from the lock, causing a massive overflow of vagus activity.

CLINICAL CORRELATION *Organophosphate poisoning most commonly results from accidental ingestion or inhalation of insecticides and is characterized by SLUDGE: salivation (drooling), lacrimation (tearing), urination (bladder incontinence), defecation (bowel incontinence), gastrointestinal upset (nausea), and emesis (vomiting), all of which are naturally turned on by the vagus. More important, patients with organophosphate poisoning experience life-threatening bronchoconstriction (tightening of the airways in the lungs) and eventually bradycardia (slow heart rate). Treatment is rapid, high doses of atropine to block the vagal effects. In addition, the drug pralidoxime, or 2-PAM, counteracts the vagus effects of organophosphate poisoning by regenerating acetylcholinesterase.*

GLANDS OF THE NECK

Thyroid

The **thyroid gland** is a butterfly-shaped gland in the front of the neck (see Fig. 2-6) that takes up iodine and produces thyroid hormone. Salt is iodized to ensure we get enough iodine.

CLINICAL CORRELATION *In urban areas, it is common to have influxes of refugees or immigrants from Third World countries who do not have sufficient iodine in their diets, resulting in goiters, or enlarged thyroid glands. Sometimes, the gland grows to be larger than a grapefruit, but only occasionally does it cause an airway compromise. Intervention before these patients arrive at the hospital usually is not necessary, but people with goiters need to be treated at the hospital.*

The function of thyroid hormone is to increase the body's overall metabolic activity level. It also works with the sympathetic system to control metabolism. A variety of thyroid diseases result in the thyroid gland's producing too much thyroid hormone, causing the patient to be **hyperthyroid,** or producing too little thyroid hormone, causing the patient to be **hypothyroid.** Size of the thyroid and thyroid function are not related.

Hypothyroid
Many thyroid diseases are best treated by the complete surgical removal of the thyroid gland, making patients hypothyroid for the rest of their lives. In addition, some thyroid diseases may cause the thyroid gland to become hypothyroid on its own. In acute or severe cases of hypothyroidism, a condition known as **myxedema coma** may ensue. Patients with myxedema have characteristically puffy faces, swelling (edema) almost everywhere, and a decreased level of consciousness that leads to coma. There is no specific treatment for myxedema before arriving at the hospital other than airway protection and respiratory support.

Hyperthyroid
In hyperthyroidism, the body is "revved-up." Hyperthyroid patients tend to sweat, to have racing heart rates and bugged-out eyes, and be hyperactive, nervous, jittery, always too warm, and skinny despite eating well. As noted, many of the effects of hyperthyroidism are sympathetic. Danger arises if the patient has an acute and severe thyroid excess known as **thyrotoxicosis,** or **thyrotoxic storm.** Thyrotoxicosis can be caused by an overdose of thyroid replacement medication (Synthroid), or it can happen spontaneously.

Patients in thyrotoxic storm develop life-threatening tachycardias (rapid heart rates). They go either into supraventricular tachycardia or ventricular tachycardia (see Chap. 3).

CLINICAL CORRELATION *The best immediate treatment for thyrotoxicosis is the administration of beta-blockers such as propranolol to stop the sympathetic effects. If this treatment is not available, treat cardiac rhythms symptomatically per normal advanced cardiac life support protocols.*

Parathyroids

Parathyroid glands are four very small glands along the back of the thyroid that regulate the body's calcium levels but have nothing to do with thyroid function. Disease of the parathyroids may result in kidney stone formation, which can be painful enough to warrant 911 calls, but you'll never need to treat the parathyroid glands directly.

Lymphatics

Lymph vessels drain the interstitial space (see Chap. 4), the fluid between cells, back into the veins. Within the lymphatics are *nodes* that harbor large collections of *lymphocytes,* a type of white blood cell whose role is to combat infection. When you have a cold or sore throat, the lymph nodes in your neck swell and are commonly called "swollen glands," though they are actually not glands at all.

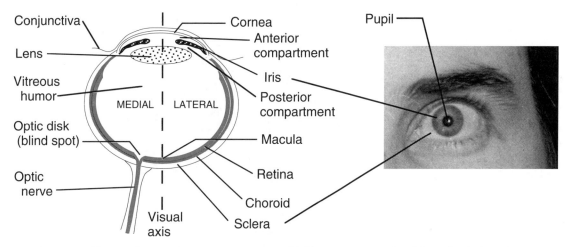

Fig. 2-29. The eye. The pupils are of greatest interest to EMTs and paramedics. They should be of equal size, be round, and constrict in response to light. Any abnormality is evidence of significant head injury or drug intoxication.

EYES AND EARS

Eyes

Light travels from the outside world through the **pupil** to the *lens*, which focuses images onto the *retina*. The *optic nerve* then collects images from the retina and sends them to the back of the brain (occipital lobe) for processing (Fig. 2-29).

The pupil is the dark center of the eye created by an opening in the *iris*. It is the iris that constricts or dilates to make the pupil larger or smaller, allowing more or less light in, even though we commonly say that the pupils are reacting to light. Normally, both pupils should constrict when a light is shined into either eye, known as a *consensual response*.

CLINICAL CORRELATION *Normally, the patient's eyes should be PERRL: pupils equal, round, and reactive to light, both direct and consensually. Anything else should be considered abnormal and noted. Typically, abnormal pupil responses are a sign of problems with the eye, the optic nerve, or the brain.*

The *cornea* is the clear surface outside of the lens. *Cataracts*, a condition in which the cornea becomes cloudy, often are corrected by surgery, which leaves the pupils in odd, asymmetric shapes.

CLINICAL CORRELATION *If the patient has an abnormal pupil, ask if he or she has ever had cataract or eye surgery, which could explain the abnormality.*

The **conjunctiva** are highly vascular membranes lining the inside of the eyelids and the surface of the eyes.

CLINICAL CORRELATION *The conjunctiva are good places to look for pallor or cyanosis, especially in dark-skinned people. The conjunctiva on the inside of the eyelids are normally quite pink and quickly turn pale, gray, or blue if deprived of oxygen or blood.*

The *sclera* are the so-called whites of the eye. Remember the battle cry of the Battle of Bunker Hill, "Don't shoot until you can see their sclera!" Yellow sclera or *jaundice* are signs of liver disease, which may be caused by *hepatitis. Always wear gloves.*

The lens focuses images on the *retina* at the back of the eye. Trauma can cause *retinal detachment*, with a sudden, painful loss of vision in that eye. Like retinal detachment, *retinal artery occlusion* is characterized by vision loss on one side; however, the vision loss is painless and is caused by thrombi becoming caught in the artery feeding the retina—actually a form of stroke. Ischemic events involving the entire brain or large por-

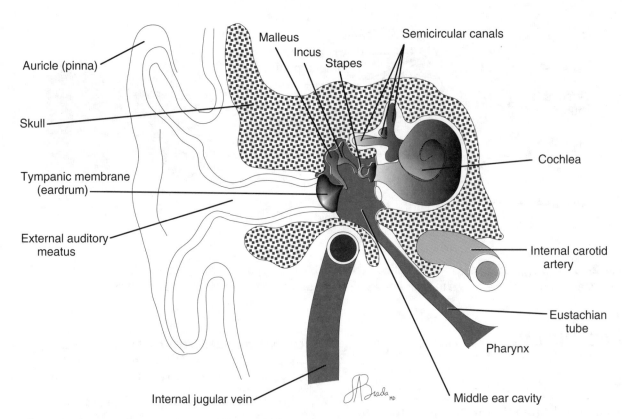

Fig. 2-30. The ear. The tympanic membrane (eardrum) can be damaged by loud noises or sudden pressure changes. The middle ear (shown in red) lies behind the eardrum and is prone to infection (otitis media) due to bacteria rising up the eustachian tubes from the pharynx.

tions of it also may be characterized by a painless loss of vision.

CLINICAL CORRELATION *Check vital signs and orthostatic blood pressures (see Chap. 3) of patients complaining of vision loss to ensure they are not hypotensive (have blood pressure that is too low).*

Glaucoma occurs when the pressure inside of the globe of the eye becomes too high. It is usually a slow, chronic process but may occur suddenly (acute glaucoma), causing severe pain in the eye. Patients usually complain of seeing halos around lights and blind spots and eventually may lose all vision.

CLINICAL CORRELATION *Eye problems may prompt calls for ambulances but are not life-threatening, and there is little to be done before arriving at the hospital unless you suspect a patient of having a retinal detachment. In this case, give the patient as gentle a ride as*

possible to the hospital; even bumps in the road can worsen retinal detachment.*

The eye muscles are yoked together in the nervous system, so both eyes move together.

CLINICAL CORRELATION *When you encounter any trauma to the eye, bandage both eyes even if only one eye is injured. Bandaging both eyes may prevent the uninjured eye from moving and dragging the injured eye with it.*

Ear

The external ear canal ends in the *tympanic membrane*, or eardrum (Fig. 2-30). Foreign objects often become stuck in the external canal, especially in children, and can be a painful, but not life-threatening, experience. The tiny bones of the *middle ear* transmit sound and are attached to the *eardrum*. The eardrum itself separates the external ear canal from the *auditory tube* (also called the *eustachian tube*), which leads down to the back of the throat. The eustachian tube is the source of ear infections that plague some children. Air pressure is equalized across the *tympanic membrane*; thus, the feeling of ears "popping" when you move to a different level of elevation in an airplane. The *inner ear*, physically separated from the middle ear by bone, helps the body determine and maintain balance.

Sinuses

Sinuses are simply cavities in the bones of the skull that make the head lighter and mechanically easier to support. The major sinuses are located in the lower forehead and the maxilla, around the nose, and behind the ear. They often become infected (*sinusitis/mastoiditis*) and may at times be extraordinarily painful, but a sinus infection is not a life-threatening condition.

VOCABULARY LIST

absence seizure	Petit mal seizures, staring spells common in children
adrenaline	(epinephrine) a predominantly beta-sympathetic stimulant produced both naturally in the body and synthetically as a medication
adrenergic	referring to the sympathetic nervous system
alpha-receptor	sympathetic receptor found mostly on blood vessels; causes vasoconstriction and increases blood pressure
angle of the mandible	the corner of the jaw
anticholinergic	anything that blocks the effects of the parasympathetic nervous system
artery	any blood vessel carrying blood away from the heart
arytenoid cartilage	a visual landmark for intubation posterior to the vocal cords
atropine	the prototype anticholinergic drug; a parasympathetic blocker
aura	a vague feeling some patients have preceding a seizure or migraine
autonomic nervous system	the part of the nervous system that controls involuntary functions
basilar skull fracture	a fracture of the bottom of the cranium
Battle's sign	ecchymosis about the mastoid; a sign of a basilar skull fracture
beta-blocker	any drug that blocks the beta responses of the sympathetic nervous system; propranolol is the prototype
beta$_1$-receptor	a sympathetic receptor found mostly in the heart; causes an increase in heart rate and force of contraction
beta$_2$-receptor	a sympathetic receptor found mostly in the lungs and bronchi; causes bronchodilation, which makes breathing easier
brain	part of the central nervous system; controls all higher functions in humans
brain stem	found at the base of the brain; connects the brain to the spinal cord; responsible for primitive body functions such as breathing and autonomic responses

carina	the point at which the trachea forks; the desired point for the end of an endotracheal tube
carotid artery	the major artery carrying blood from the heart to the head
carotid body/ carotid sinus	found just below the angle of the mandible; can be stimulated to produce a vagal response
carotid sinus massage	a vagal maneuver performed by briskly massaging the carotid body to slow the heart
central nervous system (CNS)	the brain and the spinal cord
cerebellum	part of the brain responsible for coordination
cerebrospinal fluid (CSF)	the clear, colorless fluid that bathes the central nervous system and acts as a shock absorber
cerebrovascular accident (CVA)	a stroke; a neurological deficit caused by an area of the brain becoming ischemic
cerebrum	part of the brain responsible for higher function
cervical spine	seven vertebrae immediately below the head
cholinergic	referring to the parasympathetic nervous system
coccyx	fused tailbone; the end of the spine
complex partial seizure	a seizure that starts in a focused area of the brain and causes an alteration in level of consciousness without necessarily becoming a grand mal seizure
conjunctiva	the highly vascular membrane covering the inside of the eyelid and the surface of the eye; the inside of the eyelid is normally pink
cranium	the bones of the head that form a rigid protective shell around the brain
cricoid cartilage	cartilage that sits anterior in the neck; lower border of cricothyroid membrane
cricothyroid membrane	a membrane stretching between the cricoid cartilage and thyroid cartilage; a good site for emergency airway access
diaphragm	the major muscle of breathing separating the chest from the abdomen
dura mater	"tough mother," the outermost meninge covering the central nervous system

ecchymosis	pooling of blood beneath the skin; bruising
epidural hematoma	collecting of blood in the epidural space secondary to trauma
epidural space	the space between the dura and the skull
epiglottis	the "flapper valve" protecting the top of the trachea
epilepsy	a diagnosis of seizures with no other known cause
epinephrine	adrenaline, the prototype sympathetic stimulator
esophagus	the "food tube" connecting the pharynx to the stomach
external jugular vein	vein that runs across the sternocleidomastoid muscle; a good site for emergency peripheral intravenous line access
frontal	the bone of the forehead; part of the cranium
glottis	the space between the vocal cords that needs to be visualized during intubation in order to pass an endotracheal tube into the trachea
grand mal seizure	a primary generalized seizure characterized by periods of muscle tension and spastic movements
heart failure	any condition in which the heart cannot pump an adequate supply of blood, causing a backup of blood behind the side of the heart that is failing
hyperthyroid	an excess of thyroid hormone; causes an overactive metabolic state
hypothyroid	a deficiency of thyroid hormone; causes an underactive metabolic state
internal jugular vein	vein best found just superior to the sternum and clavicle
intracranial pressure (ICP)	the pressure inside the head; is elevated by any bleeding inside the cranium
ischemic	deprived of blood
jugular venous distention (JVD)	engorgement of the jugular veins, especially the internal jugular; a sign of right-sided heart failure
larynx	the voice box, protected in front by the thyroid cartilage; contains the vocal cords
lucid interval	a period of normal consciousness between an initial loss of consciousness and a coma; characteristic of epidural hematomas

lumbar spine	the large spine of the lower back
mainstem bronchi	the two principle airways leading to each lung and arising just proximal to the carina
mandible	the jaw
mastoid process	the bony prominence at the base of the skull behind the ear
maxilla	the facial bones below the nose
meninges	the coverings of the brain and spinal cord
meningitis	inflammation of the meninges; may be caused by an infectious agent
myxedema coma	loss of consciousness accompanied by facial swelling; caused by hypothyroidism
nares	nostrils, the openings of the nose
nasal septum	the internal divider between the left and right side of the nose made mostly of cartilage
nasopharynx	the airway passage through the nose
neurogenic shock	a shock state caused by widespread vasodilation due to loss of sympathetic tone, secondary to spinal trauma
occipital	the bone on the back of the cranium
orbits	eye sockets
organophosphates	common poisons found in most insecticides
organophosphate poisoning	poisoning characterized by overactive parasympathetic tone and treated with atropine
oropharynx	the airway passage through the mouth
parasympathetic blocker	any drug that blocks the effects of the parasympathetic system; atropine is the prototype
parasympathetic nervous system	the part of the autonomic nervous system that tends to slow the body down, decrease heart rate, bronchoconstrict, and vasodilate
parietal	the bones on the top of the cranium on each side
pharynx	the upper "throat"; the airway passage connecting the mouth and nose to the larynx
phrenic nerve	the major nerve of respiration coming off of the spinal cord at C3-4-5; innervates the diaphragm

postictal	a period of confusion or decreased level of consciousness immediately following grand mal seizures
pulse pressure	the difference between the systolic and diastolic blood pressures; may widen with increased intracranial pressure
pupil	the normally round, dark circle in the center of the eye; both pupils should become smaller when light is shined into either eye
raccoon eyes	ecchymosis about the orbits; a sign of basilar skull fracture
sacrum	the "butt bone," a fused bone of the spine between the lumbar spine and the coccyx
scalp	the layers of skin stretched across the head; tends to bleed profusely if cut
spinal cord	the major nervous pathway connecting the brain and the body; is protected by the spine
spine	the backbone or spinal column; a long series of vertebrae
status epilepticus	seizures that will not stop or seizures that recur before the patient can regain consciousness
sternocleidomastoid muscle	the large strap-like muscle of the neck; a landmark for the carotid artery and the internal jugular vein
subdural hematoma	bleeding into the subdural space that is usually caused by even minor trauma
subdural space	the space below the dura mater outside the brain
sympathetic nervous system	the part of the autonomic nervous system representing the body's "fight or flight" response; its general effect is to speed the body up, increase heart rate, bronchodilate, vasoconstrict, and raise blood pressure
sympathetic tone	activation of the sympathetic nervous system, a baseline that can be increased or blocked (decreased)
sympathomimetic	any drug that mimics the sympathetic nervous system
temporal	the bones on the side of the head; the temples
temporal lobe epilepsy	a common type of epilepsy that results in complex partial seizures characterized by bizarre behavior and activity not necessarily accompanied by grand mal seizures
thoracic spine	the spine of the chest and rib cage between the cervical spine and the lumbar spine

thrombus a blood clot

thyroid cartilage the "Adam's apple"; cartilage in the neck that protects the larynx

thyroid gland butterfly-shaped gland to the side of the thyroid cartilage that maintains the body's metabolic rate

thyrotoxicosis/ thyrotoxic storm an emergency caused by hyperthyroidism usually resulting in life-threatening tachyarrhythmias

trachea the windpipe; airway passage leading from the larynx to the mainstem bronchi

transient ischemic attack (TIA) a "mini-stroke" similar to a cerebrovascular accident but lasting only minutes to hours and producing no permanent deficit

turbinates plates on the lateral side of the nose that warm and filter air

vagal maneuvers procedures that increase the body's vagal tone, or level of parasympathetic stimulus

vagal response a response that stimulates the parasympathetic nervous system

vagus nerve the major nerve of the parasympathetic nervous system

vallecula the soft tissue anterior to the epiglottis that must be displaced forward during endotracheal intubation

Valsalva maneuver a vagal maneuver performed by bearing down as if having a bowel movement

vasovagal a response occurring after parasympathetic stimulation that causes vasodilation and usually results in a sudden drop of blood pressure and syncope (fainting)

vein a blood vessel that carries blood back to the heart

vertebra one of the bones of the spine; plural: vertebrae

vocal cords cords within the larynx that allow us to speak, appear to be a white inverted V during endotracheal intubation

SELF-ASSESSMENT QUESTIONS

1. You have been called to aid a man who has been shot in the face at close range. The police have secured the scene. On initial assessment, you find the man moaning in pain. His jaw is barely recognizable, his face is grossly distorted, and he is gurgling blood. What are your initial priorities, and how would you manage this patient?

2. You are called to the home of an elderly woman who reportedly collapsed to the ground. On initial assessment, she appears alert and in no acute distress but does not speak. Her mouth is draining sputum. Her breathing is regular and unlabored, and her vital signs are all within normal limits. She is able to follow commands but only with her left arm and leg. What is your initial diagnosis, and how would you manage her?

3. You are called to a street corner by police for a man displaying "bizarre behavior." On arrival, you see an approximately 25-year-old slender man, clearly pale and diaphoretic, drop to the ground and become very stiff in a tonic contraction. What do you do?

4. A motorist calls you to the aid of a bicyclist found sitting by the side of the road. The bicyclist clearly has been in an accident: His bicycle is severely damaged, and he has numerous cuts and scrapes. He was not wearing a helmet. He is alert but does not remember what happened. He is generally uncooperative and does not wish to be examined or treated. What are your thoughts, and what should you do?

5. You are called to a farm where a young worker is reportedly "sick, dazed, and confused" after cleaning a storage shed. Firefighters report cleaning a white powder off of him and assure you that he is not a contamination risk. On arrival, you find an otherwise healthy-appearing young man lying on the ground responsive to voice but completely disoriented. He is draining copious fluids from his mouth and nose. What are your greatest concerns regarding this patient?

3

Thorax, Cardiovascular System, and Respiratory System

THE CHEST WALL

The term **thorax** refers to the chest and all of its contents. The chest is a well-armored cage designed to protect the body's vital organs. The **chest wall** consists of the bones and muscles making up the cage.

Bony Structures of the Chest

In the back, 12 **thoracic vertebrae**, the thoracic spine, define the backbone of the chest. Each thoracic vertebra gives rise to a pair of **ribs**; thus, there are 12 pairs of ribs. The first seven pairs, the *true ribs*, join by *costal cartilage* to the **sternum**, or breastbone, in front. The eighth, ninth, and tenth ribs, or *false ribs*, each join to the rib above it in front. The eleventh and twelfth ribs, the *floating ribs*, are not connected to anything in front. The space between each rib is known as **intercostal space** (Figs. 3-1 and 3-2).

The superior-most (top) part of the sternum is the **sternal notch**. The sternum also forms an angle, known as the **sternal angle**, at the point where the second rib joins it. The bottom, or inferior-most part, of the sternum is the **xiphoid**, made of cartilage at birth but eventually hardening (calcifying) into bone with age.

CLINICAL CORRELATION *The best place to look for tracheal deviation is in the sternal notch. Always feel for the trachea in the sternal notch of any patient who has sustained trauma to the chest or of any patient you suspect of having a tension pneumothorax. If the trachea is not in the midline, it is deviated, a sign of a tension pneumothorax (see the section on Respiratory Injuries).*

CLINICAL CORRELATION *The xiphoid, although made of cartilage in young people, is almost always hard and sharp in older people, the patients who most often need cardiopulmonary resuscitation (CPR). Proper hand position is essential during CPR to avoid breaking the xiphoid, which can lacerate (jaggedly cut) the liver directly underneath it. When performing CPR, your hands should be a distance of two finger widths above the xiphoid.*

45

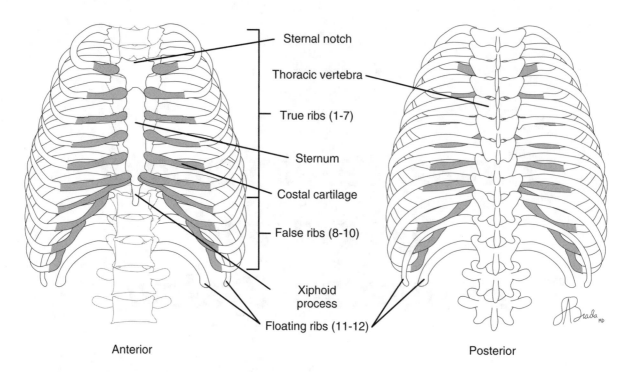

Fig. 3-1. The bony thorax. The 12 pairs of ribs, thoracic vertebrae, and sternum form a protective shell for both the chest and upper abdomen.

CLINICAL CORRELATION *In elderly people, bones and cartilage generally are brittle and easy to break. When performing CPR, it is very common to either separate the costal cartilage or break ribs when you start compressions, even when correctly performing CPR. It is an awful feeling and sound, so don't be surprised or alarmed. Just recheck your hand position to make sure you are still in the right place.*

CLINICAL CORRELATION *The sternal angle is an important and easily palpable landmark—that is, it is easy to feel when running a finger down the sternum, even on obese people (see Fig. 3-2). (Try to find it on yourself.) When you feel the sternal angle, you know you are at the level of the second rib. The space below that rib is the second intercostal space, which you may need to find if you need to do a needle decompression of a tension pneumothorax (see the section on respiratory injuries).*

The **clavicle**, or collar bone, and **scapula**, or shoulder blade, are bones found on the chest actually of the upper extremity, or arm (Fig. 3-3). The clavicle and scapula anchor the arm to the rest of the body and with the muscles of the upper extremity form the *shoulder girdle*, discussed in more detail in Chapter 6.

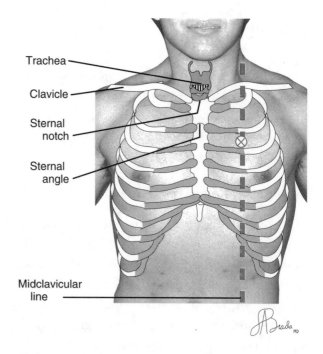

Fig. 3-2. Surface anatomy of the chest. The best place to perform needle thoracentesis is at the second intercostal space along the midclavicular line.

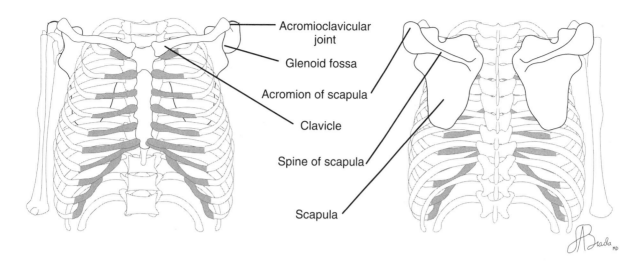

Fig. 3-3. Clavicle and scapula. Located on the anterior and posterior surface of the ribcage, the clavicle and scapula are the only connections between the bone of the upper arm (humerus) and the axial skeleton.

Muscles of the Chest

The muscles of the chest support the arms, head, and back and help with breathing. An anatomically important feature of the chest muscles in the back is the **triangle of auscultation**. This area is not covered by extra muscle layers but forms a bare triangle from the edges of three muscles (Fig. 3-4).

CLINICAL CORRELATION *The best spot to listen for (or auscultate) lung sounds is the triangle of auscultation, where you can hear the lungs more directly, rather than through thick muscle layers. The spot is located just medial and inferior to the bottom corner of the scapula and enables you to listen to the base, or bottom, of the lungs, where fluid can accumulate when a person's heart fails (see section on The Circulatory Pathway Through the Heart).*

THE CIRCULATORY PATHWAY THROUGH THE HEART

The heart is a hollow muscle and is the main part of the **cardiovascular system** (cardio = heart, vascular = blood vessels). The cardiovascular system, also known as the **circulatory system** and the "C" of the "ABCs," includes

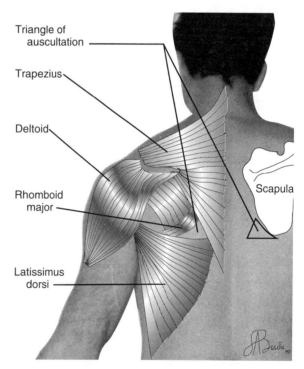

Fig. 3-4. Triangle of auscultation. Located between the borders of the trapezius, latissimus dorsi, and rhomboid major, the triangle allows stethoscope access to the lungs without the interference of any overlying muscles.

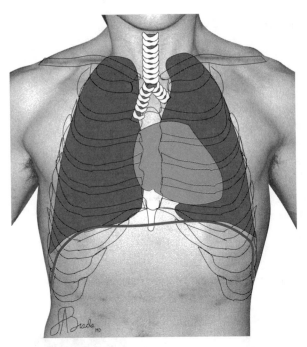

Fig. 3-5. Surface projection of the heart and lungs.

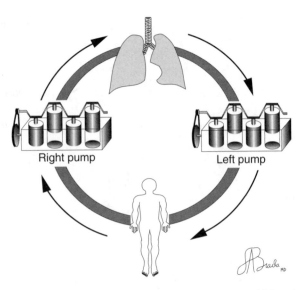

Fig. 3-6. The circulatory cycle. Deoxygenated blood returning from the body enters the right side of the heart, which pumps it to the lungs to be oxygenated. Oxygen-rich blood then enters the left side of the heart, which pumps it under high pressure throughout the body.

the heart, blood vessels, and the blood carried throughout the body. The function of the system is to bring blood everywhere in the body. When the system fails either from injury or illness, life-threatening emergencies occur.

The heart is located in the middle of the chest, slightly leaning to the left (Fig. 3-5) and sandwiched between the lungs. It rests on top of the **diaphragm**, the muscle separating the chest from the abdomen.

When considering the anatomy of the heart, it is important to remember the heart's function. The heart is nothing more than a pump, a muscle that simply squeezes blood out when it beats. Blood returns from all over the body to the *right side* of the heart, which pumps the blood into the lungs. The blood then flows from the lungs to the *left side* of the heart, which pumps it back out to the rest of the body again (Fig. 3-6).

Physically, the heart is shaped like a globular cone. The *base* of the heart (or cone) happens to be up and to the right, and the *apex*, or point, of the heart/cone is down and to the left.

The heart has four chambers: the **right atrium** and **right ventricle,** making up the *right heart,* and the **left atrium** and **left ventricle,** making up the *left heart.* The atria (plural for atrium) sit on top of the ventricles (Fig. 3-7).

The detailed circulatory pathway through the heart is as follows: Blood from the head and arms returns through the **superior vena cava** ("upper big vein"); blood from the lower body returns through the **inferior vena cava** ("lower big vein"). This is **venous blood,** which has little **oxygen** (O_2) and a lot of **carbon dioxide** (CO_2). The two venae cavae drain venous blood into the right atrium. The right atrium **contracts,** pumping blood into the right ventricle, which is separated from the right atrium by the **tricuspid valve.** (Valves exist in the heart and veins to keep blood from flowing backward. When working correctly, all the valves are "one-way valves.") When the right atrium contracts, the tricuspid valve is blown open and blood enters the ventricle.

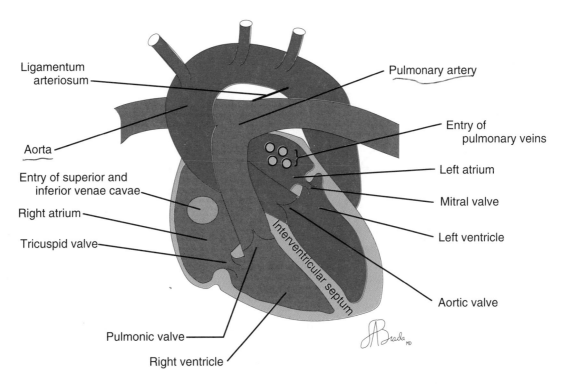

Fig. 3-7. The heart. The atrium and ventricle of the right side of the heart work in series with the two chambers on the left to circulate blood between the lungs and body tissues. Each chamber contains a one-way valve at its exit to ensure blood flows in only one direction. The right side pumps deoxygenated blood (gray) to the lungs via the pulmonary arteries. The left side of the heart pumps the newly oxygenated blood (red) through the aorta and to the rest of the body.

The tricuspid valve is anchored by **chordae tendinae** (tendinous chords), which connect the leaflets of the valves to **papillary muscles** inside the right ventricle. When the right ventricle contracts, the papillary muscles also contract, or shorten, preventing the tricuspid valve from being blown backward into the atrium and holding it closed so that blood does not go backward (Fig. 3-8).

Blood leaves the right ventricle through the **pulmonic valve,** blown open when the ventricle contracts. This blood must travel only as far as the lungs, which normally do not offer much resistance to blood flow. Hence, the right ventricle need not produce much pressure to pump blood into the lungs, making the right side of the heart a *low-pressure* pumping system.

Blood from the right ventricle then enters the **pulmonary artery,** which splits right and left to supply the lungs. In the lungs, blood releases CO_2 and picks up O_2. The blood, now described as **oxygenated** or **arterial,** returns through the **pulmonary veins** to the **left atrium.**

(Note: A favorite trick question on paramedic tests makes the point that the pulmonary *vein* carries oxygenated blood, and the pulmonary *artery* carries deoxygenated blood. The reverse is true everywhere else in the body. The term artery refers to a blood vessel leaving the heart, and a vein is a blood vessel returning to the heart.)

The left side of the heart is very similar to the right. Blood leaves the left atrium through the **mitral valve,** entering the left ventricle. The mitral valve, like the tricuspid valve, is anchored with its own set of chordae tendinae and papillary muscles. The left ventricle is the largest, and by far the most important chamber of the heart because it has the duty of pumping blood throughout the

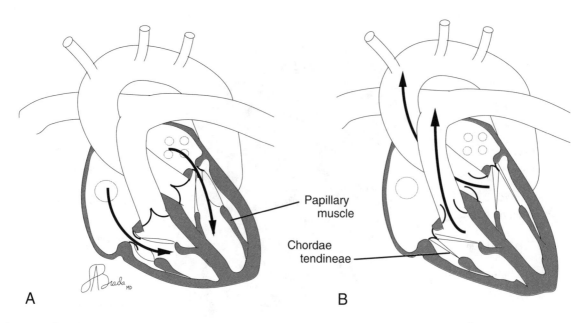

Fig. 3-8 Cardiac contraction. A. The heart during the diastolic (relaxation) phase. Pressures in both atria are higher than the corresponding ventricles, allowing blood returning from the vena cavae and pulmonary veins to flow through the open tricuspid and mitral valves. B. The ventricles contract simultaneously, increasing the pressure within the ventricles and closing the tricuspid and mitral valves, which are kept from blowing back into the atria by chordae tendineae. The increased pressure forces open the pulmonic and aortic valves and ejects blood into the pulmonary artery and aorta.

body. In order to do this, it must pump using a lot of pressure, making the left side of the heart a *high-pressure* pumping system.

The left ventricle pumps blood through the **aortic valve**, which is very similar in function to the pulmonic valve on the right side, to the **aorta**, the giant blood vessel that eventually branches into arteries throughout the body. The blood then collects in the veins and returns to the heart, completing the circuit.

Heart Failure

Heart failure occurs when the heart does not pump sufficiently to circulate blood. Just as in a mechanical pump, failure of either side of the heart to pump causes fluid to back up *behind* the pump. *Left heart failure* occurs when the left side of the heart fails and fluid backs up into the lungs because the left ventricle cannot pump it out of the lungs (Fig. 3-9).

CLINICAL CORRELATION *Fluid in the lungs, most often caused by left heart failure, is known as pulmonary edema. Pulmonary refers to circulation in the lungs; edema means fluid collecting where it doesn't belong. Pulmonary edema is diagnosed clinically by listening to lung sounds and hearing a wet sound known as rales or crackles (the two terms are largely interchangeable) that is similar to the sound made by rubbing hair together next to your ear. The best place to hear lung sounds is the triangle of auscultation because you are listening to the bottom of the lungs, where gravity tends to pull fluid. Severe pulmonary edema is a life-threatening emergency that initially can be rapidly and effectively treated by sitting the patient up to prevent fluid from spreading throughout the lungs, dangling the feet to help fluid pool in the legs instead of in the lungs, and giving oxygen. In addition, giving nitroglycerin, morphine, and/or furosemide (Lasix) usually are warranted (see sections on Cardiovascular Dynamics and Anatomy of the Respiratory System).*

The left side of the heart usually is considered more important because when it stops functioning, the brain begins to lose blood and the lungs fill with fluid. Either of these events can lead

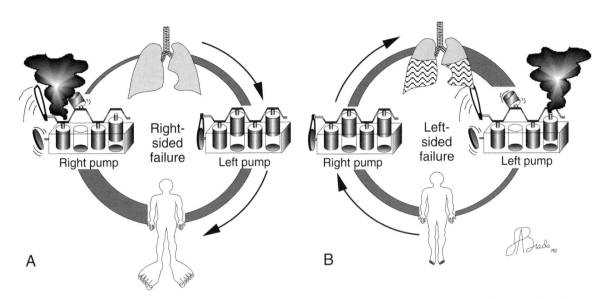

Fig. 3-9. Heart failure. A. The mechanism of right-sided heart failure. Blood returning from the body is not pumped to the lungs and pools in the veins. Systemic venous pressure increases while pulmonary arterial pressure falls. Increased venous pressure causes fluid to seep into body tissues and collect in dependent regions, producing pedal edema. B. The scenario is similar, except left-sided heart failure produces a backlog of blood in the pulmonary veins that results in pulmonary edema and a fall in systemic arterial pressure.

rapidly to death. The right side of the heart can fail too. When it does, fluid backs up behind it and the whole body collects fluid (see Fig. 3-9).

CLINICAL CORRELATION *The classic sign of right heart failure is pedal edema. Pedal means foot; edema still means fluid where it doesn't belong. The feet, usually the lowest part of the body, collect fluid. Both feet and ankles tend to swell, often dramatically. The term dependent edema also is used to refer to the fact that the feet are the most "dependent," that is, the lowest point in the body. You can tell an ankle is swollen (and not just fat) when you push a finger into the skin and leave behind a small indention, or pit, that does not spring back for some time, warranting the term pitting edema. Pitting edema is rated on a scale of "1 plus" to "4 plus" (+, ++, +++ ,++++) depending on the severity of the edema or how high up the leg the edema goes. One plus refers to edema in the foot, "++" the ankle, "+++" the knee, and "++++" up to the waist or higher. Remember: The more plusses, the more severe the edema.*

CLINICAL CORRELATION *The other classic sign of severe right heart failure is jugular venous distention. When the right side of the heart cannot pump, blood backs up into the internal jugular vein. Jugular venous distention is best seen in the notch between the two heads of the sternocleidomastoid muscle (see Chap. 2).*

Heart failure has a variety of causes and can come on suddenly (*acutely*) or be an ongoing, *chronic* problem (or both). Chronic patients also are prone to acute, sudden attacks of pulmonary edema. Patients with chronic heart failure often tell you they have a history of **congestive heart failure,** often used as a catch-all term for any type of heart failure.

The most common cause of left heart failure is damage to the heart muscle over time from **ischemia,** meaning not enough blood getting to where it's needed. As described in the next section, if the heart is prevented from getting the blood it needs, it eventually will be damaged, not pump well, and fail. Heart failure also can be caused by a heart attack, where heart muscle dies and can no longer pump. Other causes of heart failure include valve problems (either not opening or allowing blood to pump backwards) or other diseases of the heart such as infections.

A patient may have either left or right heart failure or both. Left heart failure from long-term damage is more common because the left ventricle is the part of the pump that does the most work by far. Left heart failure may lead to right heart failure. The most common cause of right heart failure is left heart failure, but right heart failure alone usually is caused by *lung disease* (see section on Anatomy of the Respiratory System). When smokers' lungs are diseased, it is virtually always more difficult for their right ventricles to pump blood through them. Recall that the right ventricle normally works under low pressure and usually does not need to exert much effort to pump blood into the lungs. With lung disease, however, the right ventricle has to work harder and harder, eventually cannot live up to the demand, and fails. This is called **cor pulmonale**, or right-sided heart failure caused by chronic lung disease.

Heart Sounds

Under the best of circumstances, heart sounds are difficult to hear accurately, and in the field with diesel engines running, it is almost impossible. If you have the chance to listen to many hearts during your hospital training rotations, you may be provided with one more diagnostic tool in your bag of tricks. Unlike lung sounds, which every emergency medical technician and paramedic should be very good at distinguishing, heart sounds are much less essential for paramedics to master.

The heart makes a variety of sounds when it beats. A regular heartbeat has two parts: the contraction of the atria rapidly followed by the contraction of the ventricles. A normal heart makes two sounds called S1 and S2. If you listen to the heart with your stethoscope, you will hear a "lub-dub." S1, the "lub," is the sound made when the tricuspid and mitral valves close after the atria contract. S2, the "dub," is the sound made when the pulmonic and aortic valves close after the ventricles contract.

An additional heart sound is the *gallop*, so named because it has the sound of a horse galloping. S3 is an extra sound heard just after the normal S2 that supposedly is caused by turbulent blood flow vibrating around the heart from excess fluid. S4 is a sound heard just before S1 that may occur because of turbulence caused by excess back pressure on the left ventricle.

CLINICAL CORRELATION *Gallops have the rhythm of saying the word "Tennessee" very quickly. They are not healthy or normal and are often a sign of heart failure. If you hear a gallop, look for other signs of heart failure you might need to treat, namely pulmonary edema.*

A *murmur* is a coarse, flowing sound in addition to the normal S1 and S2 that may represent only a large amount of blood flow (such as in a young athlete) or, more seriously, disease of the heart valves. There are a wide variety of murmurs of differing significance, so if someone tells you he or she has a murmur, do not necessarily be alarmed.

The single best place to listen to the heart is in the midclavicular line on the left side, below the nipple, and between the ribs—the fifth intercostal space, also called the *point of maximal impulse* because it is over the apex of the left ventricle, normally the hardest pumping part of the heart (Fig. 3-10).

THE HEART MUSCLE

The tissue of the heart itself has four layers: the **pericardium, epicardium, myocardium,** and **endocardium.** The pericardium, or **pericardial sac,** is a tough, fibrous sac surrounding the heart (peri = around, cardia = heart) (Fig. 3-11). The outermost layer of the heart wall is called the **epicardium** (epi = outside), the bulk of the heart muscle is called the **myocardium** (myo = muscle), and the innermost layer of the heart is called the **endocardium** (endo = within).

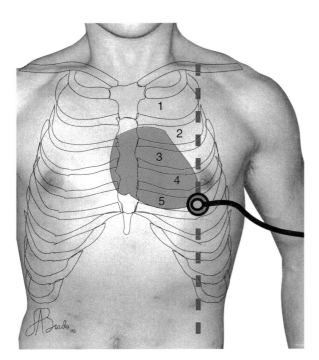

Fig. 3-10. Point of maximal impulse.

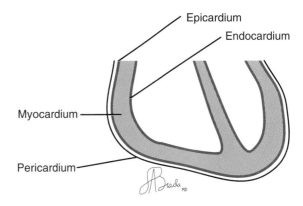

Fig. 3-11. The layers of the heart. The wall of the heart consists of the innermost endocardium, the myocardium, and the outermost epicardium. The heart is surrounded by a double-layered fibrous sac closely applied to the epicardium called the pericardium (shown in black).

If the heart suffers direct trauma, either penetrating trauma, such as a knife or gunshot wound, or blunt trauma, such as a motor vehicle accident, the myocardium (heart muscle) can bleed. When the myocardium bleeds, however, blood tends to become trapped in the pericardium, which cannot stretch well and squeezes the heart muscle, a life-threatening condition known as a **pericardial tamponade** (Fig. 3-12). As blood in the pericardium compresses the heart, the inside of the heart cannot fill with blood, preventing the heart from pumping any blood out and possibly leading to **heart failure**, **cardiogenic shock** (see section on Shock), or **pulseless electrical activity** (see below).

CLINICAL CORRELATION *To diagnose a tamponade, you must be highly suspicious of any significant chest trauma. The classic signs of tamponade are jugular venous distention, a narrowing pulse pressure (that is, the systolic and diastolic blood pressure become very close) (see section on Cardiovascular Dynamics), heart sounds that become "distant" or hard to hear, and eventually, low blood pressure and shock (see section on Shock).*

The treatment for a pericardial tamponade is to drain the blood out of the pericardial sac. This is best done at the hospital. As an act of sheer desperation, it is possible to drain the pericardial sac through the chest wall with a needle, a procedure known as *pericardiocentesis.*

CLINICAL CORRELATION *To perform a pericardiocentesis in the field, you need a long needle, a syringe, and a patient with nothing to lose (seriously). Insert the needle below the xiphoid at an angle upward and backward toward the left shoulder. The key is to aspirate (or pull back on) the syringe while you approach. When you get a return of blood, presumably you have reached the pericardial sac. Always monitor the patient's electrocardiogram (ECG) closely because the needle's hitting the myocardium is likely to cause abnormal beats. Pericardiocentesis is an extremely risky procedure under the best of circumstances and can be recommended only as a last resort.*

Blood Supply to the Heart

The heart, like everything else in the body, needs oxygenated blood to survive. The heart cannot pull much blood from the inside, so it is fed by two arteries coming off the base of the aorta known as **coronary arteries**, namely, the *right*

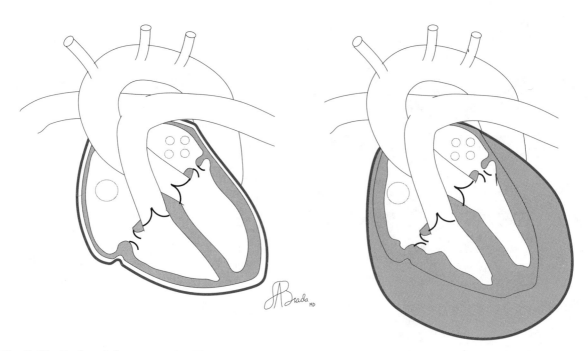

Fig. 3-12. Pericardial tamponade. The figure on the left shows the normal relation of the pericardium (in red) to the exterior of the heart. Rupture of a coronary artery or of the heart muscle itself can cause the pericardial space to become distended with blood, as seen on the right. Notice how this distension compresses the heart and limits the amount of blood that can fill each chamber.

and *left main coronary arteries.* (Coronary means like a crown, as in "coronation," and the coronary arteries sit like a crown on top of the heart). The left main coronary artery rapidly splits into the *left anterior descending (LAD) artery* and the *circumflex.* The right coronary artery, LAD, and circumflex arteries then branch into numerous smaller arteries supplying blood to the heart (Fig. 3-13).

The coronary arteries are prone to disease. In fact, coronary artery disease is by far the leading cause of death in the United States. In young, healthy vegetarians, coronary arteries are wide open and blood easily flows through them to the heart muscle. As people become older and eat too many cheeseburgers, deposits of fat and cholesterol known as *plaques* accumulate in their coronary arteries. The formation of plaques is known as *atherosclerosis,* or hardening of the arteries (Fig. 3-14). Smoking is one of the most significant contributors to arterial disease.

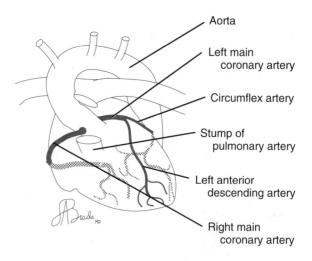

Aorta

Left main coronary artery

Circumflex artery

Stump of pulmonary artery

Left anterior descending artery

Right main coronary artery

Fig. 3-13. The coronary circulation. Blood supply to the heart is provided by three major vessels: the right main coronary artery, which supplies the right atrium and part of the base; the left main coronary artery, which divides into the left anterior descending artery and supplies the anterior aspects of the heart and septum; and the circumflex artery, which loops around the back of the heart and supplies the left atrium and ventricle.

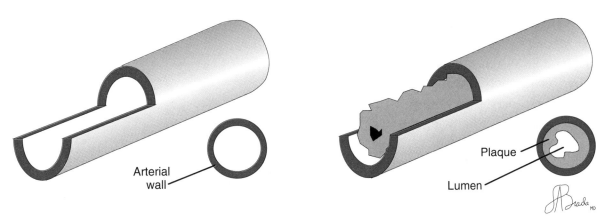

Fig. 3-14. Atherosclerosis. Cholesterol and fatty deposits form plaques in arteries. Plaques limit blood flow downstream by reducing the size of the arterial lumen and interfering with the wall's normal elasticity.

When an artery "hardens" (becomes atherosclerotic), two things occur: The internal passage, or lumen, becomes more narrow so that less blood can flow through it, and the artery loses its flexibility, preventing it from stretching out (dilating) to meet higher needs downstream.

Angina

Working, exercising, or stress of any sort all make the heart work harder. When the heart works hard, it needs more oxygen and therefore more blood. If coronary arteries are narrow and hard, the heart cannot get the blood it needs. When the heart requires more blood than the coronary arteries can deliver, the heart muscle becomes *ischemic*. As stated previously, ischemia means not enough blood being delivered to a tissue that needs it—in this case, the heart. This condition is known as **angina** (or *angina pectoris)*, characterized by dull, aching, or crushing chest pain below the sternum (substernal) that comes on after some exertion (e.g., shoveling snow, climbing stairs). The pain also typically is relieved by rest. When the heart is at risk of being damaged (as in an anginal attack), the body's response is to push the "panic button"; thus, it is not uncommon for the sympathetic nervous system to be activated (see Chap. 2). Therefore, sympathetic

nervous system responses can occur with angina: pale, cool, clammy skin, fast heart rate, etc.

CLINICAL CORRELATION *Angina typically presents as chest pain, but many patients present with "anginal equivalents" such as shortness of breath or abdominal pain as their chief complaints. Do not be too quick to disregard someone as not having a cardiac problem just because they do not present with classic symptoms. Up to one-fourth of elderly patients with angina do not complain of chest pain.*

CLINICAL CORRELATION *The treatment of choice for angina is oxygen, nitroglycerin, and/or morphine. Many patients carry their own nitroglycerin tablets, and emergency medical technicians can encourage them to take their own medicine. It is important to remember that these tablets need to dissolve under the tongue— they are useless if swallowed. Also remember that nitroglycerin loses its effectiveness quickly if exposed to light. If patients don't tell you that the tablet burned or tingled under their tongues or that they have a headache, the tablet may have been useless.*

Myocardial Infarction

A tissue that is ischemic long enough dies, and becomes infarcted. A **myocardial infarction**, or heart attack, is death of myocardial (heart muscle) tissue from a lack of blood supply (Fig. 3-15). When heart muscle dies, it cannot grow back. A heart attack is not, however, the same thing as cardiac arrest (death from the heart stopping). A person can have a heart attack and have some of his or her heart muscle die, yet the person can survive. It is even possible for a person to have a "silent heart attack" without ever knowing that part of his or her heart muscle has died.

Heart attacks usually are caused by blood clots that form in the coronary arteries along the rough surfaces of the cholesterol plaques found in everyone with coronary artery disease. A blood clot (or **thrombus**) then can break off, float downstream, become stuck, and completely block blood flow to the rest of the heart normally supplied by that artery.

CLINICAL CORRELATION   *A clot's becoming stuck in an artery is a random event. Thus, heart attacks can occur suddenly without warning and without any relationship to exercise, as seen in typical angina.*

Heart attacks, like angina, involve damage to myocardial tissue. Therefore, symptoms are very similar, except that heart attacks tend to be worse because heart muscle actually is dying rather than being overworked. Naturally, there is an area of overlap between angina and myocardial infarctions; what appears to be angina at first may indeed progress into an infarct.

The best chance a patient with an infarct has for survival is prompt therapy with *thrombolytic agents* such as streptokinase and tissue plasminogen activator (TPA), which are not routinely used before arriving at the hospital but eventually might be. A thrombolytic agent dissolves blood clots. Because damage in the heart usually is caused by a clot's blocking flow, dissolving the clot can restore blood flow and save the tissue. This therapy obviously is not without risks because any blood clot anywhere in the body will dissolve, and patients tend to bleed. The worst complication of thrombolytic therapy is a stroke (see Chap. 2).

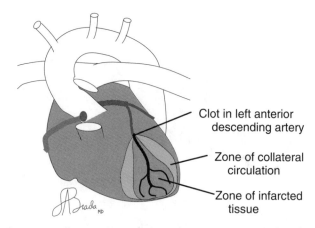

Clot in left anterior descending artery

Zone of collateral circulation

Zone of infarcted tissue

Fig. 3-15. Myocardial infarct. Occlusion of a coronary artery either by blood clot or atherosclerotic plaque interferes with blood flow downstream. If the blockage is not cleared within a period of minutes, the myocardial tissue supplied by the artery (shown in gray) will die. Some of the surrounding area (light pink) may receive blood supply from more than one artery. It will experience diminished blood flow but may not perish if collateral circulation is adequate.

CLINICAL CORRELATION   *The current treatment of choice for anyone suspected of having an infarct is oxygen, an aspirin (chewed for rapid absorption to help prevent clot formation), beta-blockers, nitroglycerin, heparin (which also prevents clot formation), thrombolytics, morphine, and antiarrhythmics (e.g., lidocaine) only if arrhythmias are present. Not all of these latter therapies are commonly used before arriving at the hospital, although they often are used when transferring patients from one facility to another.*

If cholesterol plaques accumulate in the coronary arteries slowly over time, the heart has a chance to develop **collateral circulation** (see Fig. 3-15). As the main pipeline slowly is closed off, multiple small bypass routes spring up to fill the need of the heart muscle being supplied. Collateral circulation does much to protect the heart from damage.

CLINICAL CORRELATION   *Younger patients in their 40s and 50s rarely have had enough time to develop collateral circulation, so when a 45-year-old has a heart attack, there is no bypass route for blood to flow. When younger people have heart attacks, they tend to have more damage to their myocardia than older people* *who have heart attacks. Don't disregard a person's chest pain just because he or she is young. In fact, chest pain in a younger person can be a life-threatening sign.*

ELECTRICAL CONDUCTION SYSTEM

Each cell in the heart contracts, stimulated by an electrical impulse, or signal. When the cells collectively contract together, the heart beats. The heart has a conduction system, like a wiring harness, that coordinates all of the cells of the heart so that they beat in a coordinated, organized fashion.

The signal starts with the heart's natural pacemaker, the **sinoatrial node**, also called the **sinus node** or **SA node**, located in the right atrium. The SA node works like a clock that pulses electrical signals at regular intervals (Fig. 3-16). When myocardial cells receive the signal, they contract. From the SA node, the signal travels along **internodal pathways** in the atria that converge at the base of the right atrium in the **atrioventricular node** or **junction** (**AV node/junction**). From the AV node, the conduction pathway travels via the **bundle of His** down into the ventricles. Important to note is that the ventricles normally receive electrical signals only through the bundle from the AV node. The bundle of His then splits into the **left** and **right bundle branches**. The left bundle branch branches further into *anterior* and *posterior fascicles*. The different branches finally split into the **Purkinje fibers**, which carry the electrical signal throughout the ventricles.

So, in a normal heartbeat, the SA node sends a signal carried by the internal pathways through the atria, causing the atria to contract. The signal then comes down to the AV node, which sends the signal on to the ventricles through the bundle of His, the bundle branches, and the Purkinje fibers. The ventricles then contract when they receive the signal. All this occurs with every heartbeat.

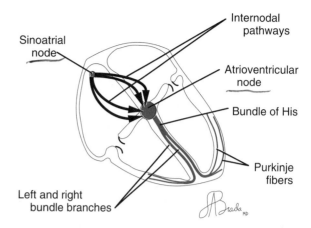

Fig. 3-16. Electrical conduction system of the heart. Impulses begin in the sinoatrial node and travel through the atrial wall to the atrioventricular node. After a short delay, they are passed down the bundle of His to the bundle branches and finally the Purkinje fibers, which run in the walls of the ventricles and signal them to contract.

The Cardiac Cell

Ordinary table salt is a molecule containing an atom of sodium (Na) and an atom of chlorine (Cl)—that is, sodium chloride (NaCl). When you dissolve salt in water, however, the two atoms split into a free sodium *ion* with a positive charge (Na^+) and a free chloride ion with a negative charge (Cl^-) (see Chap. 4). The fluid outside cells is mainly full of Na^+; the fluid inside cells is mainly full of a different ion, potassium (K^+). Every cell is surrounded by a cell membrane that works to keep sodium out and potassium in, with the net effect of forming an *electric potential* across the cell membrane similar to the charge across the poles of a car battery.

When a cardiac cell gets an electrical signal from the SA node, the cell **depolarizes** (like a spark plug firing). This depolarization causes the cell to contract and the electrical signal is passed down to the next cell in line. When a cell depolarizes, Na^+ rushes into the cell (a common question on the paramedic boards.) After the signal has been passed, the cell then needs to **repolarize** to be ready for the next signal and therefore ready to contract again. When the cell repolarizes, K⁺ ions move out of the cell (Fig. 3-17). While the cell is repolarizing, it is in a **refractory phase**—that is, it is not yet ready for the next signal to come along. The depolarization and repolarization of cardiac cells are what we see on the ECG (see section on The Electrocardiogram).

The SA node has the ability to make itself depolarize, creating its own electrical signal, which is why the SA node is the body's natural pacemaker. The truth is, however, *any cell in the heart has the ability to act as a pacemaker*, a quality known as **automaticity**. In other words, every cardiac cell can run itself automatically.

CLINICAL CORRELATION *Cardiac cells normally depolarize (beat) only when the SA node tells them to. When they depolarize (beat) on their own, arrhythmias can result.*

The Electrocardiogram

The ECG (popularly called EKG) is the electrical signal from the heart we can monitor that corresponds to the depolarization and repolarization of the heart's cells. The ECG has three parts: the **P wave**, corresponding to the depolarization of the atria, the **QRS complex**, the sharply peaked set of waves corresponding to the depolarization of the ventricles, and the **T wave**, corresponding to the repolarization of the ventricles. The repolarization of the atria is lost in the QRS complex (you can't see atrial repolarization) (Fig. 3-18). A late *U wave* sometimes appears after the T wave. The significance of the U wave is unclear and its presence or absence need not be considered abnormal.

As mentioned previously, when a heart cell is repolarizing, it is in a refractory period during which it is not ready to receive another sig-

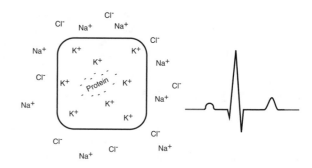

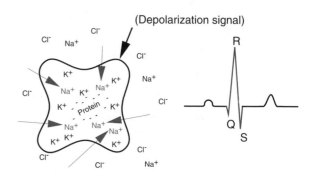

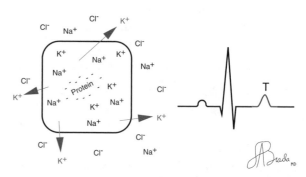

Fig. 3-17. Cardiac cell cycle. When a depolarization signal reaches the myocardial cell, sodium channels in the cell membrane open, allowing positively charged sodium ions to rush into the negatively charged intracellular space. This depolarization, signified by the QRS-wave on the ECG, makes the cell contract. Afterward, potassium channels open and positively charged potassium ions rush out (T-wave), repolarizing the cell and causing it to relax until the next depolarization signal.

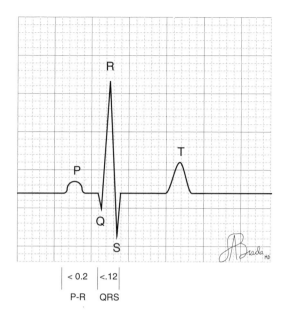

Fig. 3-18. The normal ECG. On standard tracings, each 1-mm box along the x-axis corresponds to 0.04 seconds (0.2 seconds/cm); each 1-mm box along the y-axis represents 0.1 mV.

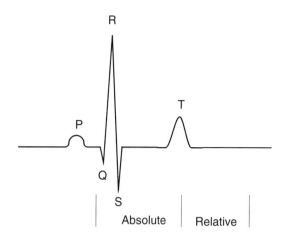

Fig. 3-19. Electrical refractory period. During the absolute refractory period, the myocardial cell is incapable of contracting in response to new electrical signals. During the relative refractory period, however, the cell can respond to a signal and contract before it repolarizes completely.

nal to beat. The refractory period actually has two parts: the **absolute refractory period** and **relative refractory period** (Fig. 3-19). During the absolute refractory period, the cell is not ready to fire again. Even if it receives another impulse, it will not fire. The relative refractory period, however, is a dangerous time during which the cell doesn't want to receive a new signal to beat. If a signal comes along, however, it can cause the cell to depolarize before it's ready. This can cause the cell can go haywire, throwing the entire heart into a life-threatening rhythm (ventricular tachycardia or ventricular fibrillation).

Ectopic Beats

Any cell in the heart has the potential to initiate its own beat—that is, all cardiac cells have automaticity. If a cell initiates its own beat, its signal will be passed along to the rest of the heart in addition to the regular signal from the SA node. An abnormal beat results in an

ectopic beat because it is not coming from the normal source, the SA node. (Ectopic means not in the normal position.) Ectopic beats can originate in the atria, from the AV junction, or from the ventricles. People with many ectopic beats are said to have **ectopy.**

There are two basic types of ectopic beats: **premature** and **escape beats.**

Premature Beats

Premature beats come earlier than expected. They occur naturally all the time. If a heart cell is irritated, however, it is more likely to produce premature beats. Heart cells are irritated by ischemia or chemical imbalances (Fig. 3-20).

Premature atrial complexes (PACs) are beats that arise from some **focus** (or point of origin) in the atria. They are extremely common and easily distinguishable because they generally have the same QRS pattern as normal beats, only they occur early. PACs have the same QRS pattern because the signal, originating somewhere in the atria, must still get through the AV junction, where it resumes its normal conduc-

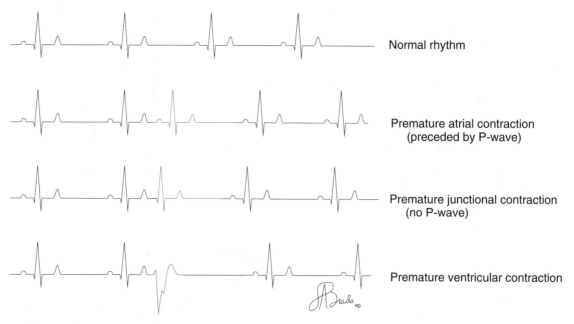

Normal rhythm

Premature atrial contraction
(preceded by P-wave)

Premature junctional contraction
(no P-wave)

Premature ventricular contraction

Fig. 3-20. ECG tracings of different premature contractions.

tion through the ventricles. **Premature junctional complexes** (PJCs) are less common and often difficult to distinguish from PACs except that the P wave is absent, too close to the QRS complex, or inverted. These characteristics can be due to conduction of a signal *backward* into the atria from the junction. **Premature ventricular complexes** (PVCs) are premature beats that originate in the ventricles. Although they can be common, they are potentially the most alarming of the premature beats in the presence of an acute myocardial infarction. PVCs are easily distinguishable as *wide and bizarre* complexes because they do not follow the normal ventricular conduction pathway.

Premature beats are generally benign; that is, they will not hurt the patient. In fact, most people occasionally have some form of premature beat. The only time premature beats are a cause for alarm is when you suspect a patient with PVCs of having a heart attack (acute myocardial infarction).

CLINICAL CORRELATION *Ischemic areas of the heart are prone to produce ectopic beats. In the context of chest pain or suspected myocardial infarction, be wary of PVCs, as they indicate damage to the heart muscle.*

CLINICAL CORRELATION *A PVC that falls in the relative refractory period of the preceding beat is called the R-on-T pattern. An R-on-T pattern is extremely dangerous and must be suppressed because it can precipitate sudden death by ventricular tachycardia or ventricular fibrillation.*

As mentioned, PACs and PJCs are rarely a problem, and PVCs are worrisome only when they accompany a suspected acute myocardial infarction. You can stop (or suppress) PVCs with drugs, but it needs to be done only if one of the following criteria is present: more than six PVCs in one minute, couplets (two PVCs in a row), salvos (three or more PVCs in a row, really a "short run of ventricular tachycardia"; see below), multifocal PVCs (PVCs from more than one focus, distinguishable by two very different PVC types on the ECG), **bigeminy** (a pattern in which every other beat is a PVC), or the R-on-T pattern (Fig. 3-21).

CLINICAL CORRELATION *Lidocaine is the antiarrhythmic drug of choice for suppressing PVCs,*

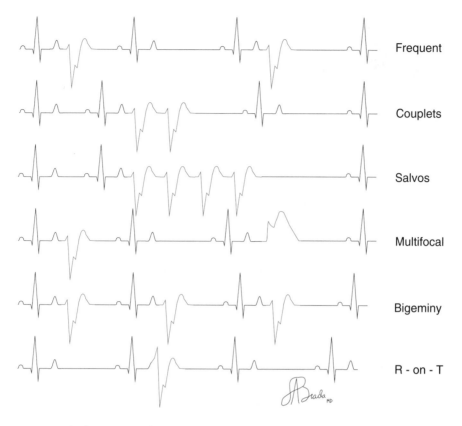

Frequent

Couplets

Salvos

Multifocal

Bigeminy

R - on - T

Fig. 3-21. Premature ventricular contractions.

although procainamide and bretylium also can be used. (Lidocaine blocks Na+ channels in cell membranes.) You should suppress PVCs (that is, administer lidocaine) only if you are worried that the patient is having a myocardial infarction. You should not routinely administer lidocaine to anyone with PVCs not having a heart attack or to anyone having a heart attack without PVCs.

Escape Beats

Escape beats, like premature beats, may originate from the AV junction or from the ventricles. The difference is that escape beats arise when the SA node has failed to provide a beat and the rest of the heart becomes impatient waiting for a signal. The SA node normally fires at a rate of 60–100 beats per minute. If the sinus node is sick or diseased (it can get ischemic damage just like the rest of the heart), then the AV node may take over as pacemaker. The AV node normally fires at a rate of 40–60 beats per minute, and if the AV node fails, the ventricles themselves may fire at a rate of 20–40 beats per minute. The heart has to be very sick before you see a ventricular escape rhythm.

CLINICAL CORRELATION *If the patient is bradycardic (has a slow heart rate), do not mistake ventricular escape beats for PVCs and treat with lidocaine. This could be a lethal error. If the patient's heart rate is less than 60, he or she should be treated with atropine instead to increase the rate (see below).*

Tachyarrhythmias

Tachyarrhythmias are the abnormally fast rhythms (tachy = fast). Any time a patient's heart rate is fast—more than 100 beats per minute—the patient is said to have a **tachycardia**. Sometimes an ectopic focus (or more than one) can be excited to beat out of control at incredible rates as in the phenomenon of *re-*

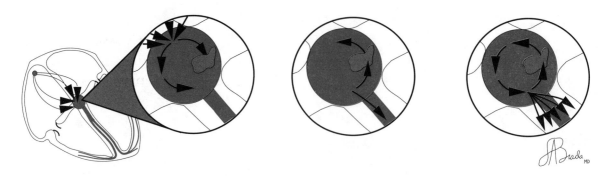

Fig. 3-22. Mechanism of re-entrant pathway. When the AV node is injured, it may conduct signals from the sinoatrial node inappropriately, resulting in blocked forward conduction of electrical signals (left) followed by delayed retrograde transmission through the injured region (middle). This may create a constant circuit of electrical activity around the diseased node (right) with transmission to the ventricles with each go-round (shown by branching arrows). The end result is a supraventricular tachycardia with normal sinoatrial node activity.

entry, when part of the normal electrical signal gets caught up in a short circuit instead of traveling all the way through the heart. The signal then loops back on itself and stimulates itself to fire again, setting up a feedback that rapidly speeds up out of control (Fig. 3-22). Re-entry can happen within the AV node or around damaged tissue in the atria or ventricles.

There are two basic types of tachyarrhythmias: those arising from the ventricles, or **ventricular tachycardia** (V-tach), and those arising from some place above the ventricles, or **supraventricular tachycardias** (SVTs).

V-tach is a **wide complex tachycardia** that is unstable, immediately life-threatening, and often incompatible with life (that is, a person can be pulseless, or temporarily dead, while in V-tach). V-tach also may degenerate into **ventricular fibrillation** (V-fib), which is definitely incompatible with life. During V-fib, cells throughout the ventricles are beating randomly, out of control, and there is no effective heart beat (Fig. 3-23). The heart in V-fib actually is like a sack of worms all wiggling about.

CLINICAL CORRELATION *V-fib is the most common arrhythmia seen immediately after sudden death. Rapid defibrillation is the treatment of choice. Do*

not delay defibrillation for anything if a patient is in V-fib. Only perform CPR until a defibrillator is ready. Seconds can count, so know your machinery cold!

There are a variety of SVTs, including **sinus tachycardia** (sinus tach), **atrial tachycardia** (atrial tach), **junctional tachycardia, atrial flutter** (A-flutter), and **atrial fibrillation** (A-fib) (Fig. 3-24). Sinus tach is perfectly natural, representing the heart's acceleration in response to anything (such as exercise or increased sympathetic tone). Atrial tach can occur **paroxysmally**—one minute heart rate is normal and the next it's racing at 200 beats a minute. In A-flutter, the atria contract 200–300 beats per minute, and in A-fib, the atria, like the ventricles in V-fib, are totally out of control. In any of the SVTs, the AV node acts as a gatekeeper to protect the ventricle from the outrageous rates the atria are producing. For clinical purposes, all of these tachycardias should have narrow QRS complexes, or be **narrow complex tachycardia.**

CLINICAL CORRELATION *The initial treatment for a patient with SVT who is stable is a vagal maneuver such as the carotid sinus massage or the Valsalva maneuver. These maneuvers increase parasympathetic tone on the AV node, which slows conduction through the node (see Chap. 2). These maneuvers may*

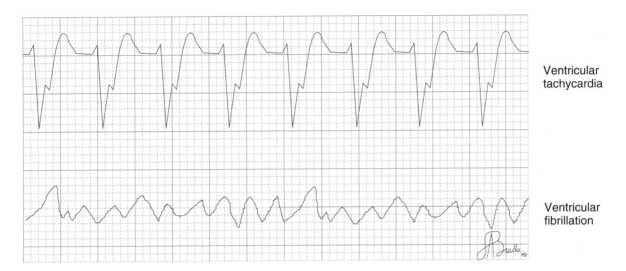

Fig. 3-23. Ventricular tachycardia and ventricular fibrillation.

Ventricular tachycardia

Ventricular fibrillation

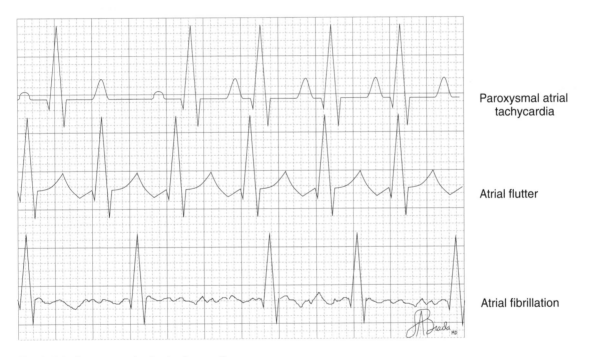

Fig. 3-24. Supraventricular tachycardias.

Paroxysmal atrial tachycardia

Atrial flutter

Atrial fibrillation

slow the heart rate or even change the rhythm back to a normal sinus rhythm. They also may have no effect at all.

SVT is not as dangerous as V-tach. As with any tachycardia, however, if the ventricles beat too quickly (i.e., more than 150 beats per minute), they may not have time to fill with blood between strokes. Thus, the heart has nothing to pump out, and blood does not circulate effectively.

CLINICAL CORRELATION *Tachycardias can lead to hemodynamic instability, or falling blood pressure, and decreased level of consciousness (from not enough blood reaching the brain). As perfusion drops, the body responds by increasing sympathetic tone, making the tachycardia worse. Rapid cardioversion is the treatment of choice for any unstable tachycardia.*

CLINICAL CORRELATION *When "shocking" a tachycardic patient, it is important to use the synchro-*

nized mode of the cardioverter. The synchronizer times the electrical discharge to fall immediately after a QRS complex, thus avoiding the relative refractory period. If you were to defibrillate without synchronization and the shock came during the relative refractory period, you could send the patient into V-fib (which is worse).

There can be abnormalities of the conduction system in the ventricles (such as bundle branch blocks, described below) that can widen the QRS complex. These often are called *conduction defects*. The problem arises when a patient has an SVT *and* a conduction defect, which will be an SVT that looks like V-tach.

CLINICAL CORRELATION *Treat all wide-complex tachycardias as V-tach. You will not hurt someone who really may have an SVT, but if you try to be really fancy and call a V-tach an SVT with a conduction defect, you could end up watching someone die.*

CLINICAL CORRELATION *Cardiovert any unstable tachycardia—wide or narrow—first, and ask questions later.*

CLINICAL CORRELATION *The drug of choice for narrow-complex SVTs is adenosine, which has anti-adrenergic properties but is not a beta-blocker, followed by verapamil or beta blockers. Each of these drugs acts to block conduction through the AV node.*

CLINICAL CORRELATION *If a patient is in an unstable tachycardia, cardioversion is not available, and you are unsure whether the rhythm is an SVT or V-tach, you can use procainamide because it affects both the atria and ventricles and treats both SVT and V-tach. Lidocaine is safe and quicker but probably will not help SVTs. Adenosine is also safe, but verapamil could be a deadly mistake in a wide-complex tachycardia.*

Another re-entrant mechanism for tachycardia worth mentioning is **Wolff-Parkinson-White syndrome** (WPW). People with WPW have a bypass electrical pathway from the atria to the ventricles that goes around the AV node. In these patients, electrical signals can travel from the AV node back up into the atria through the bypass tract and then back down through the AV node again. They also may

lose the benefit of the AV node as being a gate-keeper of atrial signals into the ventricles. People with WPW are prone to tachyarrhythmias, often wide-complex, because of conduction problems accompanying the syndrome. It is hoped your patients will know they have WPW.

CLINICAL CORRELATION *Ask a patient with what appears to be an SVT, especially what looks like A-fib with a slightly wide QRS, if he or she has a history of WPW before you begin treatment. Verapamil is contraindicated in these patients because it can lower blood pressure, causing a rebound increase in sympathetic tone that further drives the tachycardia through the bypass pathway. Use adenosine or a beta-blocker instead if possible, and cardiovert if unstable.*

Bradyarrhythmias

Brady means slow. Thus, **bradyarrhythmias** are abnormally slow rhythms, and **bradycardia** refers to an abnormally slow heart rate. Bradycardias arise when the normal conduction system is diseased or damaged and can be either chronic or acute. An infarct that destroys the sinus node may produce a bradycardia (likely a junctional or ventricular escape rhythm). Some bradycardias are normal, such as those as in young, well-trained athletes (especially women), who can have normal resting heart rates in the 40s. A **sinus bradycardia** is simply a sinus rhythm with a rate less than 60.

If the AV node becomes damaged or under the influence of certain medications (such as beta-blockers, calcium channel blockers, or digitalis), conduction through it can be slowed or *blocked* (Fig. 3-25). AV blocks are rated by degrees. A **first-degree AV block** is characterized by conduction through the node that is only slightly delayed, as witnessed by an increase in the P-R interval. In a **second-degree AV block type I** (Wenkebach), the block through the AV node varies. The P-R interval progressively widens until there is P wave with

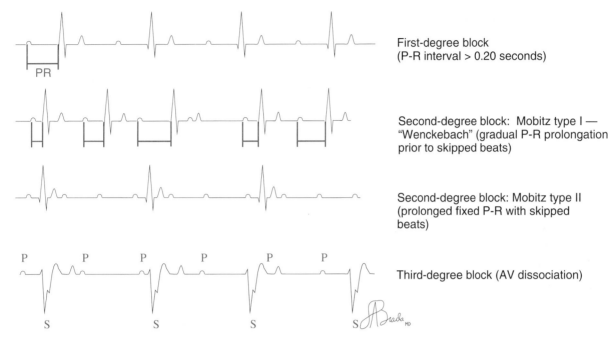

Fig. 3-25. Varieties of heart block.

no following QRS (a "dropped beat"). Neither of these rhythms is urgently alarming.

A **second-degree AV block type II** is seen only in sick hearts. The AV node is not able to transmit all of the atrial impulses, and the P waves often are not followed by QRS complexes. When the P waves are conducted, there is a uniform delay, so the P-R interval is constant, unlike the P-R intervals seen in second-degree type I and third-degree blocks. In a **third-degree**, or **complete**, **AV block**, the AV node is so sick that no communication between the atria and ventricles exists whatsoever; each is doing its own thing. There is no correlation between P waves and QRS complexes (see Fig. 3-25). In either of these blocks, the damage is usually below the AV node in the His fibers, the reason these bradycardias tend to have wide QRS complexes.

CLINICAL CORRELATION *The important point about bradycardias and AV blocks is that if the heart pumps slowly enough, it can cause hemodynamic instability because it is not pumping enough blood. It doesn't matter what rhythm someone is in: If the patient's heart rate is slow and unstable, speed it up. The treatment of choice is atropine, an antiparasympathetic agent (see Chap. 2) to reduce vagal tone, "take the foot off of the brakes" and, it is hoped, speed up the heart.*

CLINICAL CORRELATION *Advanced blocks, second-degree type II and third-degree, may not respond to atropine because the AV node is too sick by that point (or the block is actually in the His fibers below the AV node, which are not affected by atropine). Patients with advanced blocks are the sickest and may need to be treated with a temporary transthoracic pacer, which artificially gives the ventricles the signal they need to beat.*

CLINICAL CORRELATION *Heart blocks often are caused by acute myocardial infarctions that deprive blood to the AV node or to His-Purkinje fibers. In these cases, bradycardia sometimes protects the heart by reducing the amount of work it has to do. If the patient with an acute myocardial infarction is hemodynamically stable, do not speed up the patient's heart rate with atropine, or you may make the heart attack worse by overworking the heart.*

CLINICAL CORRELATION *If atropine fails to improve a symptomatic bradycardia and pacing is not available, the next drugs of choice are dopamine and epinephrine. These drugs are adrenergic, raising blood pressure and stimulating the heart to pump faster. The drug of* *last resort is isoproterenol, a pure beta-agonist. The problem with isoproterenol is that it greatly increases myocardial demand for oxygen because it makes the heart muscle work harder. A damaged heart may not be able to tolerate an increase in oxygen demand, so isoproterenol can be harmful at high doses.*

The ultimate bradycardia, so to speak, is **asystole**, meaning no contraction. Asystole is the infamous "flat line" that occurs when the heart is not doing anything at all. These patients are dead, and unfortunately, most of them stay dead. More unfortunately still, these are perhaps the most common cardiac arrest patients you are likely to see.

CLINICAL CORRELATION *Always confirm asystole in at least two different leads (such as lead II and lead III). Some patients may not produce a very good electrical signal, which can look like asystole, especially in lead I, so double-check!*

The treatment of choice for asystole is epinephrine and atropine. Put your foot on the gas, take your foot off the break, and hope the heart starts again.

CLINICAL CORRELATION *If there is the slightest doubt about whether a person's heart is still beating, defibrillate a patient in asystole because he or she actually may be in a "fine" V-fib.*

In addition to blocks at the AV node, patients can have blocks further along in their conduction systems. *Bundle branch blocks* cause slow conduction in whichever bundle is blocked. By slowing the conduction in part of the ventricle, the QRS complex widens. A person also can have *aberrant conduction*, or abnormal conduction pathways through the heart.

CLINICAL CORRELATION *A wide complex with a normal rate is not necessarily a ventricular rhythm. Look for a P wave associated with the QRS.*

Pulseless Electrical Activity

Pulseless electrical activity (PEA) is just that—electrical activity you can see on the monitor that does not have a palpable pulse or blood pressure. In this case, the electrical control system may be intact, but the heart isn't working. PEA actually is a "grab bag" of phenomena including **electromechanical dissociation** (EMD) and other rhythms (e.g., "idioventricular," "agonal") the heart produces without a pulse.

CLINICAL CORRELATION *Any rhythm that is not V-tach or V-fib and does not have a pulse is PEA by definition.*

EMD has been the term traditionally used for organized electrical activity without a pulse. For example, the patient may show a normal sinus rhythm on the monitor yet not have a pulse. The other rhythms often have wide, unrecognizable complexes.

There are several common causes of PEA, some of which are potentially reversible (Table 3-1). They include hypovolemia (too little fluid), hypoxia (too little oxygen), acidosis (too much acid, often caused by too much carbon dioxide from not breathing), tension pneumothorax, hypothermia (too cold), and pericardial tamponade.

CLINICAL CORRELATION *Treat any obvious causes of PEA. Give patients intravenous fluids (in case they are hypovolemic), intubate and hyperventilate them with 100% oxygen (to correct hypoxia and acidosis), warm them (if appropriate), and treat for a pneumothorax if necessary (see section on Anatomy of the Respiratory System). These are the things you can do in the field.*

CLINICAL CORRELATION *Treat the patient, not the monitor. This is true for any of the arrhythmias. Don't forget it!*

CIRCULATORY ANATOMY

The circulatory pathway is fairly straightforward. The heart pumps blood out of the left ventricle through the **aorta**. The aorta forms a small arch, ascending then descending. At the base of the aorta are the right and left **coro-**

Table 3-1. Causes and treatment of pulseless electrical activity (PEA)

Cause	Treatment
Hypovolemia	Intravenous fluids
Tension pneumothorax	Needle chest decompression
Hypoxia	Oxygenation/ventilation
Acidosis	Ventilation, intravenous bicarbonate
Hypothermia	Rewarming, ACLS protocol
Pericardial tamponade	Pericardiocentesis*
Pulmonary embolus	Thrombolytics*
Massive myocardial infarction	Thrombolytics, ACLS protocol
Drug overdose	Appropriate antidote (e.g., naloxone, atropine)*
Metabolic abnormalities	*

ACLS = advanced cardiac life support.
*Some conditions are difficult or impossible to treat before arriving at the hospital.

nary arteries, which feed the heart muscle itself (Fig. 3-26).

The aorta, like all larger arteries, has three layers in its wall: the *tunica intima*, *media*, and *adventitia* (Fig. 3-27). Sometimes, these layers separate, and blood flows *between* the layers rather than through the center of the aorta, where it should. This is known as an **aortic dissection** because blood is "dissecting" through the walls of the aorta. It can be a life-threatening emergency because individual layers of the aortic wall are not strong enough to hold blood in and may split open. Consequently, the patient will bleed internally.

CLINICAL CORRELATION *The hallmark of aortic dissection is a sharp chest pain radiating between the shoulder blades or lower back. Pulses in the neck, arms, or groin may be unequal because the dissection selectively blocks flow to either the left or the right side. If you suspect a dissection, get large-bore intravenous access because if the dissection opens up, the patient will bleed rapidly.*

The aorta gives rise to three major arteries: the *brachiocephalic* ("arm-and-head"), left common **carotid**, and left **subclavian** ("under the clavicle"). The brachiocephalic artery quickly forks into the right common carotid and the right subclavian arteries.

The common carotid arteries travel up the neck into the head (see Chap. 2). They each branch into internal and external carotid arteries that feed the brain and the rest of the head. The subclavian artery (one on each side of the body) travels into the arm where it becomes the **brachial artery.** The brachial artery travels along the humerus, a bone of the arm, and can be felt between the muscles of the upper arm (the biceps and triceps) (Fig. 3-28).

CLINICAL CORRELATION *The brachial artery is a good pulse point. It is the best pulse point in infants and also can be used as a pressure point. If someone is bleeding from the arm, you can apply pressure over the brachial artery to help control the bleeding. (You are probably better off, however, finding the site of the bleed and applying direct pressure right at that point.)*

At the elbow, the brachial artery divides into the **radial artery**, which follows the radius (one of two bones in the forearm), and the *ulnar artery*, which follows the ulna (the other bone in the forearm) (Fig. 3-29) (see Chap. 6). The radial pulse can be felt in the wrist just proximal to the thumb.

The aorta loops over the top of the **pulmonary artery** (which leaves the right ventricle on its way to the lungs). The aorta and the pul-

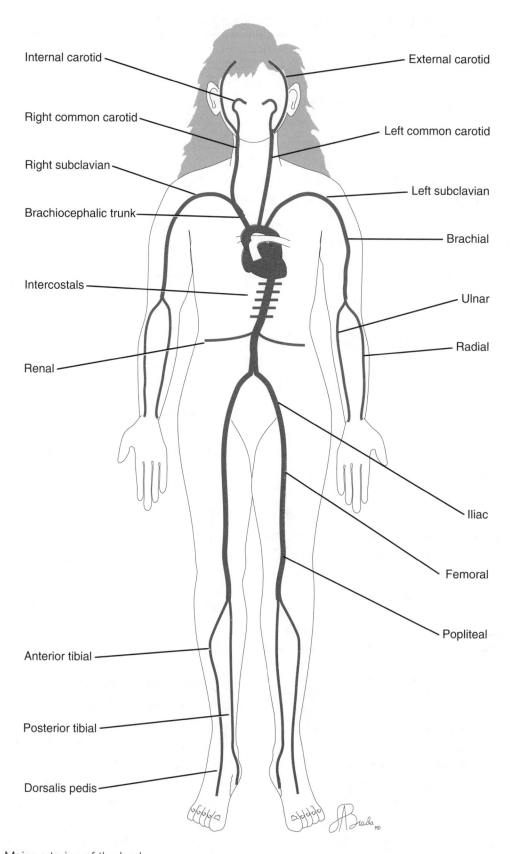

Fig. 3-26. Major arteries of the body.

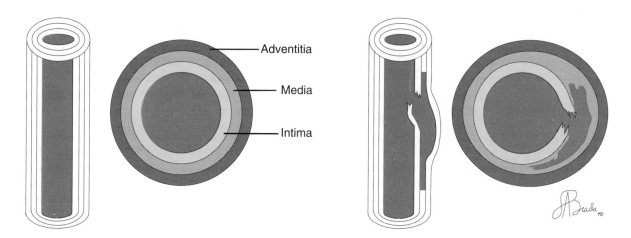

Fig. 3-27. Aortic dissection. A tear in the intima of the aorta (right) allows blood under pressure to dissect through the media, creating a false passage that may distort the aortic wall enough to occlude smaller branches at their origins.

monary artery actually are attached to one another by a small fibrous cord called the *ligamentum arteriosum* ("ligament of the arteries"). This ligament tethers the aorta in place, preventing it from moving.

CLINICAL CORRELATION *In rapidly decelerating trauma (as in a very sudden stop) internal organs slosh forward inside the body. The aorta, being tethered down by the ligamentum arteriosum, cannot move and thus can be torn open. You never will see this trauma on the outside of the patient, but it can cause sudden, massive internal bleeding and shock. Always be careful with patients who have had deceleration injuries. They may look all right but suddenly start to die. The treatment of choice for a torn aorta is to administer massive fluids and quickly get the patient to a trauma center.*

The aorta continues to descend down the chest, giving rise to pairs of **intercostal arteries,** one pair for each pair of ribs. The intercostal arteries travel along the bottom side of each rib (Fig. 3-30).

CLINICAL CORRELATION *If you are sticking a needle into the chest to relieve a tension pneumothorax, always slide the needle just over the top of the rib to avoid being anywhere near the intercostal arteries.*

After the aorta gives rise to its last pair of intercostal arteries, it passes through the diaphragm into the abdomen. In the abdomen

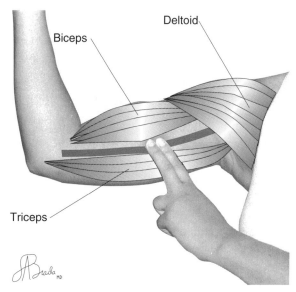

Fig. 3-28. Palpation of the brachial artery.

it gives off three major arteries that feed all of the gastrointestinal tract: the *celiac, superior mesenteric,* and *inferior mesenteric arteries* (see Chap. 4). The aorta also gives rise to a pair of *renal arteries* that feed the kidneys, which are toward the back.

As the aorta drops lower, it forks into the *iliac arteries* just as it enters into the pelvis (see Chap. 5). At this point in the aorta, blood flow tends to be very turbulent (just like traffic at a fork in the road—there's always someone changing lanes at the last minute). Conse-

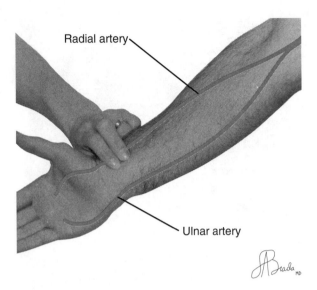

Radial artery

Ulnar artery

Fig. 3-29. Palpation of the radial artery.

quently, in the abdomen, the aorta is prone to **aneurysms**, an outpouching of a weak spot in the wall of the aorta, sometimes referred to as abdominal aortic aneurysms (AAAs) (Fig. 3-31). Like dissections, AAAs can rupture and suddenly bleed. A big AAA sometimes can be felt as a mass in the middle of the belly pulsing along with the heartbeat.

CLINICAL CORRELATION *If a patient (usually an older guy who smokes and eats lots of cheeseburgers) has abdominal or back pain and a large, pulsating mass right around the navel, he or she may have an AAA about to burst. Get large-bore IV access, and move quickly!*

The iliac arteries branch out to feed everything in the pelvis. They eventually cross out of the groin and become the **femoral arteries** (Fig. 3-32).

CLINICAL CORRELATION *The femoral artery is an important pulse point. While doing CPR, it is a good idea to have someone monitor the patient's pulse during compressions to check for spontaneous pulses. Ideally, this should be done at the carotid pulses, but often it is crowded at the patient's head. The femoral pulse is nearly as good as the carotid pulse and often much easier to find. Keep a hand on it.*

CLINICAL CORRELATION *The femoral pulse can be used as a pressure point to control bleeding in the leg when direct pressure fails. If a patient is bleeding so badly that direct pressure won't stop it, he or she could probably use military antishock trousers (MAST trousers).*

The femoral artery becomes the *popliteal artery* behind the knee and eventually splits to feed the foot. In the foot, two common pulses

Fig. 3-30. Intercostal neurovascular bundle. Each rib has an associated vein, artery, and nerve running together along a notch in the underside of the bone. When performing a needle pleurocentesis, make sure you slide the needle along the superior surface of the rib to avoid damaging these structures.

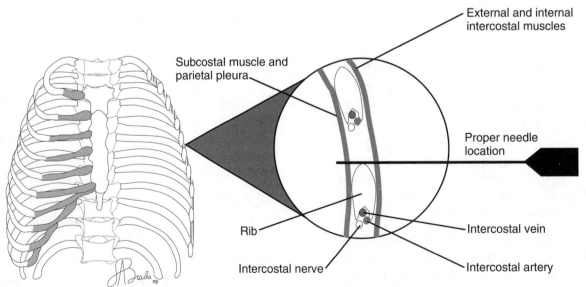

Subcostal muscle and parietal pleura

External and internal intercostal muscles

Proper needle location

Rib

Intercostal nerve

Intercostal vein

Intercostal artery

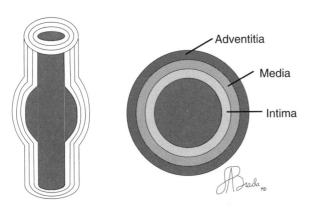

Fig. 3-31. Abdominal aortic aneurysm. Notice how, unlike the aortic dissection, an aneurysm involves the stretching of all three layers of the aortic wall. Blood flow remains within the true lumen, though slowed blood flow through the widened portion can lead to clot formation. Abdominal aortic aneurysms more than 5 cm wide are at risk of bursting.

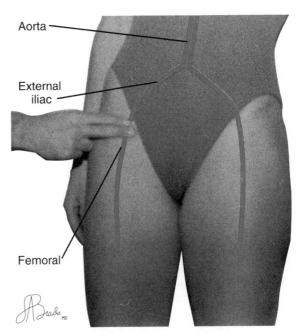

Fig. 3-32. Palpation of the femoral artery.

can be found: the **dorsalis pedis** ("back of foot"), found, interestingly enough, on the back of the foot, and the **posterior tibial** ("behind the tibia"), found on the medial side of the ankle behind the tibia sticking out to the side (Figs. 3-33 and 3-34)

CLINICAL CORRELATION *Whenever a patient has trauma to an arm or a leg, you need to check distal pulses—that is, the dorsalis pedis and posterior tibial in the foot or the radial pulse in the arm (see Chap. 6). Anyone who does not have one of these pulses may have an artery squeezed off somewhere upstream. The artery cannot remain squeezed off long, or the hand or foot will necrose—that is, all the tissue will die.*

Arteries, wherever they end up, continue to branch until, at a certain point, they become very small *arterioles* and eventually **capillaries**, blood vessels so small that only one red blood cell can fit through them at a time (Fig. 3-35). All of the action takes place in the capillaries, that is, where the red blood cells drop off O_2 into the tissues and pick up CO_2. *Plasma* (the liquid part of the blood not including cells), also brings nutrients to the tissues and picks up waste.

O_2 turns blood bright red, whereas CO_2 turns it much darker (nearly blue). Capillaries

give skin, mucous membranes (such as the lips and conjunctuva in the eyes), and nailbeds their pink/red or bluish color, depending on the blood's levels of O_2 and CO_2.

CLINICAL CORRELATION *Pink skin/nailbeds/ mucous membranes is a sign of oxygenated blood reaching the tissues. Cyanosis, blue skin/nailbeds/mucous membranes, indicates the blood reaching the tissues is not well-oxygenated, a sign that something is wrong with the respiratory system. Pale or white tissues indicates blood is not reaching the capillary beds, a sign of cardiovascular failure.*

Blood from the capillaries then enters venuoles, or small veins, which rapidly become big veins. There are a variety of veins that drain blood from the foot, a major one being the *saphenous vein*, which runs up the medial side of the leg (Fig. 3-36).

CLINICAL CORRELATION *Sometimes patients have massive trauma to their arms and necks, especially because of burn injuries. These people may go into shock (see section on Shock) but have no easy venous access for intravenous lines. Given a choice between MAST trousers covering both legs or an IV in the lower leg or foot, you are*

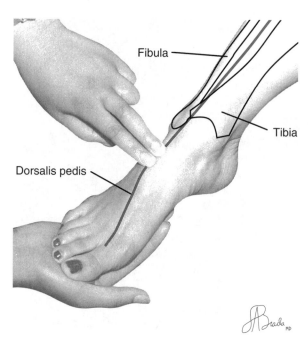

Fig. 3-33. Palpation of the dorsalis pedis artery.

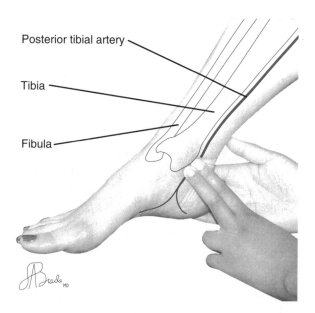

Fig. 3-34. Palpation of the posterior tibial artery.

probably better off using the IV, which is much more important in the long run. Do not be afraid to start IVs in the foot or leg; just clean the site well if you can.

Blood throughout the leg eventually collects in the *femoral vein*, which follows the same basic course as the femoral artery in reverse. Not surprisingly, the femoral vein turns into the *iliac vein* in the pelvis, eventual-

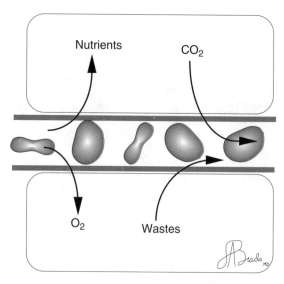

Fig. 3-35. Capillary exchange. At the capillary level, red blood cells release oxygen and pick up carbon dioxide from tissues. At the same time, nutrients diffuse into the cells from plasma and waste products diffuse into plasma to be transported to the kidneys or liver for removal.

ly leading into the **inferior vena cava** (IVC). The IVC travels near the aorta close to the spine and eventually drains into the right atrium. The IVC is important in that it acts as a major storage pool for the body's blood supply.

Blood from the gastrointestinal tract, unlike the legs, does not drain directly into the IVC. Instead, it collects into the **portal vein,** which collects everything the body has absorbed from what a person has just eaten (see Chap. 4). Blood then goes into the liver, which acts as the body's detoxifier. Blood actually must go through a second capillary system in the liver before the liver drains it back into the IVC through the *hepatic vein.*

Blood from the arms travels up a variety of veins including the *basilic* and *cephalic* veins found on the back of the forearm. They wrap around the front and cross, forming the **antecubital veins** (actually different-angled branches of the cephalic and basilic), which cross in the crease of the elbow. They usually are easy to find (Fig. 3-37).

CLINICAL CORRELATION *It's better to start IVs distally if possible. That way, if you miss (or if the vein infiltrates) you can move up and try again proximally.*

CLINICAL CORRELATION *The best veins to start IVs in are the veins you can feel, not the blue lines you see.*

CLINICAL CORRELATION *When starting an IV, put the tourniquet on and find the healthiest vein. Remembering where the vasculature is supposed to be usually is not helpful except when you are desperate to start an IV and cannot find a vein (often in obese patients). In this situation, you can try "anatomical sticks"—that is, starting an IV in a place where you know a vein should be even though you can't find one. There are two good target spots: the proverbial "intern's vein" in the wrist just proximal to the dorsal aspect of the thumb, and the antecubital vein (see Fig. 3-37).*

The veins of the arm eventually condense into the *subclavian vein*, a vein that, surprisingly enough, follows the subclavian artery just below the clavicle. The subclavian veins join the **superior vena cava** (SVC), which drains into the right atrium.

Blood from the brain (fed by the internal carotid arteries) collects in the **internal jugular vein** (see Chap. 2). Blood from the scalp and face collect in the **external jugular vein**. Both of these veins eventually join up with the SVC.

As mentioned above, the right atrium sends blood into the right ventricle, which pumps it into the **pulmonary artery**. The pulmonary artery splits, sending a branch into the left and right lungs. Across the pulmonary capillaries in the lungs, the blood trades the CO_2 picked up throughout the body for fresh O_2. The freshly oxygenated blood then collects into the **pulmonary veins** and drains into the left atrium. The cycle continues.

Virtually every part of the body also drains fluid from between cells not in the bloodstream. This fluid, *lymph*, collects in little vessels known as lymphatic vessels, which eventually drain back into the venous system. You cannot see them unless they are infected, characterized by bright red streaks running up the body.

Blood

The average adult has about 5 liters of blood equaling 10 units that are each 500 ml (or nearly one pint each). Blood contains many things—most important, red blood cells (*erythrocytes*) full of *hemoglobin*, an iron-containing molecule that carries oxygen in the blood.

CLINICAL CORRELATION *Carbon monoxide (CO) (not to be confused with carbon dioxide—CO_2) is the infamous odorless, colorless gas that comes out of cigarettes, car exhaust, and faulty furnaces. It irreversibly binds to hemoglobin, preventing oxygen from binding. Thus, a person breathing CO eventually becomes oxygen-starved. Classically, textbooks say people turn "cherry red" from breathing carbon monoxide. This, however, usually happens after a person has been dead for a while. In the field, what you will see is a sick, possibly cyanotic patient with vague symptoms and probably a headache (if he or she is still conscious). Your job simply is to provide ventilation and oxygenation (100%), but keep your suspicions up and get a fire marshal or a hazardous materials expert to inspect the place for carbon monoxide.*

Red blood cells are normally round, almost doughnut-shaped, which helps them slip through the narrow capillaries. In *sickle cell disease*, a genetic disease found in people of African decent, red blood cells are shaped like sickles, sometimes making if difficult for the cells to get through capillaries. (For those of you who have never harvested wheat by hand, a sickle is a curved blade.) The cells become stuck, causing a lot of pain (a sickle cell crisis). Patients with sickle cell anemia are common in major cities, but there is nothing you can do for them except control the pain.

Also found in blood are white blood cells (leukocytes, lymphocytes, monocytes, and others). The white cells make up a large part of the *immune system*, which is responsible for

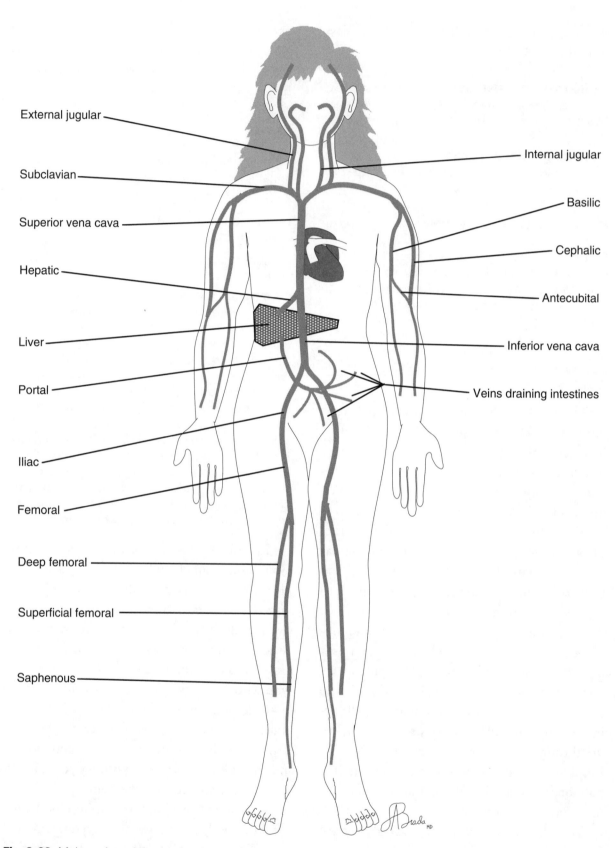

Fig. 3-36. Major veins of the body.

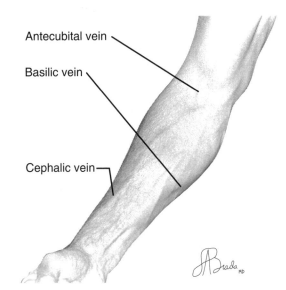

Fig. 3-37. Major veins of the forearm.

fighting off disease. The human immunodeficiency virus (HIV), the virus that causes AIDS, infects a type of lymphocyte that in turn cripples the immune system. Thus, AIDS patients are susceptible to all types of infections a healthy person would be able to fight off. Most AIDS patients die of pneumonia.

CLINICAL CORRELATION *HIV can be transmitted by blood. Assume all patients have HIV, and wear latex gloves whenever you suspect you might come in contact with a patient's blood. When you're at work, always keep an extra couple of pairs on your person so you can reglove when your gloves tear. No patient ever died in the amount of time it takes to put on a pair of gloves.*

Platelets are specialized cell fragments that work with specific clotting factors to let the blood clot; there is a variety of clotting factors at work. *Hemophilia*, an inherited disease of which there are several types, results when a person is missing specific clotting factors and has difficulty clotting. Hemophilia does not cause a person to bleed to death with every little scratch; however, it does mean hemophiliacs require more time to clot and are thus more prone to bleeding.

CLINICAL CORRELATION *There are two things you need to worry about when patients tell you*

they have hemophilia. First, they are more likely to bleed from any given trauma, including internal bleeding and strokes. Second, they are at a higher risk for carrying HIV because most hemophiliac patients receive blood transfusions, and until the mid-1980s, there was no screening of blood for HIV.

CLINICAL CORRELATION *Aspirin prevents platelets from clumping into clots. Anyone suspected of having an acute myocardial infarction should take an aspirin right away because it helps reduce clot formation in the coronary arteries, the most likely cause of the infarct.*

Plasma is the part of the blood that remains when all of the cells and platelets are removed. Plasma includes proteins such as *antibodies*, part of the immune system, that help fight disease. Removing the proteins leaves *serum*, which contains various salts, ions, and glucose found in blood.

CARDIOVASCULAR DYNAMICS

Blood Pressure

Blood pressure is the measure of how much pressure blood has in the arteries when the heart pumps. Think of water in a hose or pipeline. The more pressure there is in the line, the more water comes out. The more pressure there is in the artery, the more blood flows through.

There are two different pressures in the **circulatory** system: **systolic** and **diastolic. Systole** (pronounced "sis-toll-ee") means contraction of the heart; therefore, systolic blood pressure is the pressure in the arteries when the heart, or more specifically, the left ventricle, pumps. It is the higher number taken when measuring blood pressure and is usually around 120 mm Hg. (mm Hg = millimeters of mercury, the unit blood pressure is measured in) **Diastole** (pronounced "die-ass-toll-ee") is the term for the heart at rest. Therefore, diastolic pressure is the pressure that stays in the system when the left ventricle is relaxing and filling. It is the lower number taken when measuring blood pressure, usually around 80 mm Hg. A person's blood pressure always is reported as two numbers, for example, 120/80 (read as "120 over 80"), meaning that systolic pressure is 120 and diastolic pressure is 80.

The difference between systolic and diastolic pressure is the **pulse pressure.**

Pulse pressure = systolic pressure –
diastolic pressure

CLINICAL CORRELATION *A narrow pulse pressure is a sign of approaching shock (see section on Shock). A wide pulse pressure is a sign of increased intracranial pressure (see Chap. 2).*

A person with high blood pressure has **hypertension** (hyper = high, tension = pressure); that is, he or she is **hypertensive.** The most common definition of hypertension is a resting blood pressure over 140/90. Some people have pressures much higher all the time.

CLINICAL CORRELATION *People with hypertension, which includes many older Americans, are at increased risk of stroke and heart disease.*

A person with low blood pressure has **hypotension,** or is **hypotensive.** Usually, we say people are hypotensive when their systolic blood pressure is less than 90, but keep in mind that some people, especially young athletes and slender women, often have normally low blood pressures.

Preload

Remember that the cardiovascular system is just a pumping system inside the body. In order for the heart to work as a pump, it must be "loaded" with blood. **Preload** is the volume of the heart before it contracts—that is, when it is full of blood. If preload is high, the heart has plenty of blood to pump. If preload is too low, the heart does not have enough blood to

pump, and the whole system can fail. Practically, preload = volume.

The heart's volume depends on the quantity of blood in the body and the body's ability to get that blood to the heart. The major veins, especially the IVC, work as the body's storage bin for blood. When veins **dilate** (that is, when they relax and get big), blood tends to pool in them. When blood pools, preload drops because blood is not getting to the heart.

CLINICAL CORRELATION *When a person stands suddenly after lying down, blood naturally pools in the veins of the legs and feet. A person can feel light-headed or even pass out because there is insufficient pre-load to pump blood to the brain. Blood pressure will drop briefly. If blood pressure doesn't return to normal after 3–5 minutes, the person has orthostatic hypotension, a sign of not having enough fluid in the body that is best treated by elevating the feet and administering IV fluids if necessary.*

Preload is affected by several factors, some of which the emergency medical technician or paramedic can control:

1. *Position*: Lying a patient supine (flat on their back) with the feet elevated (the *Trendelenburg position*) *increases* preload simply by allowing blood to more easily flow back to the heart by using gravity. Likewise, sitting up or standing *decreases* preload.
2. *Sympathetic/parasympathetic tone*: The predominant effect of sympathetic tone is to *increase* preload by causing constriction of the blood vessels (through alpha-receptors). When veins are constricted, blood is unable to pool in the body and is returned to the heart. Parasympathetics, or the vagus nerve, tend to do the opposite of the sympathetics, causing vasodilation, blood pooling, and a *decrease* in preload.
3. *Nitroglycerin/morphine/furosemide (Lasix)*: Each of these medications tends to *decrease* preload by vasodilation. Furosemide also is a diuretic, meaning it will

cause a person to urinate and therefore lose fluid.

A patient may need his or her preload increased or decreased, depending on the situation.

CLINICAL CORRELATION *When a patient is in heart failure and has pulmonary edema, you need to lower his or her preload because the heart cannot handle the fluid. The best drug for the job is furosemide (Lasix) because it has an early effect of vasodilation, which lowers preload and helps clear the lungs by allowing fluid to pool in the veins. Furosemide then turns on the kidneys, allowing excess fluid to be urinated. Always carry a urinal in the ambulance.*

CLINICAL CORRELATION *The heart of a patient with angina is asked to work harder than it is able; thus, reducing preload reduces the amount of work the heart has to do. One reason nitroglycerin and morphine are the drugs of choice for angina is because both decrease preload. Be careful when you administer these, however, because they also lower blood pressure! Always know your patient's vital signs before administering any drug. If your patient is hypotensive, avoid these drugs.*

Remember that the autonomic nervous system doesn't just send *out* signals controlling the body—it senses what is going on as well. For example, a drop in preload will be sensed and the body will respond by turning on the sympathetic nervous system, raising blood pressure (see Chap. 2).

Heart Dynamics

The amount of blood the heart actually pumps out is known as **cardiac output**. Cardiac output depends on two things: **stroke volume**, or how much blood is pumped with each stroke, and heart rate, or how quickly the heart beats.

Cardiac output = stroke volume × heart rate

The actual number is not important, but the concept is. Emergency medical technicians and paramedics have the ability to control both stroke volume and heart rate (to a certain extent) to keep the patient's cardiac output high enough.

The heart itself has several important characteristics: *Starling's law of the heart*, **inotropy**, and **chronotropy**. Starling's law of the heart states that the more the heart is stretched (by filling it with blood), the stronger it will contract. This is the body's natural way of adapting to increases in preload. As preload increases, so does stroke volume. Thus, a person with a healthy heart can handle extra fluids.

Inotropy refers to how strong, or how hard, the heart is able to beat. The harder the heart beats, the higher the stroke volume. Things that make the heart beat harder are said to have a **positive inotropic effect**; things that make the heart beat less hard are said to have a **negative inotropic effect**. The sympathetic nervous system and all of the sympathetic drugs (epinephrine, isoproterenol, dobutamine) have a strong positive inotropic effect. Using a positive inotrope makes the heart beat harder and do more work, thereby increasing the heart's demand for oxygen, which may not be a good thing. Calcium channel blockers (like verapamil and nifedipine) have a negative inotropic effect.

The other major characteristic of the heart that sometimes can be controlled is **chronotropy**, which refers to heart rate, governed mostly by the SA and AV nodes. Anything that speeds up the heart has a **positive chronotropic effect**; anything that slows it down has a **negative chronotropic effect.** Not surprisingly, sympathetics all have a positive chronotropic effect. Parasympathetics have a negative chronotropic effect, as do calcium channel blockers (especially verapamil). Atropine, a parasympathetic blocker, is a positive chronotrope.

The faster the heart beats, the higher the cardiac output. The slower the heart beats, the lower the cardiac output.

Afterload

The pressure load on the heart's outflowing side is the **afterload**, largely determined by how much resistance blood vessels give to blood flowing through them (*peripheral vascular resistance*). Practically speaking, afterload is best reflected by blood pressure. If the pump has a lot of pressure to pump against, it must work harder to keep the water flowing. At the same time, if there is no pressure in the system at all, the system has failed.

Preload = volume

Afterload = pressure/resistance

Afterload is set in the arteries (specifically, the small arterioles). Things that cause vasodilation in the arteries lower afterload by reducing the resistance to blood flow (lowering peripheral vascular resistance). The sympathetic nervous system increases afterload. Calcium channel blockers (like verapamil and nifedipine) reduce afterload, as do nitrates (like nitroglycerin and nitroprusside), which are all vasodilators.

Most patients with hypertension take some afterload-reducing agent, such as the calcium channel blocker nifedipine, or drugs known as angiotensin-converting enzyme (ACE) inhibitors. All cause arteriole dilation through different mechanisms, thus lowering blood pressure.

Arteriole blood vessels are also sensitive to CO_2. As levels of CO_2 increase, these blood vessels dilate, a reflex designed to help bring more blood into a tissue so that CO_2 can be carried away. Hyperventilate patients bleeding inside their heads because it reduces intracranial pressure by reducing CO_2 levels, resulting in vasoconstriction of the artioles in the brain (see Chap. 2). Hyperventilation, however, probably will not change the patient's blood pressure measurably.

SHOCK

Treating shock is one of the most important ways emergency medical technicians and paramedics save lives.

Shock means cardiovascular failure. A person in shock is unable to get enough oxygenated blood to important body tissues. That is, the person's tissue perfusion is inadequate. You can define shock in one word: hypoperfusion (hypo = low, perfusion = getting oxygenated blood to the tissues that need it).

There is nothing mystical or magical about shock. Nonmedical people are quick to say, "Oh! He's going into shock," but please don't misunderstand shock. It all has to do with the cardiovascular system—the pump, pipes, and volume. When any one of these things fails, the whole system fails, and shock results. It's that simple.

Imagine, if you would, the mythical little town of ECNALUBMA. You may have seen one of the town's many emergency vehicles driving toward you. The water company in this town is charged with making sure that everyone living there gets enough water. The town has a big storage tank full of water (the blood supply), a pumping station (the heart), and a system of pipes (blood vessels) carrying water to all of the houses so the townspeople can shower in the morning (can get adequate tissue perfusion) (Fig. 3-38). If a townsperson doesn't get a morning shower, he or she will be underperfused and go into shock.

There are three basic ways for the water company to fail the townspeople; that is, there are three basic types of shock: inadequate fluid (**hypovolemic shock**), a failing pump (**cardiogenic shock**), or problems with the pipes (**vasogenic shock**).

Hypovolemic Shock

Hypovolemia means not enough volume (hypo = low, volemia = volume). If someone punctures the ECNALUBMA town storage tank, all of the water will pour out, and the townspeople won't get their showers (Fig. 3-39). Likewise, a person who is stabbed and has blood pouring out will begin to lose volume and will soon go into shock. Shock from blood loss, or hemorrhage, is also known as *hemorrhagic shock*.

Blood loss is not the only way to lose fluids; prolonged vomiting or diarrhea also can result in fluid loss. It is not unusual to take a person with the flu to the hospital. Dehydration from sweating, either due to the environment or from fevers, is a source of fluid loss as well (see Chap. 6).

CLINICAL CORRELATION *The treatment of choice for hypovolemia is IV fluids. Even basic emergency medical technicians should be allowed to start IVs to give fluids.*

CLINICAL CORRELATION *Flulike illnesses, especially in children and the elderly, can cause life-threatening hypovolemia from a combination of vomiting, diarrhea, and sweat loss from fevers.*

CLINICAL CORRELATION *It's usually not worth trying to rehydrate someone orally on an ambu-*

lance unless you're doing a standby at a road race or similar event. Anyone sick or injured should not get anything orally because it may make things worse if the patient has a problem with his or her gastrointestinal tract (see Chap. 4).

The body's response to fluid loss is predictable. The early loss in cardiac output usually is sensed in places such as the carotid sinus, which has pressure sensors known as *baroreceptors*. When the body senses a drop in cardiac output (*not* a drop in blood pressure), it responds by pushing the internal "panic button"—that is, the body activates the sympathetic nervous system, pouring out adrenaline in the classic "fight or flight" response (see Chap. 2). The role of the sympathetic nervous system is to maintain perfusion to the brain.

So, the symptoms of hypovolemic shock are predictable, keeping in mind that the sympathetic nervous system is in full swing: vasoconstriction of the peripheral blood vessels, which keeps blood out of useless places such as skin and saves it for important organs, and sweating from the effects of adrenaline. Thus, skin is *pale* and *cool* from reduced blood flow to it and *clammy* (or moist) from sweat.

CLINICAL CORRELATION *One of the earliest signs of shock is delayed capillary refill. Fingernails are normally pinkish (no matter how dark the skin) from blood in the capillaries underneath the nails. If you pinch a person's nail, it will blanch (turn white) because you have squeezed out the blood. The nail should become pink again in less than three seconds. If it takes longer, there is a problem. The sympathetic nervous system already has begun to clamp down on the capillaries and shunt blood away from the skin. Capillary refill is the best quick test for early hypoperfusion (shock)—it only takes three seconds to do!*

As the patient loses more fluid, the sympathetics push even harder; consequently, the heart starts to beat faster. The pulse, however, may not be that strong because each heart beat has very little stroke volume (because there is no volume). As a result, the pulse becomes *rapid* and *thready* (a thready pulse is supposed

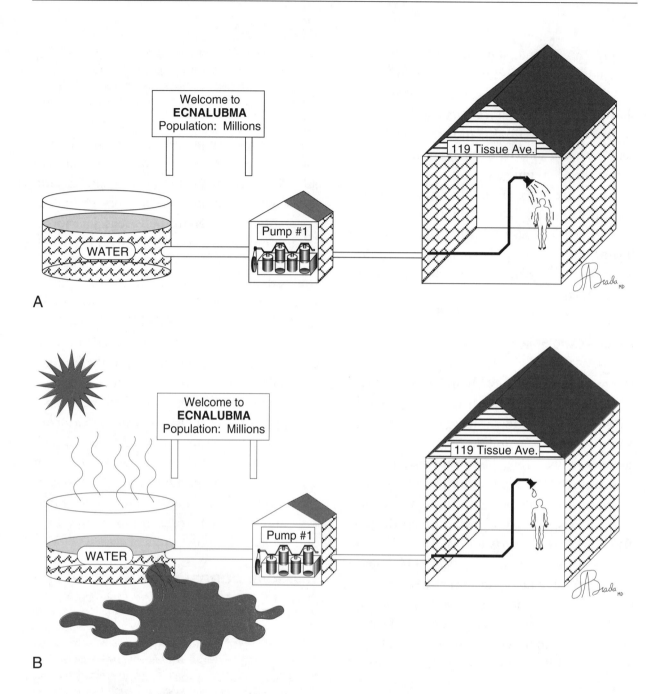

Fig. 3-38. A. The Ecnalubma town water supply. The water tank represents venous capacity, the pumping station symbolizes the heart, and the figure in the shower represents a single cell in the body. As the goal of pumping blood is to maintain perfusion in the cells, which require oxygen and nutrients, adequacy of cardiovascular function is measured on the microvascular level. In short, the ultimate evaluation of the system depends on whether the figure gets an adequate shower. B. Hypovolemic shock. If the Ecnalubma water supply fails for any reason—by rupture of the storage tank (massive hemorrhage), evaporation, or lack of rainfall (dehydration)—the station will have nothing to pump and Mr. Cell will not get his shower.

to feel like a thread with little knots in it being pulled under your finger; it will be weak).

Likewise, adrenaline causes faster breathing; thus, respiratory rate increases, and the patient may begin to have *rapid, shallow respirations.*

If the sympathetic system cannot keep enough cardiac output going to the brain, the patient will begin to experience *altered mental status* or *decreased level of consciousness.* Intelligent thought in the brain is the first thing to go as the brain shuts down; therefore, patients can become *disoriented.*

Eventually, as more and more fluid is lost, the heart may not have much fluid to fill with between beats. The difference between the pressure of the heart while it's beating and while it's at rest becomes smaller and smaller— a narrowing pulse pressure.

Notice that nothing about low blood pressure has been mentioned. So far, the body has been able to compensate for fluid loss by using the sympathetic nervous system, referred to as *compensated shock.* The time you need to intervene is *before* blood pressure drops and the patient goes into *decompensated shock* and the blood pressure starts to fall.

To quote Dr. M. Kamper: "Using blood pressure to watch for shock is like using an altimeter to watch for a waterfall. By the time you see a change on the gauge, it's really late in the game" (Fig. 3-40). It is absolutely imperative to detect the early signs of shock: delayed capillary refill; pale, cool, and clammy skin; rapid, shallow pulse and respirations; and disorientation.

CLINICAL CORRELATION *Any single set of vital signs is only a little useful. Repeat vital signs often and look for changes. A patient with a heart rate of 90 may not alarm you, but if it was only 60 five minutes ago, the patient may have a problem.*

CLINICAL CORRELATION *Do not rely solely on blood pressure! Be alert and look for the early signs of shock before it's too late.*

The treatment for shock is fairly straightforward. Do what you can to treat the underlying cause. For example, if you can stop an active bleed, do so, but keep in mind that definitive treatment may be surgical. *So don't waste time*!

CLINICAL CORRELATION *If you are treating a trauma patient you think is going into shock, take him or her to a shock-trauma center, not just an emergency room.*

CLINICAL CORRELATION *Supportive care for hypovolemic shock is straightforward: oxygen, Trendelenburg (elevated feet), MAST (may be helpful), but more important, fluid, fluid, fluid. Get bilateral, large-bore (14-gauge) IV access and quickly transport the patient to the treatment center. (That's what helicopters and V8 engines are for!)*

The heart can survive with surprisingly few red blood cells, but it needs fluid to maintain perfusion.

Cardiogenic Shock

Cardiogenic means originating from the heart. Imagine that something has gone wrong with the ECNALUBMA pumping station. If the pump quits, no water is pumped. Consequently, the townspeople won't get their showers (Fig. 3-41). Likewise, the heart cannot pump, the body is not able to perfuse all of its organs and goes into cardiogenic shock.

The major reasons for a person to go into cardiogenic shock are outlined in this chapter's section describing heart failure. Cardiogenic shock is the end stage of heart failure and usually is seen in medical patients with heart disease (myocardial infarctions) rather than in trauma patients.

In cardiogenic shock, the heart isn't pumping, so stroke volume and cardiac output are low. The body's response in cardiogenic shock is the same as it is for hypovolemic shock— that is, an outpouring from the sympathetic nervous system leading to poor capillary refill;

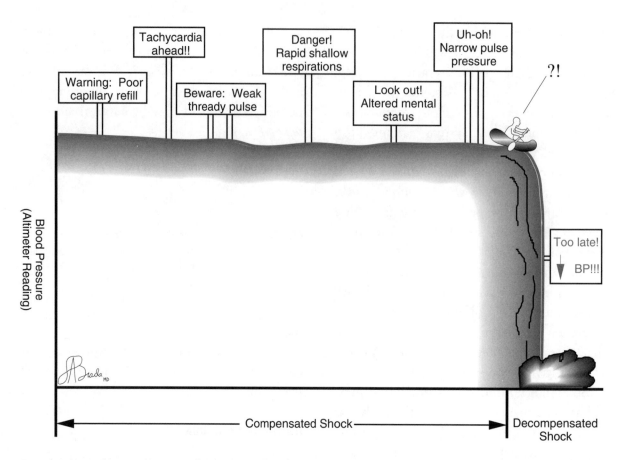

Fig. 3-40. The warning signs of shock. Many warning signs alert you that the patient is going into shock long before the bottom falls out of the blood pressure readings. If you do not consider the possibility of shock in every patient, by the time the patient's blood pressure begins to fall, it may well be too late, as he or she already is decompensating.

pale, cool, clammy skin; tachycardia (rapid weak pulse); and eventual drop in pressure. The difference is that there is plenty of fluid in the system, but the pump is just out.

CLINICAL CORRELATION   *The treatment of choice for cardiogenic shock is inotropic support with dopamine (usually called a "pressor" because it also causes peripheral vasoconstriction) and/or dobutamine, a positive inotrope.*

CLINICAL CORRELATION   *Cardiogenic shock also can be treated with fluids, especially in cases when cardiogenic shock results from traumatic causes such as pericardial tamponade or direct injury to the myocardium, but remember that heart failure can lead to pulmonary edema. Don't forget the ABCs— breathing before circulation. Do not give large volumes of fluids to patients with pulmonary edema.*

CLINICAL CORRELATION   *If the heart is damaged, as from a heart attack, the electrical system may be damaged too; thus, the patient may not be able to speed up his or her heart rate. A person who is bradycardic and looks as though he or she is going into shock is the ideal candidate for atropine or external pacing.*

Vasogenic Shock

The last way the town of ECNALUBMA's water system can fail is if there is a problem in the distribution of water to the shower. Let's say, for example, that every person in this town of millions turns on their showers and flushes just as you are about to start your shower. You're not going to get much water in your shower. You will be underperfused. It's not

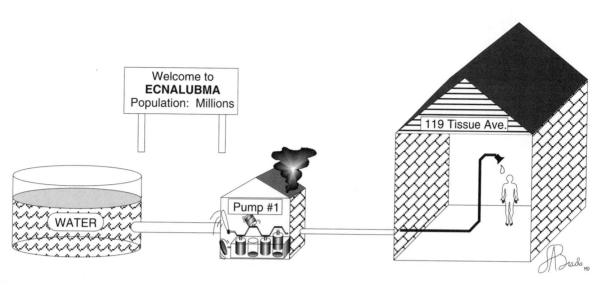

Fig. 3-41. Cardiogenic shock. When the Ecnalubma pump station fails (left-sided heart failure), the water pressure drops, and showers dry up all over town.

because there isn't enough water, and it's not because the pump isn't doing its job—both can be fine. You don't get enough water because there are too many open water lines for the amount of available water and pump pressure.

The body works the same way. When too many blood vessels open up (dilate) and demand blood at once, important organs (such as the brain) don't get enough, a problem of poor distribution. This type of shock is often referred to as *distributive shock*, more commonly known as **vasogenic shock**, because the problem rests in the control of blood vessels (Fig. 3-42).

Why would a person go into vasogenic shock? One common reason is because of a spinal cord injury. Remember, it is the sympathetic nervous system that keeps all of the blood vessels constricted. If the spinal cord is cut (such as in a motorcycle accident), all sympathetic ability below the point where the spine is cut is lost. All of the blood vessels will dilate inappropriately (just as when all of the townspeople flush at once—it's inappropriate when you want your shower). Blood pools in useless places such as the skin, and the body can do nothing about it because it has lost con-

trol of the nervous system. This particular type of vasogenic shock is commonly known as **neurogenic shock** because it is brought on by a failure in the nervous system.

CLINICAL CORRELATION *Unlike patients in hypovolemic or cardiogenic shock, a patient in neurogenic shock is red and warm rather than pale, cool, and clammy. Remember, it's the sympathetic nervous system that causes a person to be pale, cool, and clammy. In neurogenic shock, sympathetic nervous system function is lost and all the skin blood vessels dilate, sending warm blood to the skin. Thus, neurogenic shock sometimes is called "warm shock." Sometimes, a line across the body—below which is red and above which is pale—actually can be seen, marking the point where the spinal cord is cut.*

When the sympathetics are lost, the parasympathetics are unopposed; that is, if you lose the gas pedal, then the brakes tend to take hold. The parasympathetics, as you may recall, arise mostly from the vagus nerve, which comes out of the brain stem, not the spinal cord (see Chap. 2). Thus, a patient with a spinal cord injury does not lose the "brakes," only the "gas pedal."

CLINICAL CORRELATION *The sympathetic nerves to the heart originate mostly from the neck. If the cord is cut high enough, sympathetic tone to the heart is lost, meaning that the patient may have a slow heart rate*

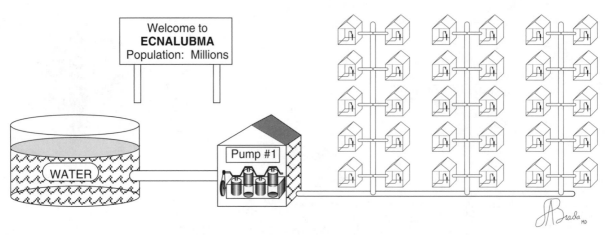

Fig. 3-42. Vasogenic shock. If everyone in the town of Ecnalubma headed for the shower at the same time, the pumping station would not be able to meet the increased demand no matter how hard it worked. Even though water pressure readings in the main pipeline heading into town may be normal, everybody would get a trickle—nobody would get a decent shower. When spinal cord injuries or anaphylactic reactions open all of the body's arterioles at once, the heart is not able to maintain adequate perfusion to all capillary beds even though it produces several times its normal cardiac output.

as well as warm, red, dry skin. The giveaway for neurogenic shock is that the patient is not be able to move or feel anything. Notice that the patient may be in shock but have none of the vital signs you would expect.

CLINICAL CORRELATION *The treatment for neurogenic shock is to administer fluids (to fill all of the useless showers being run) and dopamine (to try to shut down some of the useless showers—that is, vasoconstriction). If the patient is bradycardic, consider atropine.*

Similar to true neurogenic shock is *psychogenic shock*, better termed **syncope**, which means fainting, or a brief loss of consciousness. Given unusual stress (fright, terror, or revulsion), people faint due to a sudden outpouring from the vagus nerve, causing vasodilation. Not enough blood reaches the brain, resulting in a faint. Because fainting is caused by vagal nerve effects on the vasculature, it also is often called a **vasovagal** response, or vasovagal syncope. Fainting often is associated with a decreased heart rate, also due to increased vagal effects.

The problem is entirely self-limiting, however. After a person faints, he or she falls to the ground, blood returns to the head, and the person is fine. The vagus nerve goes mostly to the gastrointestinal tract, which is why the person also may feel nauseated. Remember, too, that the vagus can slow the heart, which adds to the problem of not getting enough blood up into the head.

Cutting the spinal cord is not the only way to bring about a true vasogenic shock. Toxins or certain chemicals in the blood can do the same thing, one way in which allergic reactions can kill a person. The extreme of allergic reactions is called **anaphylaxis**. There are billions of cells known as mast cells everywhere in the body that are filled with chemicals—for example, *histamine*. When mast cells are stimulated, they release histamine, which causes vasodilation, capillary leakage, and bronchoconstriction (squeezing the air passages in the lungs; see the section on Anatomy of the Respiratory System). Almost anything can cause mast cells to release. Ever wonder why skin turns red when it is slapped? The impact of the slap causes mast cells to release histamine, which temporarily causes local vasodilation and capillary leakage.

In **anaphylactic shock**, a toxin, such as the venom of a bee or snake, causes mast cells throughout the body to release histamine. Blood vessels dilate, and capillaries leak everywhere. Imagine trying to get water in the shower if all the pipes leaked! Anaphylactic shock, therefore, is a form of vasogenic shock. More important, anaphylaxis results in breathing difficulty as well.

CLINICAL CORRELATION *The treatment for anaphylaxis is subcutaneous epinephrine to relieve constriction of the airways and also to help pressure. Emergency medical technicians should be able to give "epi shots." Additional treatment includes antihistamines such as diphenhydramine (Benadryl), which block the actions of histamine, and IV fluids if necessary.*

Finally, metabolic failure found in profoundly ill, hospitalized patients and widespread infection (*sepsis*) also can cause vasogenic shock through a variety of toxins in the blood. These patients are very sick and are usually already hospitalized.

CLINICAL CORRELATION *If you don't have a clue about what is wrong with sick patients who appear to be going into shock, by all means treat them. As long as a patient's lungs are clear, use Trendelenburg (feet elevated) and IV fluids.*

The three major types of shock—hypovolemic, cardiogenic, and vasogenic—all eventually deteriorate into a final common pathway with features of all three. A person can lose fluid, the heart will stop working well, and capillaries will open and leak. These patients do not often survive. They have passed from *compensated shock* to *decompensated shock* and are now entering *irreversible shock*. They need care in an intensive care unit. Do your best and move quickly.

THE ANATOMY OF THE RESPIRATORY SYSTEM

The **respiratory system** refers to everything in the body related to breathing and getting O_2 into the blood, starting with the airway (see Chap. 2). Air is inhaled through the mouth and nose and travels into the naso-oropharynx, the larynx, and down the trachea. At the carina, the trachea *bifurcates* (forks) into the **left** and **right mainstem bronchi**. Each bronchus then divides repeatedly into smaller and smaller bronchi, eventually becoming small enough to be called bronchioles. The bronchioles finally end in grapelike clusters called **alveoli** (Fig. 3-43). The collection of alveoli and the airway passages feeding them make up the **lungs**. Think of the lungs as being similar to a building: The main entrance is the airway, the hallways are the bronchi and bronchioles, and all of the individual rooms are the alveoli. The walls themselves are the *interstitium* of the lungs that hold everything together.

There are three major *lobes* of the lung on the right side and two on the left, where the heart sits. The top of the lung is known as the **apex**, which reaches surprising high up in the chest and is just below muscles of the shoulders (Fig. 3-44; see Fig. 3-5). The bottom of the lung, the **base**, sits on top of the **diaphragm**, a large, flat, dome-shaped muscle separating the chest cavity from the abdomen. Although people tend to think of the chest as being defined by the ribs, lungs are defined by where the diaphragm is. The diaphragm moves up and down with breathing, so its position does not correspond exactly to the ribcage at any given time.

CLINICAL CORRELATION *It is important to appreciate where the lungs are inside the chest. Seemingly minor trauma to the top of the shoulder actually can puncture a lung, and a gunshot to the belly easily can travel upward and puncture the diaphragm and injure the lung.*

Both lungs are surrounded by two membranes: the **visceral** and **parietal pleura**. The visceral pleura, closely attached to the surface of the lungs, is closer to the gastrointestinal tract (viscera = guts). The parietal pleura, outside the visceral pleura, lines the inner surface of the ribcage and defines the *pleural cavity*,

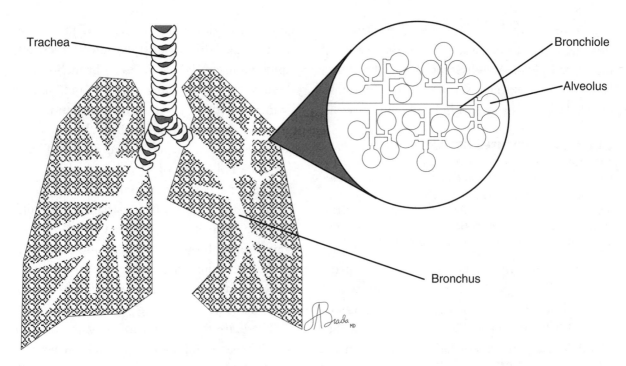

Fig. 3-43. Air spaces of the lung. Air enters the lungs via the trachea, which splits into the left and right main-stem bronchi. The bronchi divide into smaller and smaller bronchioles until they reach microscopic size. Alveoli are tiny air sacs at the end of bronchioles where exchange between air and capillary blood occurs.

the space within the chest where the lungs are. The body has two pleural cavities, one on the left and one on the right. Normally, there is no free space between the layers (Fig. 3-45).

Lung Sounds

The sounds heard by listening to the lungs with a stethoscope depend on anatomy and any underlying disease. Normally heard are *vesicular lung sounds*, corresponding to the normal movement of air into and out of the bronchioles and alveoli. If you listen closer into the midline, you should hear louder, *bronchial sounds*. These sounds are very similar to vesicular lung sounds but tend to be louder and deeper because you're listening to air moving in the big bronchi.

Stridor is an inspiratory high-pitched wheezing sound resulting from obstruction in the upper airway, as in the larynx/epiglottis (see Chap. 2). **Rhonchi** are coarse, raspy

sounds heard with either inspiration or expiration that result from fluid in the bronchi. **Rales,** or **crackles,** are sounds made from alveoli with fluid in them and are heard when you would expect to hear normal vesicular sounds, mostly during inspiration. Rales sound like hair being rubbed right next to your ear or Velcro tearing apart. **Wheezes,** usually expiratory, are sounds made by obstruction or constriction in the lower airways (the smaller bronchi and bronchioles).

BREATHING MECHANICS AND CONTROL

Breathing Mechanics

When a person inhales, either a signal comes down from the brain (voluntarily) or automatically starts in the brain stem, which normally controls breathing. The signal is passed into

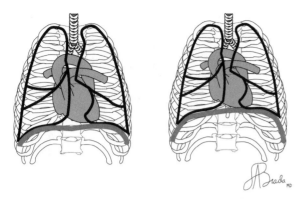

Fig. 3-44. Projections of the lung and diaphragm with inspiration (left) and expiration (right).

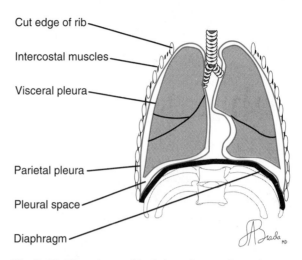

Cut edge of rib

Intercostal muscles

Visceral pleura

Parietal pleura

Pleural space

Diaphragm

Fig. 3-45. The pleura. Each lung is enveloped completely by a two-layered pleural membrane. The pleural space is a potential space between the two layers that helps the lungs inflate as the ribcage moves outward and the diaphragm descends.

the spinal cord and down through the phrenic nerve (see Chap. 2). The phrenic nerve's function is to stimulate the diaphragm, the primary muscle of respiration or breathing.

When the diaphragm is stimulated, it contracts just as any other muscle. When it contracts, it drops down, flattens out, and increases the internal size of the chest cavity, creating *negative pressure* inside the chest (Fig. 3-46). Air then rushes in, sucked in by the negative pressure. **Inspiration,** or breathing in, is normally an active process brought on by creating negative pressure inside the chest. The body "pulls air in" to breathe.

Although the diaphragm is mostly responsible for breathing, **accessory muscles of respiration** help, including the *intercostal* muscles between the ribs, the abdominal muscles, and the muscles of the neck, shoulders, and back. Each of these muscles help expand the ribcage. The more the ribcage expands, the larger internal volume of the lungs becomes, and the more negative pressure is created with each respiration, allowing more air to be sucked in.

CLINICAL CORRELATION *The body normally does not use the accessory muscles of respiration; the diaphragm is enough. The use of accessory muscles is an indication of respiratory distress. Look for intercostal retractions, during which the muscles between the ribs are sucked in with each breath; suprasternal contractions, during which the muscles of the neck above the*

sternum are used; and paradoxical movement of the abdomen, during which the abdominal muscles contract, pulling in with each breath. The abdomen is desperately trying to help increase the size the chest. Each of these are dangerous warning signs of impending respiratory failure. You may need to begin assisting with ventilations.

In contrast to normal inspiration, *positive pressure* is used to ventilate patients in respiratory distress by *pushing* air into the lungs with a bag-valve mask or other device. Normally, when a person breathes, he or she *pulls* air into the lungs with the *negative pressure* created by the diaphragm's lowering.

CLINICAL CORRELATION *The important thing to remember about positive pressure ventilation is that it is not the natural way to breathe. Subjecting the lungs to too much pressure actually can injure them (e.g., you can create a pneumothorax as described below). Always ventilate patients with an Ambu-bag of some sort and avoid mechanical pressure devices, which tend to horribly overinflate the lungs.*

When a person inspires, air travels into the bronchi and eventually into the alveoli, which are only one cell thick and completely covered by the capillaries of the pulmonary arteries (Fig. 3-47). The capillaries themselves are also only one cell thick. Remember, the pulmonary

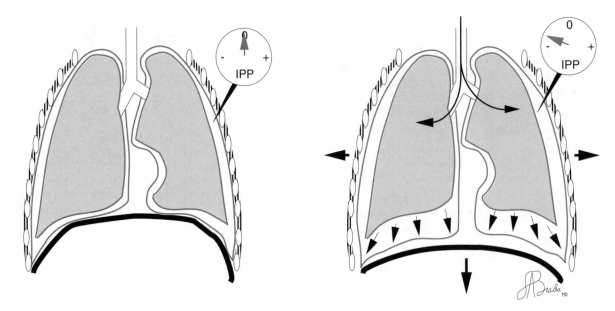

Fig. 3-46. Intrapleural changes during respiration. As the diaphragm descends and the ribcage expands, the parietal pleura is pulled away from the visceral pleura, resulting in negative intrapleural pressure (IPP), as measured by the meter. Since this pressure is now lower than the atmospheric pressure at the mouth and nose, air rushes down the trachea and into the lungs, which expand until IPP returns to zero.

arteries carry deoxygenated blood into the lungs. In the alveoli on the capillary level, blood exchanges the CO_2 it is carrying for fresh O_2 from the air. The air is approximately 21% O_2 (the other 79% is mostly nitrogen), some of which is picked up by the capillaries from the alveoli after it is inhaled. The alveoli in return take CO_2 from the capillaries. An exhaled breath contains about 17% O_2 and 3–4% CO_2. The remainder is still nitrogen, which is normally unaffected by circulation.

CLINICAL CORRELATION *Just because there is some CO_2 in an exhaled breath doesn't make it useless. An exhaled breath still contains a lot of O_2 in it, which is why mouth-to-mask resuscitation works.*

CLINICAL CORRELATION *Mouth-to-mouth resuscitation, the basic standby, should be avoided if at all possible. In addition to being extremely tiring, there is a risk of passing infectious disease from the patient to you. A patient vomiting during resuscitation also is not uncommon.*

CLINICAL CORRELATION *The fact that people exhale CO_2 can be used to the paramedic's advan-*

tage. When you intubate a patient, you can place an end-expiratory CO_2 monitor on the endotracheal tube, which indicates whether or not CO_2 is being exhaled. Only the lungs release CO_2, so if you inadvertently intubate the esophagus, you will not get any CO_2 back from the stomach. Therefore, this is an extremely reliable test for proper placement of endotracheal tubes, especially when there is too much noise to hear lung sounds well (such as in traffic or helicopters).

It is absolutely critical to understand the difference between **ventilation** and **oxygenation**. Ventilation refers to moving air in and out of the lungs (as in normal breathing). After airway management, ventilation is the most important thing for the patient. Oxygenation refers to getting O_2 into the blood. You generally cannot oxygenate blood well without good ventilation. Even with good oxygenation, ventilation is critical to remove CO_2 from the blood.

CLINICAL CORRELATION *If a patient is not breathing well—that is, if he or she is not able to take in a good breath—assist ventilations with an Ambu-bag if necessary or intubate the patient and breathe for him or her. Someone who is not able to take a good breath can be in a room full of pure O_2 that won't do them any good* *without good ventilations. Don't merely stick an oxygen mask on a patient and forget about it.*

CLINICAL CORRELATION *Transtracheal jet insufflation, or ventilating through a needle cricothyrotomy (see Chap. 2), oxygenates well but does not ventilate well. If you are desperate enough to do this, move quickly to a trauma center.*

Using a *pulse oximeter*, or *"pulse-ox"* for short, is a great way to measure oxygenation easily. This machine clips onto the patient's fingernail or earlobe and emits a light that shines across the capillaries in the fingernail or skin. The amount of light absorbed is proportional to the percentage of red blood cells that are *saturated* with O_2—the **oxygen saturation,** or "O_2-sat." Oxygen saturation should be considered a routine vital sign along with pulse, blood pressure, and respiratory rate. A healthy person will have a 94–100% oxygen saturation. Patients with chronic lung disease may have baseline O_2 saturation in the low 90s.

CLINICAL CORRELATION *Cyanosis, or blue fingertips and mucous membranes, is a result of low oxygen saturation.*

The important thing to remember about oxygen saturation is that it is not rated according to a linear scale, meaning that a 50% saturation is not half as good as a 100%. Once saturation drops below 90%, the patient may develop a problem; a saturation below 80% is definitely dangerous. Anyone with a saturation lower than 70% is facing a life-threatening emergency.

CLINICAL CORRELATION *When giving O_2 to patients, give them enough to keep oxygen saturation at least above 90%, the major exception being patients with chronic lung disease (described below). Patients with saturations over 95% do not need extra oxygen. Not everyone needs a non-rebreathing oxygen mask.*

Expiration, or the act of exhaling, is naturally a passive process. A person need only relax to exhale, and air will flow out of the lungs. Expiration should occur whether the inhalation was natural or a forced ventila-

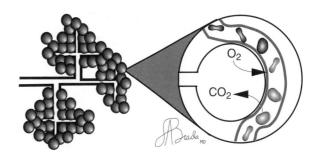

Fig. 3-47. Alveolar gas exchange. Both capillaries and alveoli have extremely thin walls that allow inspired air to come into very close contact with circulating red blood cells, which exchange carbon dioxide for oxygen in the lungs.

tion—that is, when you ventilate patients, they should exhale on their own, even if they are unconscious. Normally, with any given breath, expiration takes a little longer than inspiration.

Breathing Control

Normally, breathing occurs automatically; a control center in the brain stem sends out a signal to breathe without a person's ever having to think about it. We do, however, have the ability to exert conscious control over breathing. Now that you're thinking about it, you're aware of your breathing, and you can make yourself breathe at almost any rate you want.

The brain stem is sensitive to many different signals telling it it's time to take a breath (Table 3-2), the most important signal being the CO_2 level in the blood. When the CO_2 level rises in the blood, the brain stem sends out a signal to take another breath. An excessive level of CO_2 in the blood is known as *hypercapnia*. Holding your breath long enough results in the body's using up all of the O_2 and CO_2 accumulating in the blood. The level of CO_2 rises until eventually the body can no longer tolerate the lack of O_2 and takes a breath.

CLINICAL CORRELATION *Small children having tantrums may hold their breath (with amazing*

Table 3-2. Regulation of breathing

Increase in respiratory rate	Decrease in respiratory rate
Increase in CO_2 (hypercapnia)	Narcotics
Decrease in O_2 (hypoxia)	Alcohol
Decrease in pH (acidosis)	Depressants (benzodiazepines, barbiturates)
Increase in sympathetic tone	Head injuries
Head injuries	O_2*

*Only in *some* patients with chronic obstructive pulmonary disease; see text.

willpower). Eventually they may pass out, and the brain stem will resume normal function. They will breathe again, so don't worry. It is possible, but highly unlikely, that a child can hold his or her breath long enough to actually have a seizure. Once they are seizing, they cannot hold their breath, so give extra O_2.

CO_2 is the most important stimulant for breathing, but it is certainly not the only one. Inadequate O_2, *hypoxia*, also signals faster breathing (hypo = low, oxia = oxygen). (*Hypoxemia* is having too little O_2 in the blood [eme = blood].) *Acidosis*, a condition in which blood is too acidic, also causes a person to breathe faster (see Chap. 4).

A person who is not able to breathe for whatever reason will become hypercapnic, hypoxemic, and acidotic (too much CO_2, too little O_2, and too much acid).

The other major stimulus to breathe faster is activation of the sympathetic nervous system, which can be a response to stress or anxiety or to early shock.

CLINICAL CORRELATION *Extreme emotional agitation is a common cause of hyperventilation, during which the patient breathes faster and faster, out of control. When a person hyperventilates, the blood's CO_2 level is lowered. Too low a level of CO_2 causes numbness and a tingling sensation in the fingers and lips, which can further raise anxiety, increase sympathetic tone, and make the hyperventilation worse. The treatment of choice is to calm the patient in a quiet, nonstimulating environment and give him or her a paper bag to breathe into. Breathing into the bag results in the patient's rebreathing his or her CO_2, bringing the CO_2 level back up to a normal level in the blood. The tingling feeling will stop, and, it is hoped,*

the patient will calm down and breathe normally again. Have the patient breathe into a bag, however, only if you are absolutely sure the patient is hyperventilating. Otherwise, rebreathing CO_2 can be disastrous.

Head injuries are interesting in that they can speed up, slow down, or completely stop respirations, depending on the exact nature of the injury. As mentioned previously, hyperventilation is good for people with brain injuries because it lowers intracranial pressure. Patients' bodies may do this naturally, but if not, you certainly should do it for them.

Just as there are stimulants that excite breathing, there are depressants for breathing—namely, drugs. Both the drugs patients take (including prescription medications) and the drugs paramedics administer can cause **respiratory depression**, during which a person is not breathing enough, or even **respiratory arrest**, during which a person is not breathing at all. Common culprits are alcohol, narcotics, and benzodiazepines (e.g., sedatives like Valium). Each of these drugs can suppress the brain's stimulus to breathe, and, when mixed, the effect is synergistic—that is, extra strong!

CLINICAL CORRELATION *When the patient is unconscious for whatever reason, administer naloxone (Narcan) to reverse the effects of narcotics. Narcan will not hurt anybody, so don't be afraid to use it. Basic emergency medical technicians should be allowed to administer shots of Narcan.*

CLINICAL CORRELATION *If you suspect a patient of overdosing on a benzodiazepine—for example,* *there is an empty bottle of Xanax or Valium next to the patient—you can reverse the effect with flumazenil (Romazicon), which also works if you oversedate a patient (for example, prior to cardioversion). Unlike naloxone (Narcan), flumazenil is not without risk, so do not use it routinely (as naloxone can be used).*

CLINICAL CORRELATION *Remember, anyone not breathing well needs to be ventilated and oxygenated. Don't wait for a person to stop breathing before you start to help.*

Breathing Patterns

Patients can have a variety of breathing patterns, each with different meaning (Fig. 3-48). **Tachypnea,** meaning rapid breathing, occurs for any reason a person might breathe fast (for example, shock, excitement, or respiratory distress). **Apnea,** meaning no breathing, is obviously life-threatening.

CLINICAL CORRELATION *The natural respiratory rate is 12–20 breaths per minute. Fewer than 10 breaths and more than 30 are clearly abnormal. Patients who fall outside the natural respiratory rate probably need ventilation support. It is possible "bag" rapidly breathing patients. If they are breathing too rapidly, they may not be taking in enough air, so you have to do it for them.*

There are several abnormal breathing patterns. **Kussmaul respirations** are very deep, rapid breaths best described as "air hunger." They may represent an attempt by the body to lower ("blow off") CO_2 and can be seen in response to acidosis, especially in diabetic patients going into diabetic ketoacidosis, or "diabetic coma" (see Chap. 4). Head injuries can cause a similar breathing pattern known as **central neurogenic hyperventilation**—also deep, rapid respiration resulting from damage or pressure on the brain stem (which normally controls respirations).

Another abnormal pattern seen in head injuries and strokes is **Cheyne-Stokes respirations,** a bizarre pattern in which a patient's breathing speeds up, slows down, stops, starts

again, speeds up, and so forth. This is a dangerous sign. Also seen with head injuries is a breathing pattern of intermittent apnea.

CLINICAL CORRELATION *Your patient's breathing pattern can change from one minute to the next. Pay attention, and support respirations when necessary. If you have the luxury of additional personnel, someone should have the sole job of airway and breathing maintenance for all seriously ill or injured patients.*

RESPIRATORY INJURIES

Pneumothorax

Lung tissue is encased in the visceral pleura. Outside the visceral pleura is the parietal pleura, which sits against the chest wall muscles. The space between the visceral and parietal pleura is called the **pleural space,** normally only a "potential space"—that is, the two pleura usually lie right next to each other but have the *potential* to separate and have a real space between them. A **pneumothorax,** meaning air in the chest, occurs when air fills the pleural space. The problem is that air is in the pleural space and not in the lungs.

There are several ways a pneumothorax can occur; the most common you are likely to see involves trauma to the chest. For example, a person hits his or her chest against the steering wheel of a car, violently breaking a couple of ribs. One of the ribs punctures the pleural membranes. Now, every time this person breathes in, not only does air rush into the lungs, it rushes through the hole in the visceral pleura, filling the pleural space with air. Unfortunately, when the person exhales, the air in the pleural space remains (Fig. 3-49). This pneumothorax is *closed* or *simple.*

A variation on the theme is penetrating trauma. For example, a person is shot in the chest and the bullet punctures the parietal pleura. Every time he or she tries to take a

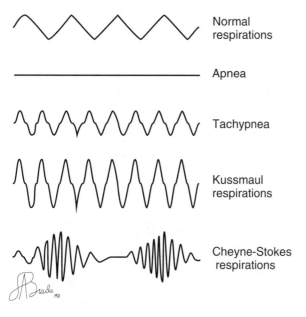

Fig. 3-48. Normal and abnormal respiratory patterns. The way a patient breathes may indicate the nature and severity of his or her illness or injury.

breath, the diaphragm drops, creating negative pressure inside the chest, which sucks air in. This time, however, air has two places to enter with every breath—through the mouth and through the hole in the chest. A damaged visceral pleura makes matters worse because even more air will tend to go into the pleural space (see Fig. 3-49). This type of injury is known as an **open pneumothorax** or **sucking chest wound.**

CLINICAL CORRELATION *The immediate treatment for a sucking chest wound is to cover the hole with an occlusive dressing—plastic or aluminum foil—that won't allow any more air to be sucked in. Try to secure the dressing on three sides to make a "flutter valve," which may let some air out of the chest but seals the hole when the patient inhales so that no more air comes in. The important thing is to not let any air into the chest, so don't get too fancy.*

CLINICAL CORRELATION *Patients with blunt trauma, such as that resulting from motor vehicle accidents and falls, are prone to pneumothoraces. People naturally respond to something awful happening (such as an impact) by gasping, or taking a sudden*

breath, which inflates the lungs like a balloon. Smash that balloon against the dashboard and pop—a pneumothorax develops, even without penetrating trauma.

The major threat of any pneumothorax is air filling the pleural space and crowding out the lung. The pneumothorax collapses the lung and pushes the contents of the chest over to the other side, creating a life-threatening **tension pneumothorax,** in which the **mediastinum** shifts. You will have a *mediastinal shift.* (Fig. 3-50). The mediastinum is the space between the lungs with everything in it such as the trachea, heart, and great blood vessels (see section on the mediastinum). Pushing the mediastinum mechanically kinks off the IVC where it comes through the diaphragm, preventing blood from returning to the heart and resulting in shock. (Effectively, the patient has almost no preload.) In addition, compression of the mediastinum also may cause jugular venous distention.

The more air in the pleural space, the more the lungs are compressed and collapse; thus, there is less usable air inside the lung. With less and less air, the patient needs to breathe more and more. The more the patient breathes, the worse the pneumothorax becomes, a viscous cycle that rapidly can lead to death.

CLINICAL CORRELATION *Suspect a pneumothorax in anyone with chest or abdominal trauma, penetrating or not. To diagnose it, remember the basics: "look, listen, and feel," or "inspection, palpation, and auscultation." Inspect the chest for evidence of trauma, look for tracheal deviation in the sternal notch, and check for jugular venous distention. (When tracheal deviation is severe enough, the trachea will be pushed away from the side of the pneumothorax.) Look at and feel the chest for equal expansion on both sides. As a pneumothorax progresses, the affected side of the chest may not rise with inspiration as does the unaffected side. Also, feel for subcutaneous emphysema, or air underneath the skin, which has a very distinct feeling similar to crunching Rice Krispies beneath wax paper. Finally, listen with your stethoscope for air movement. If the patient has a pneumothorax, you will not hear good breath sounds; they will be diminished or decreased (quieter) because air is not moving in and out of the lung.*

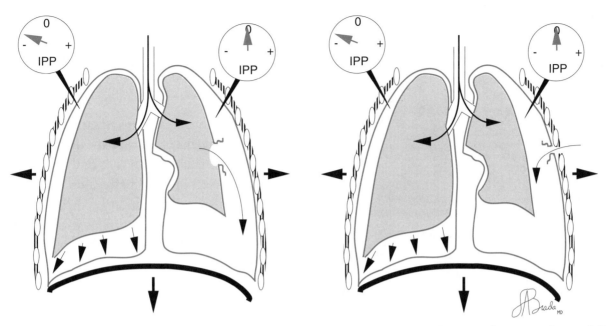

Fig. 3-49. Pneumothoraces. Rupture of the visceral pleura creates a simple (or closed) pneumothorax (left), whereas penetrating trauma through the parietal pleura produces an open pneumothorax (right). In either case, the introduction of air into the pleural space interferes with the ability to generate negative intrapleural pressures (IPP). When this happens, the affected lung does not expand well, and respiration is compromised.

CLINICAL CORRELATION *Suspect a tension pneumothorax in trauma patients who have trouble breathing, are going into shock (remembering that a tension pneumothorax compresses the IVC and prevents blood from reaching the heart), or patients going into PEA.*

CLINICAL CORRELATION *Treatment of a tension pneumothorax is chest decompression. The quickest way to do this is with a 14-gauge IV catheter inserted either in the second intercostal space in a mid-clavicular line or in the fifth intercostal space in the midaxillary line (Fig. 3-51). Remember, the sternal angle marks the second rib, so the second intercostal space is below that. Also remember to always slide the needle over the top of the rib to avoid cutting the intercostal blood vessels running on the bottom of the ribs.*

CLINICAL CORRELATION *A sucking chest wound, if it becomes a tension pneumothorax, needs to be decompressed with a needle. Make sure the original wound has an occlusive dressing. There are a variety of ways to make a "flutter valve" for needles, such as sticking the needle through a sterile rubber glove or condom. The important thing is that if someone is near death from a pneumothorax, letting the air out of the chest is the only possible life-saving procedure.*

A **spontaneous pneumothorax** can occur without any evidence of trauma. As its name implies, a spontaneous pneumothorax occurs on its own, often with no warning. Basically, a weak spot in the lung (in part of the visceral pleura) simply pops. Typical patients are young (late teens), tall, very thin, white males who play a lot of basketball (no kidding). For some reason, they are prone to spontaneous pneumothoraces. One theory is that they jump up and down so much that they make small tears in their lungs that eventually burst. Additionally, elderly patients with severe emphysema (see below) are more prone to pneumothoraces of any sort because their lungs are badly diseased and structurally weaker.

A similar injury to the pneumothorax is the **hemothorax**, the only difference between the two being that blood rather than air fills the pleural space. Hemothoraces most commonly are caused by trauma that would break a rib

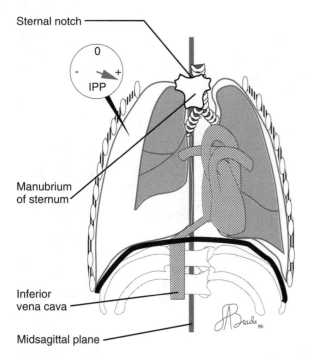

Fig. 3-50. Tension pneumothorax with mediastinal shift. If a pneumothorax is severe enough, the air pressure within the pleural space may become so positive that it not only collapses the lung on that side but also begins to compress the opposite lung and push mediastinal structures away from the midline of the body. A mediastinal shift can be detected by feeling for the trachea at the sternal notch to see if it is deviated to the side opposite the pneumothorax. A mediastinal shift also can crimp the inferior vena cava as it passes through the diaphragm, reducing blood return to the heart and sending the patient into a kind of hypovolemic shock.

and/or cut an intercostal artery. Blood does not expand as quickly as air, so a hemothorax is not as critical as a pneumothorax. Most injuries, however, have some element of both hemothoraces and pneumothoraces (a hemopneumothorax). If you must decompress a tension pneumothorax and get some blood back, don't be surprised.

Flail Chest

A **flail chest** is defined as two or more ribs broken in two or more places (Fig. 3-52). It is

a classic injury when the chest hits the steering wheel in an automobile accident. The problem with a flail chest, unlike a simple broken rib, is that it interferes with the normal mechanics of breathing.

A normal breath requires negative pressure generated inside the chest from the diaphragm's dropping to create suction that pulls in air. A free-floating section of ribs resulting from a flail chest also creates negative pressure, so instead of pulling in air, a person with a free-floating island of ribs sucks in the ribs, losing the sucking ability to get a good breath.

CLINICAL CORRELATION *Look for paradoxical movement of a section of ribs to determine whether a patient has a flail chest. Breathing in expands the chest— except for the free-floating section of the flail chest that is sucked in. Likewise, the chest collapses during exhalation—except for the flail segment that is blown outward. The flail segment moves in the opposite direction that it is supposed to (paradoxical movement).*

CLINICAL CORRELATION *The best treatment for a flail chest is to stabilize the flail segment as best you can. People have used tape, laid the patient on the affected side, or propped up sandbags. (I would avoid lying sandbags on top of the chest; it will be too difficult for the patient to breathe.) If the patient's condition worsens, intubate and ventilate, which uses positive pressure and avoids the complications of the flailing segment.*

CLINICAL CORRELATION *Don't forget that the ribs on the back can be broken and flail as easily as the ribs on the front. The sternum also can form a flail if the ribs around it break.*

RESPIRATORY DISEASES

Chronic Obstructive Pulmonary Disease

Two diseases make up **chronic obstructive pulmonary disease (COPD): emphysema** and **chronic bronchitis** (Fig. 3-53). Smokers develop COPD, and many die from it if they don't die from heart disease or cancer first. Most COPD patients have symptoms of each.

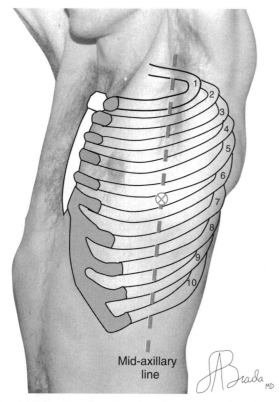

Mid-axillary
line

Fig. 3-51. Proper location for placement of a chest tube. Chest tubes should be inserted at the fifth intercostal space (between the fifth and sixth ribs) along the midaxillary line.

Emphysema is characterized by irreversible destruction of lung tissue (see Fig. 3-53). Recall the analogy of the lungs as a building: The hallways are the bronchial air passages, the rooms the alveoli, and the walls the interstitial lung tissue. Emphysema destroys a lot of the walls, resulting in collapsed hallways and less surface area. (You can't take out the wall and expect the hallway to stay open!) Without healthy lung tissue around them, bronchioles tend to collapse. Patients with emphysema can suck air in, but then it becomes trapped and cannot be exhaled. (Remember, inhalation is active, during which the chest expands to open the passages, but exhalation is passive, during which the chest collapses.) Thus, emphysema is an *obstructive* disease because the ability to exhale is obstructed.

A person with emphysema has fewer, larger rooms instead of having many little rooms (alveoli); thus he or she loses alveolar surface area. Remember, O_2 and CO_2 are exchanged on the surface of alveoli. A person who has lost a lot of alveoli has lost much of the ability to pick up O_2 and blow off CO_2. In other words, patients with emphysema lose effective lung space.

The net result is that patients with emphysema cannot take big breaths because they are unable to exhale, yet they need to breathe more because they effectively have less lung to work with. Thus, they tend to take very shallow breaths, breathe very rapidly, and often are short of breath. In fact, they can be so short of breath that they become malnourished because they can't stop breathing long enough to eat. The classic portrait of a patient with emphysema is the "pink puffer" who tends to be pink, very thin, and constantly puffing to breathe. Additionally, this patient often has loud, bronchial-type breath sounds on inspiration because he or she has no good lung tissue left to make normal vesicular breath sounds. Air moving through the larger bronchi is all that is heard.

Patients with chronic bronchitis, the other component of COPD, tend to have a lot of inflammation of their bronchi or lower airways. Thus, their "hallways" are swollen and irritated and tend to be inundated with dry mucus that they forever are trying to cough up, the proverbial "smoker's cough" (see Fig. 3-53). Irritation in the airways tends to narrow the airway passage. As with emphysema, in which the airways can't be held open, chronic bronchitis creates an obstruction mostly apparent with expiration, not inspiration. Chronic bronchitis patients are prone to having a "smoker's rattle" heard in their lungs caused by rhonchi from all the mucus stuck in their bronchi.

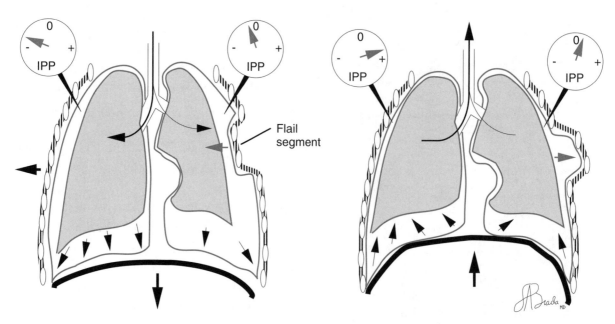

Fig. 3-52. Flail chest. When two or more ribs are broken in more than one place, a flail segment is created. The flail segment moves inward as the rest of the ribcage expands during inspiration (left) and outward as the ribcage recoils during expiration (right), a process known as paradoxical motion that interferes with the generation of appropriate intrapleural pressures (IPP). As a result, the lung does not inflate or deflate properly.

CLINICAL CORRELATION *The hallmark of COPD is expiratory wheezing. Patients usually can breathe in, but their expirations are prolonged, often three to four times the length of inspiration. The patient wheezes during expirations, sometimes so loudly that you don't need your stethoscope. Wheezing comes from air trying to blow by the tightly closed bronchioles; not all COPD patients have pronounced wheezes, however (especially the emphysemic "pink puffers"). COPD patients tend to purse their lips when they exhale, making it easier for them to exhale by keeping back pressure in the airways to hold them open.*

Additionally, COPD patients tend to overinflate their lungs with time because they can never exhale. COPD patients who have more severe chronic bronchitis than emphysema tend to be large, round, and blue because they are holding onto excess CO_2 they are unable to blow off. Thus, chronic bronchitis patients often are called "blue bloaters." Thin and pink or big and blue are the two extremes of COPD, the former being "classic" emphysema and the latter chronic bronchitis. Patients can be any-

where along the spectrum between these two extremes.

Another important physiologic change can occur in COPD patients. Normal patients get an urge to breathe when their CO_2 levels become too high. COPD patients, on the other hand, often have outrageously high CO_2 levels all of the time. Their bodies adapt so that they no longer breathe in response to high levels of CO_2; instead, they breathe when their O_2 levels are too low. These patients breathe when they are hypoxic (when they don't have enough O_2); in other words, they have a **hypoxic drive** to breathe.

CLINICAL CORRELATION *Giving COPD patients 100% O_2 to breathe could cause them to go into respiratory arrest because they will sense only the fact that they have plenty of O_2 and therefore not breathe (if they are dependent upon hypoxic drive to breathe). Therefore, don't haphazardly give patients high-flow O_2. Monitor the patient's mental status, respiratory rate, and oxygen saturation closely. If you give too much O_2 to a*

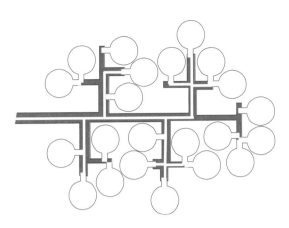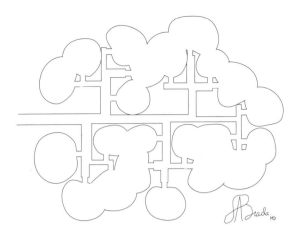

Fig. 3-53. Chronic obstructive pulmonary diseases. Chronic bronchitis (left) is characterized by deposits of thick mucus in the bronchioles that make it difficult for the patient to exhale through the narrowed passages. Emphysema (right) is characterized by the destruction of alveolar walls and loss of elasticity, resulting in troubled exhalation and gas exchange as alveolar surface area decreases.

COPD patient who is dependent on hypoxic drive, they may stop breathing.

CLINICAL CORRELATION *In spite of the above, never withhold O_2 from someone who needs it. If the COPD patient is in severe respiratory distress, badly cyanotic, or in shock, give the patient plenty of O_2, keeping in mind that you may need to ventilate him or her (or even intubate the patient if necessary).*

Long-term COPD patients often are very tenuous—that is, their lungs are barely making it, and the slightest provocation can push them into a "flare," or acute exacerbation of their COPD, which is extremely common. For example, simple infections (a common cold) that a healthy person would quickly shake off, can send a COPD patient to the intensive care unit. Some COPD patients are so sick, they require a small amount of extra O_2 at home all of the time.

Remember, the main acute problem is that a COPD patient's lower airways (bronchi and bronchioles) are too narrow. Treatment, therefore, primarily is aimed at opening the bronchi.

CLINICAL CORRELATION *Standard therapy for COPD exacerbation is any beta-agonist drug such as albuterol, a selective beta$_2$-agonist. Stimulating beta$_2$-receptors in the lungs results in bronchodilation. Albuterol usually is given via a nebulizer, which makes the*

drug easy to inhale and sends it straight to the lungs where it is needed.

CLINICAL CORRELATION *Most COPD patients have inhalers at home for their own use and virtually all will have some form of beta-agonist drug (such as albuterol). Although these drugs are supposed to be beta$_2$-specific, many have beta$_1$ effects, meaning the patient may have a racing heart rate from using the inhaler, especially if he or she is overusing it. Because some of these patients also have damaged hearts (from smoking), they may have angina (chest pains) when their hearts are overworked. Always carefully check vital signs before giving the patient any drug. If the patient's heart rate is too high, you may have to avoid using an albuterol nebulizer.*

CLINICAL CORRELATION *Other medications given intravenously, especially steroids such as methylprednisolone, are useful in COPD flares but rarely are given before arriving at the hospital. Aminophylline is a bronchodilator and smooth-muscle relaxant that opens airway passages. Aminophylline at one time was more widely used than it is today, but it is a potentially toxic drug with questionable benefit over beta-agonists such as albuterol.*

Pneumonia

Few think of pneumonia a as life-threatening emergency; however, in the days before antibiotics, pneumonia was one of the leading causes of death. A pneumonia, simply put, is an infection of the lungs. It can start with a simple virus, causing a little shortness of breath and cough, but can progress to a very serious infection caused by bacteria.

The patient may be sick and complain of a cough, often producing a lot of green-yellow phlegm. When you listen to the patient's lungs, you may hear rhonchi, rales, or wheezes. If you suspect underlying COPD, treat him or her as you would other COPD patients, with nebulized beta-agonists and appropriate O_2.

CLINICAL CORRELATION *Tuberculosis, a type of pneumonia, is making a big comeback in major cities. If you are called to see a patient with a bad cough and you have the slightest worry, wear a mask to protect yourself or, more important, place a mask on the patient. Tuberculosis can be spread by respiratory droplets, especially in tight places such as overcrowded apartments, shelters, and the backs of ambulances.*

Asthma

Asthma is a disease of chronic inflammation of the airways characterized by sensitive, hyper-reactive airways that tend to constrict with little provocation, causing an airway obstruction similar to that of airway obstruction in patients with COPD.

CLINICAL CORRELATION *Asthma patients, like COPD patients, experience a lot of shortness of breath and wheezing. As with COPD patients, the treatment for asthma patients is to open the airways with nebulized albuterol or other beta-agonist and O_2.*

The major difference between asthma patients and COPD patients is that it takes years of smoking to acquire COPD, whereas even young children can have asthma. (A sad truth is that a lot of children develop asthma from the second-hand smoke of their parents.) Triggers of an asthma attack include smoke, allergic reactions, dust, cold air, and exercise; asthma patients don't tend to have the hypoxic drive to breathe as COPD patients do. Thus, emergency medical technicians don't have to

worry as much about administering O_2. Don't forget, however, that older asthma patients may have COPD as well.

Status asthmaticus is a potentially disastrous complication of asthma in which the attack cannot be stopped regardless of the medications administered. If the attack is severe enough, it can be potentially fatal. The patient may reach a point where the only course (other than that you drive really fast) is to intubate and ventilate, which may require paralyzing the patient.

Anaphylaxis

Anaphylaxis is the extreme of allergic reactions. As discussed in the previous section, the body is full of mast cells containing histamine. When an allergen, or *antigen* (e.g., a drug, shellfish, or the venom of a bee sting) enters the body, the antigen binds to mast cells and causes widespread release of histamine. As noted, histamine causes vasodilation and can lead to shock, but more important, can result in bronchoconstriction and collapsing of the airways, especially pronounced in the upper airways. Patients having an anaphylactic reaction may develop stridorous respirations as a result of airway compromise.

CLINICAL CORRELATION *Full-blown anaphylaxis can be fatal within minutes due to airway obstruction. The treatment of choice is subcutaneous epinephrine (1:1000 concentration). Emergency medical technicians should be trained to give this type of shot.*

Anaphylaxis can sneak up on a person; it does not have to be life-threatening within moments. Warning signs of anaphylaxis are hives (red, raised spots that can appear suddenly) and itching, which are effects of histamine.

CLINICAL CORRELATION *Once you've treated the airway with epinephrine, don't forget the rest of the ABCs. The patient is still at risk of continued breathing difficulty or going into shock.*

Pulmonary Edema

Pulmonary edema is fluid in the lungs that results in respiratory difficulty and shortness of breath and can lead to respiratory failure and arrest. The cause is nearly always failure of the heart to pump effectively to clear fluid from the lungs. The hallmark of pulmonary edema is hearing rales when you listen to a patient's lung sounds. Rhonchi and wheezes also can be heard.

Cardiac asthma is a variation of pulmonary edema. Heart failure promotes fluid retention in the lungs (the normal mechanism for pulmonary edema), but instead of pooling in the alveoli, fluid swells in the interstitial space. Remember the building comparison: Normally, in pulmonary edema, rooms of the lungs flood with fluid, resulting in rales (sounds you can hear). In cardiac asthma, however, fluid is stuck in the walls, which swell, causing airway constriction. In this case, you hear mostly wheezes.

Mild pulmonary edema can be seen in a variety of diseases other than left heart failure. COPD patients often have some rales. Infections (pneumonias), cancer, and other forms of lung disease all may produce some fluid in the lungs, but acute heart failure is the most serious and potentially life-threatening problem.

CLINICAL CORRELATION *Give a wheezing patient in acute respiratory distress a brochodilator. Remember, however, that there's no reason a person can't have bronchoconstriction as well as pulmonary edema. (Smoking causes both lung and heart disease.) You may need to treat a patient with furosemide (Lasix, a diuretic) as well as albuterol. Both are relatively benign treatments as long as the patient is hemodynamically stable.*

Pulmonary Embolus

It is not uncommon for people to develop clots in their legs called *deep venous thromboses* (blood clots in the deep veins, typically of the

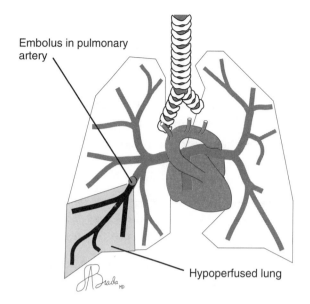

Fig. 3-54. Pulmonary embolus.

calf and thigh). These clots are *not* the superficial, spidery varicose veins that plague many women and are harmless. People prone to getting clots in their veins are smokers, obese people, sedentary people, or people who recently have been sitting still for a long period of time (such as a person who has been riding in a car for hours).

These big blood clots can break off and float downstream. Anything free-floating in the bloodstream that gets stuck somewhere else is called an **embolus**. Blood flows from the femoral vein into the iliac vein (which is bigger than the femoral) into the IVC (which is bigger still) into the right atrium (which has plenty of room) out the right ventricle and into the pulmonary artery. The pulmonary artery, however, gets smaller and smaller. A blood clot traveling this path eventually becomes stuck in the pulmonary circulation, resulting in a **pulmonary embolus**, which can be *instantaneously fatal* if the clot is big enough (Fig. 3-54).

The problem now arises that no blood can get to the lungs. Even if the patient is breathing well, there's no blood for the newly inhaled O_2, and he or she can become rapidly hypoxic (low in O_2). Soon the patient becomes short of breath, has a very low oxygen saturation, and even can go into shock due to failure of the heart to fill and pump out blood (blood can't get past the clot). Notice that there is nothing wrong with the lungs themselves. When you listen to them, they may sound fine, yet the patient will be short of breath.

CLINICAL CORRELATION *The only thing you can do for a pulmonary embolus is give O_2 and move quickly. Be on the alert for it, and don't waste time.*

Blood clots from the legs are the most common reasons for pulmonary emboli but not the only ones; patients with chronic atrial fibrillation are prone to them as well. Because the atria no longer are beating effectively, blood tends to become stagnant and clot. Emboli also can be caused by fat droplets found in bone marrow that can end up in the bloodstream when the bone breaks.

CLINICAL CORRELATION *Anyone with a fracture is at a risk of having a pulmonary embolus, especially older people who slip and break their hips. The riskiest time usually is several hours to days after the event, but remember that some people do not call an ambulance immediately and may have waited several hours or days. Be on the lookout for respiratory distress in patients with fractures or patients who recently had a fracture fixed.*

Another cause of pulmonary emboli is amniotic fluid in women who have just delivered a baby (see Chap. 5).

CLINICAL CORRELATION *Never, never, never reinsert a needle into an IV catheter once it is inside the patient's vein. With one slip you'll shear off the tip of the catheter, and then it's off to the lung. This is about the only way you can hurt (or even kill) someone with bad technique when starting an IV.*

CLINICAL CORRELATION *The medication warfarin (Coumadin) is an anticoagulant used to treat*

patients with clots. Be suspicious of respiratory distress in any patient who takes Coumadin or who fits the description of someone who would be prone to having blood pool and clot in the legs.

The current treatment of choice for pulmonary emboli is intravenous heparin, which stabilizes the clot and prevents further clot formation. Thrombolytics are sometimes used in cases of hemodynamic instability (like shock).

Pulmonary emboli are easily missed—you have to be thinking about them to pick them up. If you don't think about them, however, the patient can wind up in PEA, and then there's little you can do to save the patient.

THE MEDIASTINUM

The mediastinum refers to the space between the two lungs in the chest containing the heart, aorta, SVC and great blood vessels, trachea, esophagus (see Chap. 4), vagus nerve and a variety of other nerves, and *thymus* gland, home of some of the lymphocytes (a type of white blood cell). The thymus is thought to help the immune system learn what belongs in the body and what should be fought off. The mediastinum also contains a wide variety of lymph nodes (which are often full of cancer in patients who smoke).

The mediastinum is of importance to an emergency medical technician or paramedic only when it is forced to move. Specifically, a tension pneumothorax (see section on Anatomy of the Respiratory System) can build up pressure on one side of the chest and force the mediastinum to shift to the other side, causing a problem when the IVC coming up through the diaphragm is kinked off. You can check for mediastinal shift by looking for tracheal deviation in the sternal notch.

VOCABULARY LIST

absolute refractory period	part of the refractory period during which the cardiac cells are repolarizing and heart cells are absolutely unready to depolarize (fire) again
accessory muscles of respiration	muscles other than the diaphragm that can assist with breathing, including intercostal muscles, abdominal muscles, and muscles of the neck and back
afterload	the pressure the heart has on its outflowing side
alveoli	small, grapelike clusters at the ends of the bronchial airways in the lungs where gas exchange occurs
anaphylaxis/ anaphylactic shock	a widespread allergic reaction that can cause airway compromise, bronchoconstriction, and vasogenic shock
aneurysms	bulging weak spots in blood vessels, especially the aorta
angina	chest pain usually brought on by exercise caused by insufficient blood supply to the heart muscle
antecubital veins	veins found in the antecubital fossa, or the arm in front of the elbow
aorta	the great blood vessel that carries blood out of the left ventricle to the body
aortic dissection	a condition in which blood flows between the layers of the aortic wall rather than inside the lumen of the aorta
aortic valve	the valve on the outflow tract of the left ventricle leading to the aorta
apex	the point of a cone, top of the lungs
apnea	not breathing at all
arterial blood	blood pumped away from the heart; when not in the lungs, arterial blood has a lot of O_2 and little CO_2
asthma	a lung disease characterized by hyperreactive airways and bronchoconstriction
asystole	absence of any heart contraction or electrical activity; "flatline"
atrial fibrillation (A-fib)	an abnormal tachyarrhythmia in which the atria have lost all electrical coordination; characteristically "irregularly irregular"

atrial flutter (A-flutter)   an abnormal tachyarrhythmia in which the atria rapidly contract in a "fluttering" pattern; characterized by the "sawtooth" pattern on the ECG

atrial tachycardia   an abnormal tachyarrhythmia arising from a site in the atria

atrioventricular node/ junction (AV node/) junction   the secondary pacemaker of the heart and the "gatekeeper" of electrical impulses to the ventricles

automaticity   a characteristic of cardiac cells that allows them each to act as pacemakers

base (of the lungs)   the bottom, or inferior-most part, of the lungs

bigeminy   a cardiac rhythm in which every other beat is a PVC

block   anything that prevents or slows normal cardiac conduction

brachial artery   the major artery that travels down the upper (proximal) arm

bradyarrhythmia   any slow cardiac rhythm

bradycardia   slow heart rate

bundle branch (left/right)   the major divisions of the bundle of His as it leads into the Purkinje fibers

bundle of His   the conduction path leading from the AV node into the Purkinje fibers

capillaries   the smallest blood vessels that connect arteries to veins; where cells exchange molecules such as O_2 and CO_2

capillary refill   the time it takes for capillaries to refill with blood after it has been squeezed out (e.g., by pressing on a fingernail bed)

carbon dioxide (CO_2)   the gas that is the normal waste product of the body's metabolism

cardiac output   how much the heart is able to pump; stroke volume × heart rate

cardiogenic shock   shock due to failure of the heart

cardiovascular system   the circulatory system; includes the heart and blood vessels

carotid arteries   the major arteries arising from the aorta that supply blood to the head and brain

central neurogenic hyperventilation	a breathing pattern of deep, rapid breaths associated with head injuries
chamber	one of the four compartments of the heart; the right and left atria and ventricles
chest wall	includes the rib cage and muscles between the ribs
Cheyne-Stokes respirations	abnormal breathing pattern in which respiratory rate speeds up, slows down, stops, starts again, and so forth.
chordae tendinae	fibrous chords anchoring the flaps of the tricuspid and mitral valves to the papillary muscles
chronic bronchitis	an element of COPD characterized by chronic inflammation and mucus secretion in the bronchi that causes airway obstruction
chronic obstructive pulmonary disease (COPD)	chronic lung disease with elements of emphysema and chronic bronchitis; a disease that obstructs the flow of air in the lungs
chronotropy/ chronotropic	referring to the heart rate
circulatory system	the cardiovascular system; the heart and blood vessels
clavicle	the collarbone; extends from the sternum to the scapula
collateral circulation	blood vessels that develop over time to help the coronary arteries feed the heart muscle
congestive heart failure	a condition in which the heart cannot effectively pump and fluid backs up behind the failing ventricle
contract	the shortening of a muscle (e.g., the lowering of the diaphragm or the beating of the heart)
cor pulmonale	right-sided heart failure secondary to chronic lung disease
coronary arteries	the arteries feeding the heart muscle
crackles	sounds heard when fluid is in the lungs; rales
cyanosis	blue extremities (fingers, lips); a sign that an inadequate O_2 supply is being circulated
depolarize	occurs when a cardiac muscle or conduction cell gets an electrical signal and then "fires" or contracts
diaphragm	the flat, dome-shaped muscle separating the thorax from the abdomen; the principle muscle of respiration
diastole	the relaxation of the heart

diastolic	during diastole
dilate/dilated/dilator	referring to the opening up, or relaxing, of a tube such as a blood vessel or a bronchus
dorsalis pedis	artery found on the back of the foot
ectopic beats	any heartbeat that does not originate from the SA node
ectopy	having a lot of ectopic beats
electrical mechanical dissociation (EMD)	a type of pulseless electrical activity of the heart (PEA)
embolus	any free-floating particle in the blood stream such as a blood clot
emphysema	an element of COPD characterized by irreversible destruction of lung/alveolar tissue
endocardium	the inside layer of the heart muscle
epicardium	the outermost layer of the heart muscle located inside the pericardial sac
escape beats	abnormal beats arising from the junction or ventricles after a long pause
expiration	exhaling, normally a passive process
external jugular vein	superficial neck vein that drains the scalp and face
femoral artery	major artery feeding the leg; can be felt in the groin
first-degree atrioventricular block	mild delay through the AV node; P-R interval lengthened longer than 0.2 seconds
flail chest	two or more ribs broken in two or more places
focus	point of origin. An ectopic focus is an abnormal point of origin for a beat within the heart
heart failure	occurs when the heart muscle can no longer effectively pump
hemothorax	blood in the pleural space
hypertension	high blood pressure
hypertensive	having high blood pressure
hyperventilation	too much ventilation; breathing too much, too rapidly and deeply, thereby reducing the amount of CO_2 in the blood
hypotension	low blood pressure
hypotensive	having low blood pressure

hypovolemia	too little fluid in the body
hypovolemic shock	shock caused by having too little fluid in the body
hypoxia	low O_2 level
hypoxic drive	a condition found in COPD patients in which they breath only in response to low O_2 levels
inferior vena cava (IVC)	the great vein that collects blood from the lower body (except from the gastrointestinal tract)
inotropy/inotropic	how hard the heart is able to beat
inspiration	breathing in; normally accomplished by contraction of the diaphragm
intercostal arteries	arteries found on the bottom of each rib
intercostal retraction	contraction of the muscles of the intercostal space that aids failing respirations
intercostal space	the space between one rib and the rib above or below it; intercostal spaces are numbered by the rib above it (e.g., the second intercostal space is below the second rib)
internal jugular vein	great vein that drains the brain
internodal pathways	conduction pathways between the SA and AV nodes going through the atria
ischemia	inadequate blood flow getting to where it's needed
jugular venous distention (JVD)	engorgement of the jugular veins; a sign of right-sided heart failure
junctional tachycardia	an abnormal tachyarrhythmia arising from the AV junction
Kussmaul respirations	"air hunger"; deep, rapid breathing pattern
left atrium	the chamber of the heart that receives blood from the lungs and passes it onto the left ventricle
left ventricle	the largest chamber of the heart; pumps blood to the body
lungs	the organs of respiration consisting of airways (bronchi, bronchioles) and alveoli
lung sounds	the sound of breathing heard when listening to lungs with a stethoscope
mainstem bronchi (left/right)	the two divisions of the trachea; large airway passages
mediastinum	the space in the chest between the lungs and the contents therein

mitral valve	the valve connecting the left atrium and ventricle
myocardial infarction	"heart attack," death of heart muscle
myocardium	the heart muscle
narrow complex tachycardia	any tachycardia with a narrow QRS complex, required to classify an SVT in the field
negative chronotropic effect	anything that makes the heart beat slower
negative inotropic effect	anything that makes the heart beat less strong
neurogenic shock	type of vasogenic shock caused from cutting the spinal cord that results in widespread vasodilation
open pneumothorax	"sucking chest wound"; air in the pleural space caused by a penetrating (open) wound
orthostatic hypotension	low blood pressure when standing or sitting up
oxygen (O_2)	the gas vital for life; 21% of the atmosphere
oxygenated blood	blood with a lot of O_2 in it
oxygen saturation	the percentage of red blood cells carrying O_2; a measure of oxygenation
oxygenation	getting O_2 into the blood; the measure of how much O_2 is in the blood
papillary muscles	the muscles inside the heart that keep the tricuspid and mitral valves closed during systole
paradoxical movement of the abdomen	"see-sawing" motion of the chest and abdomen accompanying respirations that occur when abdominal muscles attempt to help with failing respirations
parietal pleura	the outside lining of the lung closer to the chest wall
paroxysmal	sudden onset, as in paroxysmal junctional tachycardia
pedal edema	fluid retained in the feet causing swelling
pericardial tamponade	a life-threatening condition in which the pericardial sac fills with blood and compresses the myocardium
pericardium/ pericardial sac	the fibrous sac surrounding the heart
pitting edema	any swelling (e.g., pedal edema) that leaves behind an impression, or "pit," when a finger is pressed into it

pleurae	the outside linings of the lungs consisting of the visceral and parietal pleurae
pleural space	the potential space between the two pleural layers that can fill with air (pneumothorax) or blood (hemothorax)
pneumothorax	air in the pleural space
portal vein	the great vein that drains from the gastrointestinal tract into the liver
positive chronotropic effect	anything that makes the heart beat faster
positive inotropic effect	anything that makes the heart beat harder
posterior tibial	artery found behind the tibia on the medial side of the ankle
preload	the volume that fills the heart before contraction
premature atrial complex (PAC)	premature beats arising from the atria
premature beats	ectopic beats that occur earlier than expected
premature junctional complex (PJC)	premature beats arising from the AV junction
premature ventricular complex (PVC)	premature beats arising from the ventricles
pulmonary artery	the artery carrying blood from the heart to the lungs
pulmonary edema	fluid in the lungs; usually caused by heart failure
pulmonary embolus	any embolus, such as a blood clot, that was free-floating and becomes lodged in the pulmonary artery system, preventing blood flow to that part of the lung
pulmonary veins	a set of veins that drain the lungs and return oxygenated blood to the left atrium
pulmonic valve	the valve on the outflow of the right ventricle leading to the pulmonary artery
pulse pressure	the difference between systolic and diastolic pressure
pulseless electrical activity	heart activity that produces some form of electrical signal but not a pulse or effective circulation
Purkinje fibers	fibers carrying electrical impulses out into the ventricular heart muscle; the last part of the cardiac conduction system

P wave	the first part of the ECG that corresponds to atrial contraction
QRS complex	the part of the ECG that corresponds to the ventricles contracting
R-on-T pattern	a pattern in which a PVC falls on the preceding beat's T wave
radial artery	major artery of the lower arm/wrist
rales	sounds from the lungs heard when fluid is present in the lungs; crackles
refractory phase/period	period during which a cardiac cell repolarizes
relative refractory period	the part of the refractory period during which heart cells are normally repolarizing/relaxing; during this period heart cells are susceptible to impulses that may cause them to depolarize (fire) prematurely
repolarization	a cell's "recharging" after it has depolarized
respiratory arrest	not breathing at all; failure to ventilate or oxygenate; apnea
respiratory depression	inadequate breathing; failing breathing
respiratory system	everything in the body having to do with breathing, delivering O_2 to the blood, and exhaling wastes such as CO_2
rhonchi	coarse, raspy breathing sounds due to congestion in the bronchi
ribs	bones of the chest; one pair is attached to each thoracic vertebra
right atrium	the chamber of the heart into which venous blood returns and is passed on to the right ventricle
right ventricle	the chamber of the heart that receives blood from the right atrium and pumps it into the lungs
scapula	the shoulder blade
second-degree atrioventricular block (types I and II)	advanced blocks through the AV node where some impulses are not conducted
second intercostal space	below the second rib; the normal point where a needle is placed to decompress a tension pneumothorax
shock	cardiovascular failure; hypoperfusion; a condition in which not enough blood is delivered to vital tissues

sinoatrial node (SA node)	the body's natural pacemaker; sinus node
sinus bradycardia	a rhythm originating from the sinus node at a rate of less than 60 beats per minute
sinus tachycardia	normal variant of sinus rhythm with a rate more than 100 beats per minute
spontaneous pneumothorax	a pneumothorax that forms without warning or obvious injury
status asthmaticus	an unstoppable, life-threatening asthma attack (bronco-constriction)
sternal angle	a palpable ridge on the sternum marking the spot where the second rib attaches to the sternum
sternal notch	the notch at the top, or superior-most part, of the sternum
sternum	breastbone; bone in the front of the chest
stridor	high-pitched inspiratory wheezing from upper airway obstruction
stroke volume	the volume pumped out of the heart in each beat
subclavian artery	a major artery arising from the aorta found below the clavicle that feeds the arm
subcutaneous emphysema	air underneath the skin that can indicate a pneumothorax
sucking chest wound	open pneumothorax
superior vena cava (SVC)	the great vein that collects blood from the arms and upper body
suprasternal retraction	contraction of the neck muscles above the sternum to aid with failing respirations
supraventricular tachycardia (SVT)	an abnormally fast rhythm arising from somewhere above the ventricles (usually a narrow complex tachycardia)
syncope	fainting; psychogenic shock; vasovagal response
systole	the contraction of the heart
systolic	during systole
tachyarrhythmia	any abnormally fast cardiac rhythm
tachycardia	a rapid heart rate

T wave	the part of the ECG that corresponds to relaxation of the ventricles
tachypnea	rapid respiratory rate (not necessarily hyperventilating)
tension pneumothorax	a life-threatening emergency in which air fills the pleural space and collapses a lung, causing a mediastinal shift
third-degree AV block	complete block in the AV node; no electrical communication between the atria and ventricles
thoracic vertebrae	the 12 bones of the spine that make up the chest
thorax	the chest, defined externally by the rib cage and internally by the organs above the diaphragm
thrombus	a blood clot
triangle of auscultation	a point just medial and inferior to the bottom tip of the scapula; the best place to hear the bases of the lungs
tricuspid valve	the valve that connects the right atrium and ventricle
vasogenic shock	shock caused by problems with the vasculature; distributive shock
venous blood	blood returning to the heart; blood from the body (not the lungs) has very little O_2 and a lot of CO_2
ventilation	moving air in and out of the lungs; required to "blow off" the body's CO_2
ventricular fibrillation (V-fib)	a potentially terminal rhythm in which the heart has lost all electrical coordination
ventricular tachycardia (V-tach)	life-threatening tachyarrhythmia arising from the ventricles
visceral pleura	the outside lining of the lung that is closer to the lung itself
Wenkebach block	second-degree AV block type I
wheezes	expiratory lung sounds made from lower airway constriction
wide complex tachycardia	any tachycardia with a wide QRS complex; to be considered V-tach until proven otherwise
Wolff-Parkinson-White syndrome (WPW)	a syndrome caused by a bypass conduction pathway around the AV node; tends to cause tachyarrhythmias
xiphoid	the lower, or inferior-most tip, of the sternum, made of cartilage

SELF-ASSESSMENT QUESTIONS

1. You are called to the aid of a patient who has been shot once in the right side of the chest. An entry wound is seen in the fifth intercostal space, just lateral to the sternal border, but there is no apparent exit wound. What major structures may have been injured, and what care should you anticipate?

2. How can a heart attack lead to shortness of breath and trouble with breathing? Can a heart attack occur without chest pain?

3. Why is morphine effective in the treatment of chest pain with pulmonary edema?

4. When are PVCs worrisome?

5. You are called to the aid of a woman who has reportedly fainted. On arrival, you find a 70-year-old woman, alert but disoriented. She has no difficulty breathing but has a heart rate of 36 beats per minute and a blood pressure of 60/40. Your monitor shows a wide and bizarre QRS complex with a rate corresponding to the pulse. What do you suspect the rhythm is, and what should you do?

6. You are called to a restaurant to the aid of a person who feels "sick." On arrival, you find a 30-year-old woman with an obviously swollen face and neck gasping for air. She has red, circular patchy marks all over her exposed skin and is otherwise pale and swollen. She is in extreme distress, has a respiratory rate of 40 breaths per minute, pulse of 110 beats per minute, and a blood pressure of 100/60. What's going on, and what should you do?

7. You are called to the home of an elderly man with troubled breathing. On arrival, you find a large 60-year-old man with pale, dusky skin. He already is breathing his own O_2 through a nasal cannula at 1 liter per minute. He is responsive to voice but completely disoriented. You hear pronounced wheezes and rhonchi without a stethoscope. He coughs up some green sputum. What's going on, and what should you do?

4

Abdomen, Gastrointestinal System, Kidneys, and Fluids

The **abdomen** is the part of the body inferior to the thorax, or chest (Fig. 4-1). Externally, the abdomen is the region below the ribcage and above the bony pelvis. Internally, the diaphragm separates the abdominal cavity below from the thoracic cavity above (see Chap. 3). You should refer to the abdomen as the "belly," not the "stomach," which is a specific organ within the abdomen. Most of the abdomen is filled with organs that make up the **gastrointestinal** (GI) tract. For reference purposes, divide the abdomen into four major quadrants: right, left, upper, and lower, with the navel (also called the *umbilicus* or "belly button") in the middle.

GASTROINTESTINAL TRACT

The GI system also is called the digestive system and includes the tract food travels through

after we eat it. (*Gastro* means stomach, and intestines are the "guts.") This pathway, known as the GI tract or alimentary canal, is essentially a hollow tube that begins with the mouth and ends with the anus. The digestive system, however, also includes several solid organs, the liver and pancreas, that aid in the digestion of food.

Anatomy

The GI tract starts with the mouth and oropharynx. The main function of these structures is to serve as air passages (see Chap. 2), but they are designed to pass food as well. When a person takes a bite of food, the teeth chew it and saliva is mixed in. Saliva contains digestive enzymes that break down the food. Food is swallowed and passed through the pharynx into the **esophagus**, while the epiglottis prevents food from going down the airway

113

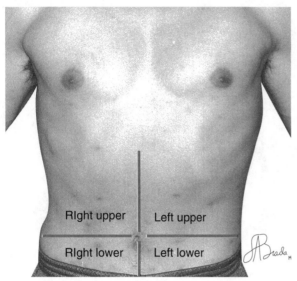

Fig. 4-1. The abdomen divided into four quadrants.

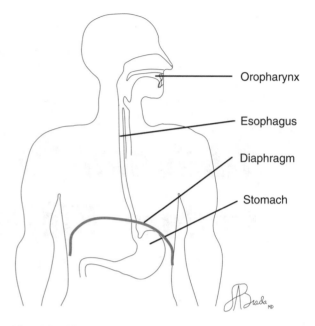

Fig. 4-2. The upper gastrointestinal tract.

(Fig. 4-2). Once food has reached the lower esophagus, it is carried along by *peristalsis*, the involuntary contraction of smooth muscle lining the GI tract. In other words, food is pushed along through the GI tract automatically.

The esophagus runs behind the trachea and empties into the **stomach**, which is below the diaphragm just below the heart and usually underneath the ribs on the left side. Inside the stomach, food is digested further by acid and enzymes.

CLINICAL CORRELATION *Fluids such as stomach contents can be aspirated into the lungs, a potentially fatal event. Acid from the stomach causes tremendous damage to the lungs. The airway should be properly maintained at all costs to prevent aspiration (see Chap. 2). Keep a patient on his or her side if necessary, always have suction ready in case the patient vomits, and intubate if necessary.*

CLINICAL CORRELATION *An esophageal obturator airway (EOA) is a large tube with a balloon on one end that can be passed into the esophagus. Inflating the balloon plugs the esophagus, preventing the contents of the stomach from being regurgitated and thus reducing the risk of aspiration. An EOA, however, should not be*

considered a reliable airway maintenance device and should be used only temporarily until endotracheal intubation is possible. EOAs are highly controversial and potentially dangerous, with risks including intubation of the trachea, trauma to the esophagus and pharynx, and decreased ability to ventilate and oxygenate. Intubate, intubate, intubate!

CLINICAL CORRELATION *Gastric tubes are small tubes designed to be passed into the stomach to suck out its contents; they may be passed through the nose (nasogastric) or the mouth (orogastric). Gastric tubes are invaluable when treating a patient who has overdosed or eaten something toxic. It is often safer to pass a nasogastric tube and suction out a stomach than it is to induce vomiting because there is less risk of aspiration with gastric tubes. When placing any tube into the esophagus or stomach, it is absolutely critical to make sure the tube is in the stomach and not the lungs! Before suctioning, inject air into the tube and listen for it over the stomach with the stethoscope.*

A *hiatal hernia* occurs when part of the stomach slides up through the diaphragm. (*Hiatus* means hole, as in the hole in the diaphragm that the esophagus passes through; *hernia* means guts poking into places they shouldn't.) Hiatal hernias are not something you need to worry about.

Food leaves the stomach and enters the **small intestine**, or **bowel**, where most of the body's digestion takes place. The first part of the small intestine is called the *duodenum*; the second, the *jejunum*; and the third, the *ileum*. If stretched out, the small intestine can be up to 6 meters (20 feet) in length. The small intestine does not stretch out, however, because it is all well attached by the *mesentery*, a large membrane holding it in place inside the abdomen. Cutting open a belly does not cause the small intestine to fall out in a 20-foot trail unless the patient has suffered extreme trauma that has torn apart the mesentery.

The muscle wall of the abdomen is lined on the inside by another membrane known as the **peritoneum**, which contains the bowels much in the same manner that the pleura contains the lungs (see Chap. 3).

The small intestine empties into the **large intestine** (or **colon**), found in the right-lower quadrant (Fig. 4-3). The large intestine absorbs water and concentrates what was undigested by the small intestine into feces, or stool. The first part of the colon is called the *cecum*. (The **appendix**, an organ with no known function, is located off the cecum near the end of the small intestine and has a tendency to become infected and rupture.) The cecum is the first part of the *right*, or *ascending*, colon, which crosses the top of the belly as the *transverse* colon. The colon then turns down as the *descending*, or *left*, colon (Fig. 4-4). The *sigmoid* colon follows the descending colon, looping back and forth in the left-lower quadrant. The last part of the GI tract is the **rectum**, which ends in the *anus*, where stool is expelled.

Hence, the GI tract, or alimentary canal, starts with the mouth and pharynx, extends to the esophagus, goes through the diaphragm into the stomach, into the small bowel, around the large intestine, and finally, out the anus.

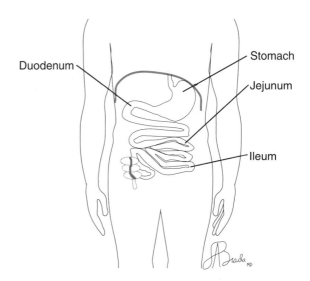

Fig. 4-3. The small intestine.

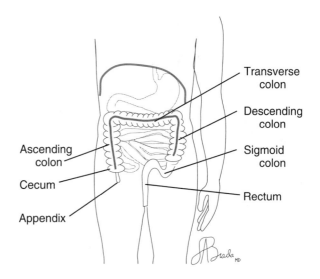

Fig. 4-4. The large intestine and rectum.

Illnesses

GI Bleeds

A **GI bleed** is the most critical medical condition associated with the GI tract. A person can bleed inside the GI tract for a number of reasons. **Esophageal varices** (see next section), which are engorged veins on the inside of the esophagus, can rupture and cause *massive* bleeding.

CLINICAL CORRELATION *Typically, patients with ruptured esophageal varices vomit copious amounts* *of blood, life-threatening from both airway management and blood loss standpoints. Keep a patient with ruptured esophageal varices on his or her side to prevent aspiration. If the patient loses consciousness, intubate and treat for shock before it's too late.*

Patients can bleed in the stomach and duodenum from ulcers, or erosions of the stomach lining or small bowel commonly caused by excess acid and digestive juices from the stomach. Many people have ulcers or erosions, although they are more common in people who both drink alcohol and smoke. Ulcers become life-threatening when they erode through the stomach wall, hit a blood vessel, and bleed. Patients with ruptured ulcers may either vomit blood (*hematemesis*) or pass it along the GI tract, passing blood mixed with stool.

CLINICAL CORRELATION   *Melena, or blood from the stomach that passes out the rectum, is jet black and tarry and has a very distinctive, unforgettable odor. Any black, red, or maroon stool may indicate bleeding from the GI tract.*

Bleeding from the small bowel is relatively rare; bleeding from the colon, however, is common. Abnormal blood vessels (arteriovenous malformations) in the colon wall can rupture and bleed. *Diverticula*, small outpouchings or defects in the colon wall, can bleed as well. Bleeding from the colon may present either as melena or as bright-red blood per rectum (rectal bleeding). Hemorrhoids also can cause rectal bleeding but normally are not life-threatening.

CLINICAL CORRELATION   *GI blood loss is treated in the same manner as any form of blood loss: appropriate management for shock (see Chap. 3) including the Trendelenburg position and intravenous (IV) fluids. You will not be able to stop GI bleeding before the patient arrives at the hospital, so get to a hospital quickly and keep up with the patient's fluid needs.*

Gastroenteritis

Gastroenteritis is inflammation of the GI tract, usually caused by some infection (gastro = stomach, entero = intestines, itis = inflamma-

tion). Gastroenteritis can be as simple as a "stomach flu" or food poisoning. A sick person may experience nausea, vomiting, abdominal pain, cramps, fever, chills, sweats, or diarrhea. You may not think of gastroenteritis as life-threatening, but remember that diarrhea is one of the leading causes of death worldwide (e.g., cholera epidemics) because of dehydration.

Vomiting, diarrhea, and fever all cause fluid loss. In children and the elderly, fluid loss can be serious. Always thoroughly evaluate patients and be prepared to treat for shock from fluid loss (hypovolemia). Remember, a person doesn't have to be bleeding to die from fluid loss.

CLINICAL CORRELATION   *"Illness" is a common 911 dispatch in some communities, especially in underserved urban areas. Always check vital signs and take a good history. Even vomiting or diarrhea can lead to shock in a fragile patient. Watch for signs of shock: altered mental status; rapid heart rate; pale, cool, and clammy skin; poor capillary refill; rapid respiration; and falling blood pressure.*

Acute Abdomen

Acute, or sudden, abdominal pain is a common complaint. "Acute abdomen" sometimes is used incorrectly as a synonym for the symptom of acute abdominal pain; "acute abdomen," however, is not a symptom but a diagnosis of *peritonitis*, or inflammation of the peritoneum, the membrane covering the outside of the bowels. Acute abdominal pain is a symptom only, not a diagnosis.

Any organ in the abdomen or pelvis can cause acute abdominal pain. Correctly diagnosing the cause in the field is nearly impossible and not essential to do. There are many contributors to acute abdominal pain, some of which are life-threatening; however, perhaps the most common culprits of abdominal pain are the appendix in the right-lower quadrant, the gallbladder in the right-upper quadrant, diverticula (in the colon) in the left-lower quadrant, and the pancreas in the left-upper quadrant.

There are a variety of physical signs indicating dangerous abdominal pain, many of which are caused by peritonitis. Indicators of dangerous abdominal pain include intense pain and tenderness, rigidity of the abdominal wall muscles (also known as "involuntary guarding"), bloating or distention of the belly, and "rebound tenderness" (so-called because the pain tends to become worse when you remove your hand from the belly, not when you press down on it). Additionally, normal bowel sounds may be absent. A patient with any of these signs needs a surgical evaluation as quickly as possible.

CLINICAL CORRELATION *A potential problem exists when the belly of someone with abdominal pain or with potential abdominal trauma is rigid, distended, and tender.*

CLINICAL CORRELATION *Use the ABCs to treat a patient with acute abdominal pain. Be prepared, as some causes of abdominal pain also can lead to shock. Movement can greatly worsen some pain, so move patients carefully (but quickly). Pain control with narcotics (such as morphine) generally is contraindicated because the emergency department will need to evaluate the patient's degree of pain.*

Injuries

The GI tract itself is relatively resistant to trauma because the bowels can move about inside the abdomen—that is, they are not fixed in place. It is much more common to injure the solid organs of the abdomen (the liver and spleen) because they are firm and fixed. It is possible, however, to puncture the bowel with penetrating trauma (such as with a knife or gun), a life-threatening injury that may develop the same signs as acute abdomen described above. Additionally, any blood vessels in the abdomen can be torn, causing bleeding inside the belly. This bleeding occurs within the peritoneum and is different from GI bleeding in that blood will not pass through the rectum.

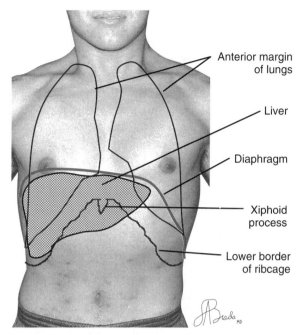

Fig. 4-5. Surface projection of the liver.

CLINICAL CORRELATION *A hard, distended abdomen is the classic sign of internal bleeding. Do not wait for the vital signs of a patient with a distended abdomen to worsen; treat for shock immediately.*

LIVER AND GALLBLADDER

Anatomy and Function

The **liver**, the largest internal organ in the body, sits primarily in the right-upper quadrant, although it does extend to the left (Fig. 4-5). It is a solid organ and highly vascular—that is, it has a lot of blood running through it. The liver is protected mostly by the ribs but is clearly an abdominal organ since it is below the diaphragm.

CLINICAL CORRELATION *Penetrating trauma (shooting and stabbing) to the liver causes a lot of blood loss and can lead to hemorrhagic (hypovolemic) shock and death. Remember that anyone with a penetrating wound to the chest or belly should be considered as having both chest and abdominal trauma.*

The liver, being solid, also is prone to blunt trauma; it can *rupture*, or break apart internally,

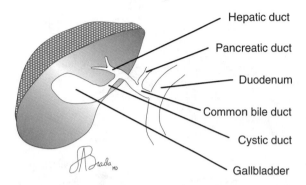

Fig. 4-6. The gallbladder. Found on the inferior surface of the liver, the gallbladder receives bile from the liver via the hepatic duct and delivers it to the duodenum by way of the cystic and common bile ducts.

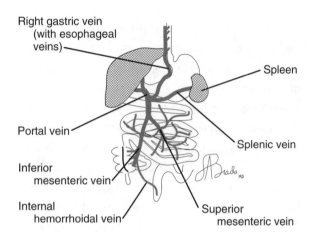

Fig. 4-7. Portal circulation. Though its main job is to accept nutrient-rich food from the intestines, the portal vein also drains the stomach, esophagus, and spleen.

and bleed profusely. The liver can rupture if a person falls from a great height or is struck by a car, even if there is no penetrating injury.

CLINICAL CORRELATION *Trauma patients may have no external evidence of trauma but have massive internal injuries and bleeding. Be suspicious of abdominal trauma, and treat for shock before the belly becomes hard and distended and vital signs begin to worsen.*

One of the liver's many functions is to make *bile*, a yellow-green liquid that helps digest fats. The liver produces bile and drains it into the **gallbladder**, a bag sitting below the liver (Fig. 4-6) whose sole function is to store bile until we eat. When food reaches the duodenum, the gallbladder squeezes and empties bile into the duodenum via a small duct. Bile can work its way back into the stomach, which is why you can vomit bile if you haven't eaten for a while.

Another major function of the liver is to detoxify what we eat. As noted above, most of what we eat, including nutrients as well as toxins and drugs, is absorbed from the small intestine into the veins of the GI tract. Blood in the GI tract passes through the **portal vein** (Fig. 4-7) to the liver, where everything that was absorbed is metabolized. Blood then returns to the blood in the inferior vena cava (IVC), back

to the heart, and to general circulation (see Chap. 3), a phenomenon known as *portal circulation*. Thus, the liver is the major detoxifier of anything bad we eat (which explains why alcoholism can cause liver damage).

CLINICAL CORRELATION *IV drugs almost always work faster than drugs taken orally because oral drugs must pass through the liver prior to circulating through the rest of the body. The liver often changes and inactivates much of a drug taken orally, which is why oral dosages are usually higher than IV dosages.*

The liver also functions as the body's biochemical factory, getting first pick of everything we eat, taking a lot of nutrients, and using them as building blocks for all the molecules the body needs to function.

Illnesses

Liver Disease and Portal Hypertension

The liver can become diseased, resulting in abnormal function; the two major causes of liver disease are alcoholism and infectious hepatitis (hepato = liver, itis = inflammation).

CLINICAL CORRELATION *Hepatitis B is a virus carried in blood and body fluids that is normally* *transmitted by IV drug use and sexual contact, as is the human immunodeficiency virus (HIV). Unlike HIV, however, hepatitis B can be prevented by an immunization.*

Cirrhosis is the end stage of liver disease, at which point the liver has been damaged for so long (commonly by alcohol) that little working liver tissue and mostly scar tissue remains. Scar tissue causes *portal hypertension*, in which blood from the GI tract draining into the liver becomes backed up in the portal vein. Portal hypertension causes back pressure on the blood in the veins that normally drain into the liver. Scar tissue in the liver prevents the blood in these veins from draining, so the veins become engorged (Fig. 4-8), resulting in esophageal varices. Blood from the esophagus normally drains into the liver, but if the liver is scarred, blood backs up in the esophageal veins. As noted above, esophageal varices are prone to tearing, which rapidly can lead to a fatal GI bleed.

A similar mechanism can create internal hemorrhoids (not the painful ones from sitting on cold benches too long). Internal hemorrhoids are varicosities (engorged veins) in the rectum that, like esophageal varices, are prone to bleeding (one type of GI bleeding).

The **spleen** (see section on Pancreas and Spleen) also normally drains blood into the liver even though it is not a digestive organ. Cirrhosis and portal hypertension can result in blood backing up in the spleen, causing it to enlarge. An enlarged spleen is very susceptible to trauma; traumatized spleens bleed profusely.

The liver is also responsible for making clotting factors in the blood. A cirrhotic liver cannot make enough clotting factors, making it more likely bleeding will occur.

CLINICAL CORRELATION *Chronic alcoholic patients are very susceptible to GI bleeding. With little warning, they may find themselves in life-threatening situations.*

Portal hypertension also creates back pressure on the veins draining the intestines, causing fluid to leak out of the blood vessels into

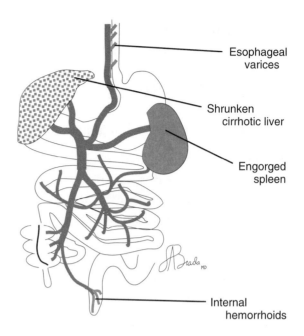

Fig. 4-8. Portal hypertension. Any disorder that reduces blood flow through the portal vein or liver will result in portal hypertension. When this occurs, blood backs up through the contributing veins, causing esophageal varices, splenic enlargement, and internal hemorrhoids.

the peritoneal cavity, a definite sign of advanced liver disease known as *ascites*. The belly can fill with literally liters of fluid (I have seen as much as 20 liters, or more than five gallons!) and become so distended that the skin over it becomes tight. This much distention below the diaphragm can make it mechanically difficult to breathe (the diaphragm can't easily contract), but little can be done for the patient before arriving at the hospital except providing supportive care.

Gallbladder Disease
Although gallbladder disease is rarely immediately life-threatening, it can be painful enough for a person to call an ambulance. The most common problem is *gallstones*. When the gallbladder squeezes, the stones can become stuck, causing a lot of pain. The pain is *classically* in the right-upper quadrant and can radiate to the right shoulder. More commonly, however, the pain is

epigastric (in the middle near the xiphoid), occurring at night between 10 P.M. and 2 A.M.

PANCREAS AND SPLEEN

Anatomy and Function of the Spleen

The spleen, a solid, round organ normally well-protected by the ribs, is a part of the circulatory and immune system that destroys old red blood cells and platelets (see Chap. 3). If the spleen is engorged—for example, from portal hypertension due to cirrhosis of the liver—it may become overactive, causing the patient to lose blood cells and become *anemic*. The patient also loses platelets, meaning he or she is more likely to bleed.

CLINICAL CORRELATION *Chronic alcoholics with advanced liver disease too have additional complications when they bleed. They are usually anemic and therefore have fewer red blood cells in the first place, and they have difficulty stopping bleeding. These patients can go into shock quickly.*

CLINICAL CORRELATION *Any trauma to the left side of the body—either blunt or penetrating—can rupture the spleen. Because the spleen is so high under the ribs, you may not see much on an abdominal exam. A person can bleed to death from a ruptured spleen, so be prepared to treat any patient with trauma on the left side for shock.*

The spleen also serves as the home of many white blood cells that fight infectious germs that may have entered the bloodstream.

CLINICAL CORRELATION *Infections such as mononucleosis (common in teen-agers) cause the spleen to enlarge in response to the increase in activity of the body's immune system. The larger the spleen, the more easily it becomes injured. Even minor bumps can cause a rupture and hemorrhage in a very large spleen.*

Anatomy and Function of the Pancreas

The **pancreas** is located mostly in the center of the belly in the left-upper quadrant with its head

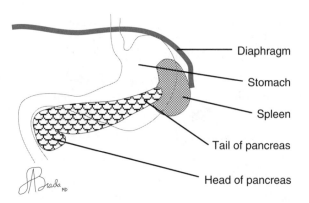

Fig. 4-9. The spleen and pancreas. Lying in close proximity to the stomach, the spleen fights infections and removes old red blood cells from the circulation; the pancreas secretes digestive enzymes and produces insulin.

against the duodenum and its tail against the spleen (Fig. 4-9). (Even though the pancreas rests against the spleen, the two organs have nothing to do with each other.) The pancreas has two major functions: to secrete juices through a duct into the small intestine (the duodenum) that help digest food and to secrete *hormones*, naturally occurring chemicals the body uses to control various functions. Like the gallbladder, the pancreas receives a signal from the GI tracts that food is coming and squirts out digestive juices. The pancreas and gallbladder normally share a common exit into the small bowel.

The pancreas's second major function is regulated by special cells known as the *islets of Langerhans*. These cells secrete hormones into the blood, the most important of which is **insulin**, which helps the body control blood sugar levels.

Illnesses

Pancreatitis

Pancreatitis, or inflammation of the pancreas, usually is caused by one of two common contributors: gallstones, which block the pancreatic duct, or alcohol. The major complication with pancreatitis is that the pancreas begins to

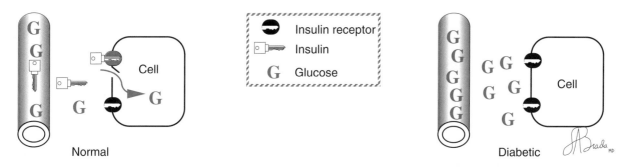

Fig. 4-10. Insulin function. For cells to receive the glucose they need as fuel, insulin (the key) produced by the pancreas must bind to cellular receptors to allow the uptake of glucose from the bloodstream (left). In a diabetic patient who does not produce enough insulin (right), this mechanism fails, and cells burn other fuels as glucose levels accumulate in the blood.

digest itself, causing *a lot of pain*, certainly enough that a person with pancreatitis will call an ambulance. *Hemorrhagic pancreatitis* is the worst case of pancreatitis because the pancreas digests into a blood vessel that then bleeds. Although pancreatitis can be life-threatening, there is nothing specifically you can do for patients except treat for shock with IV fluids.

Diabetes Mellitus

Diabetes mellitus (or just diabetes), is a common problem of sugar regulation in the body. Much of the food we eat is sugar (starch, breads, etc. are mostly complex sugars). When sugar is absorbed from the GI tract into the bloodstream, the islet cells in the pancreas secrete insulin, whose function is to unlock the body's cells to allow sugar in (Fig. 4-10). Without insulin, sugar cannot get into most cells. Every cell needs sugar to survive.

In *type I* diabetes, the body destroys all of its own islet cells so the pancreas no longer can make insulin. Because type I diabetes usually develops during youth, it commonly is called *juvenile diabetes*. Because patients with type I diabetes also are absolutely dependent on insulin injections for their survival, it also is called *insulin-dependent diabetes*. (Both terms are misleading, however, because type I diabetes can develop during adulthood, and type

II diabetics, although not insulin-dependent, often take insulin as well.)

Type II diabetes, or adult-onset diabetes, commonly develops in middle-aged, overweight adults. The body may produce less insulin, and the body's cells can be resistant to it (the insulin does not work as well). This type of diabetes occurs gradually and often is controlled by diet alone, which is why it also is called *non-insulin-dependent diabetes* (a deceiving term because some type II diabetics require large doses of insulin, as their bodies are resistant).

When the body does not have any insulin (or not enough working insulin), sugar cannot get into cells. Blood sugar, called **glucose**, becomes stuck in the bloodstream, leading to high levels of blood sugar, or **hyperglycemia** (hyper = high, glyc = sugar, emia = blood). The major immediate complication of hyperglycemia is that blood becomes overly concentrated with sugar. To reduce sugar concentration, the bloodstream pulls water into it from the rest of the body. Thus, the body "waters down" blood, similar to watering down a drink so that it is not as strong. The body then clears the extra water (and some sugar with it) through the urine, known as **osmotic diuresis** (see section on Kidneys and Fluids). Thus, a patient who is hyperglycemic from uncontrolled diabetes loses water, resulting in massive dehydration.

CLINICAL CORRELATION *Patients with severe hyperglycemia actually can go into hypovolemic shock due to dehydration. The treatment of choice is IV normal saline.*

Patients with severe hyperglycemia have dry, warm, red skin due to dehydration. The body normally loses heat by sweating (see Chap. 6), but with little water left, a dehydrated body loses heat by vasodilating the skin's blood vessels and radiating heat off.

Normally, cells use sugar (glucose) as fuel. Without insulin, however, they cannot get sugar, in which case, they switch to a backup and begin to run on proteins in the body. Proteins are not as "clean burning" a fuel as sugar, so when the body is forced to use them, waste products called *ketoacids* develop, which smell like acetone, the principle ingredient in nail polish remover (they have a kind of sickly sweet smell).

CLINICAL CORRELATION *Diabetic patients who are hyperglycemic may have fruity, acetone-like breath because their bodies are trying to get rid of ketoacids through the respiratory system. Ketoacids smell different from alcohol, although patients who are stuporous from hyperglycemia may look and act similarly to patients who are stuporous from alcohol.*

Type I diabetics can accumulate enough ketoacids to cause metabolic acidosis (see section on Kidneys and Fluids). Essentially, the body becomes too acidic, a situation commonly referred to as **diabetic ketoacidosis** (DKA). The brain is very sensitive to acid and also can be "sucked dry" to some extent by dehydration in the body; thus, patients with DKA may have altered mental status and eventually become unconscious. (*Diabetic coma* is an older term for hyperglycemia-induced unconsciousness.)

One way the body responds to too much acid is to increase the breathing rate (see Chap. 3), which produces the classic Kussmaul respirations, an attempt by the body to "blow off" carbon dioxide to reduce acidity in the body.

CLINICAL CORRELATION *The signs of hyperglycemia (or its worst form, DKA) are straightforward and related either to dehydration or ketoacids in the body: dry, warm, red skin; rapid heart rate; altered mental status; Kussmaul respirations; and fruity odor. The treatment of choice is IV fluid rehydration.*

The long-term management of patients with diabetes requires the use of insulin. Type I diabetic patients take shots of insulin daily to lower their blood sugar levels and avoid becoming hyperglycemic. Type II diabetics also may take oral medicines that stimulate the body to release more insulin. The net effect of either treatment is to increase insulin levels and lower blood sugar levels.

A blood sugar level that becomes too low, however, creates problems too. **Hypoglycemia,** or low blood sugar, can come on suddenly and be a life-threatening but easily reversible problem. It is caused by having relatively too much insulin; thus, the older term for hypoglycemia is *insulin shock*.

CLINICAL CORRELATION *A common scenario for hypoglycemia is a diabetic patient who took his or her normal morning insulin dose but skipped breakfast or did some extra physical exercise. The patient therefore has too little sugar in the blood for the amount of insulin, and all of the available sugar has been quickly used up.*

The major organ affected by having too low blood sugar levels is the brain, which needs two things to function: oxygen and sugar. Taking too much insulin and not enough food results in inadequate sugar for the brain.

CLINICAL CORRELATION *The major sign of hypoglycemia is altered mental status, which can occur very rapidly and even lead to seizures.*

The body does its best to combat hypoglycemia by releasing adrenaline (epinephrine). Adrenaline, aside from mimicking sympathetic messengers, also works as a hormone-affecting sugar, having the opposite effect of insulin. It raises the body's blood sugar level by causing the liver to kick out stores of sugar.

CLINICAL CORRELATION *Hypoglycemia always has been called insulin shock because the signs of hypoglycemia are similar to the signs of shock: pale, clammy skin, rapid pulse, rapid breathing, and altered mental status (from not enough sugar). The similarities exist because adrenaline is being poured into the body in both conditions. Keep in mind, however, that insulin shock is not true shock. The treatment of choice is sugar, not fluids.*

CLINICAL CORRELATION *Always check a patient's blood sugar level to make sure he or she is not hypoglycemic. Checking takes merely a finger prick. If you are unsure whether or not your patient is hypoglycemic, give sugar.*

CLINICAL CORRELATION *If a hypoglycemic patient is conscious, have him or her eat; orange juice with extra sugar packets is especially effective. If the patient is losing consciousness, don't risk the airway by giving food or drink; administer IV sugar.*

CLINICAL CORRELATION *The standard IV solution is 50% dextrose (D50) (D-Glucose, or normal blood sugar) in which 50 ml of the solution has 25 g of sugar. Using D50 is like pouring maple syrup into the veins. To avoid damaging veins from the high sugar concentration, infuse D50 slowly in a large vein with normal saline flowing "wide open," which is very important for elderly patients who have poor veins.*

Another hormone that fights the effects of insulin is *glucagon*, which, like adrenaline, causes blood sugar levels to rise. If IV access is not available, it is possible to give intramuscular shots of glucagon.

Hypoglycemia can occur quickly and can be fatal. Most patients have early warning signs and know when a problem is coming. Many patients, however, lose that ability to detect the onset of hypoglycemia over time, so it really sneaks up on them. You may wonder why diabetics keep their blood sugar levels low rather than letting them stay high. It makes hypoglycemia easier to avoid, but the closer to normal diabetics keep their blood sugar levels, the fewer complications they have later in life.

Diabetic patients are prone to a variety of long-term complications, most of which stem from damaged blood vessels, including heart disease (diabetics are more likely to have heart attacks), strokes, peripheral vascular disease (diabetics often have amputations and nerve disease because blood is not adequately circulated to their toes and feet, which end up becoming injured and even dying), kidney disease (diabetics are commonly on dialysis; see the section on Kidneys and Fluids), and eye disease (diabetes is a leading cause of blindness).

CLINICAL CORRELATION *Diabetics occasionally are referred to as "brittle," a term that usually refers to difficulty maintaining normal blood sugar (patients' blood sugar levels are always too high or low). Keep in mind that anyone with a history of diabetes is at higher risk for all sorts of problems, especially cardiovascular disease. Stay alert.*

Diabetes insipidus is very rare and totally unrelated to diabetes mellitus, which is very common. Diabetes insipidus is caused by a malfunction in either the pituitary gland or kidney that causes the body to urinate excessively. (*Diabetes* in Greek means "to run through.") The only thing diabetes insipidus and diabetes mellitus have in common is that both are characterized by frequent urination but for completely different reasons.

KIDNEYS AND FLUIDS

Anatomy and Function

The body has two **kidneys**—one on each side (Fig. 4-11) sitting high in the flanks and protected by the ribs. They are in back and *retroperitoneal*—that is, they sit behind the peritoneum and are not inside the peritoneal cavity as the intestines are. Each kidney is supplied by an artery from the aorta. Blood enters the kidney, where it is filtered, and then returns to the IVC. From fluid taken from filtered blood, the kidneys produce urine, which leaves the kidneys through tubes known as **ureters**.

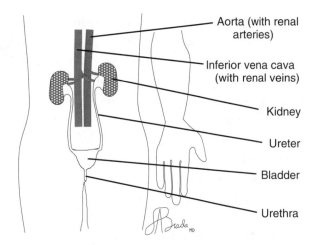

Fig. 4-11. The urinary system.

The ureters travel down the back of the abdomen on each side and enter the **bladder** deep in the pelvis (see Chap. 5).

The major function of the kidney is to regulate the body's fluid, electrolyte, and acid-base status. Electrolytes are the different salts found in the body. Body fluids also normally have a certain amount of acid. The kidneys and lungs work together to regulate the amount of acidity in the body fluids.

Patients who do not have working kidneys survive by *dialysis*, an artificial, mechanical means of replacing the kidneys' normal filtering function. Dialysis usually is accomplished by either filtering blood *inside* the belly (peritoneal dialysis) or more commonly by surgically creating a *shunt* between an artery and vein in the patient's arm. These patients then visit a dialysis center three times a week for *hemodialysis*.

CLINICAL CORRELATION Do not start IVs in shunts. *Shunts are obvious tubes below the skin that feel like one-half inch thick veins. Resist the temptation to put a needle into it, no matter how sick the patient is. The shunt is vital for hemodialysis, and without hemodialysis, the patient may soon die.*

Patients on dialysis can be very sick with a wide variety of health problems associated with the loss of normal kidney function, including metabolic and electrolyte problems, anemia, and bone loss. Kidney failure commonly is caused by the long-term complications of diabetes mellitus, so these patients are often "diabetics on dialysis" ("DD"). Avoid casually giving them fluids or drugs unless necessary to keep them alive, as their problems are far too complex to be managed effectively in the field.

Fluid and Electrolyte Balance

Bodily fluids are either **intracellular** (inside of cells) or **extracellular** (outside of cells). Extracellular fluid is either **intravascular** (fluid inside blood vessels) or **interstitial** (fluid in spaces outside of and between cells but not inside an artery or vein) (Fig. 4-12).

Fig. 4-12. Distribution of total body water.

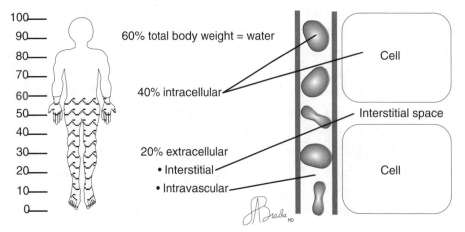

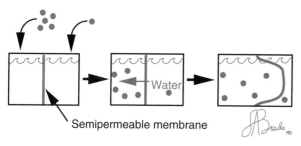

Fig. 4-13. Osmosis. When two compartments having unequal concentrations of particles dissolved in solution are separated by a membrane that allows water to diffuse through it, water will move from the side of lower concentration to the side of higher concentration until both concentrations are equal.

Sixty percent of the body's weight is water—that is, if you weighed 100 pounds, 60 pounds of it is water. Forty percent of the body's total water weight is intracellular; thus, 20% of the body's total water weight is extracellular (interstitial and intravascular).

We have access to the intravascular world, so it is important to think about what we're pouring into someone's veins when we start a bag of IV fluid.

The principal electrolytes in the extracellular space are sodium (Na^+) and chloride (Cl^-). (Sodium chloride [NaCl] is ordinary table salt.) The normal concentration of extracellular NaCl is 0.9 g in 100 ml of water, or 0.9%.

CLINICAL CORRELATION *Normal saline is 0.9% NaCl, salt water that very closely approximates normal extracellular fluid. Other mixtures of saline exist, so pay attention when stocking the ambulance.*

It is important to understand how fluids move in the body. Imagine two tanks of water beside each other connected by a membrane that allows water to pass through it (Fig. 4-13). The membrane may or may not, however, allow particles through. Five particles are put in the left tank and only one in the right. It is a law of nature that since water can pass

between tanks, both tanks will end up with the same concentration.

$$Concentration = \frac{amount}{volume}$$

The left tank is five times more concentrated than the right because it contains five times more particles. To correct that, water will be sucked into the left until the concentrations of both tanks are equal (see Fig. 4-13), a process known as **osmosis**. Simply put, osmosis is a process in which water flows from a less concentrated compartment into a more concentrated one, "watering down the drinks" until water concentration is equal throughout.

Osmotic pressure is the pressure created by particles to suck water into a concentrated compartment. Each particle is actually an individual molecule. **Oncotic pressure** describes osmotic pressure created by molecules of proteins such as albumin or plasma proteins rather than salt molecules. The degree of concentration is termed *osmolarity* or *osmolality*. Describe osmolarity caused by salts using the term *tonicity*.

A fluid more concentrated than normal body fluid is **hypertonic**, a fluid with close to the same concentration is **isotonic**, and a fluid more dilute than normal body fluid is called **hypotonic** (Fig. 4-14). A hypertonic fluid sucks water into it from an isotonic fluid. An isoton-

Fig. 4-14. Fluid tonicity. Solutions with particle concentrations equal to blood are said to be isotonic. Those with fewer particles than blood are hypotonic; those with higher concentrations are hypertonic.

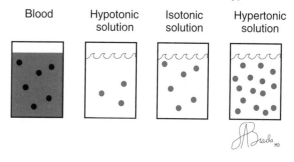

ic solution, being more concentrated than a hypotonic fluid, sucks water in from the hypotonic solution.

Compare the bloodstream and the body's cells. Raise the concentration of blood by adding a lot of sugar, as in a diabetic patient who is hyperglycemic. The kidney normally can reabsorb much of the glucose in blood, but when the concentration of glucose becomes high enough, it will exceed the kidneys' capacity to reabsorb it. The extra glucose in blood increases the blood's concentration, creating osmotic pressure that sucks water into the bloodstream from the cells. When blood volume increases, the kidneys do not tolerate it and remove extra fluid and sugar through urination, an increase of which is called **diuresis.** In this case, an increase in osmotic pressure in the blood started diuresis, which is why hyperglycemia leads to **osmotic diuresis** (Fig. 4-15).

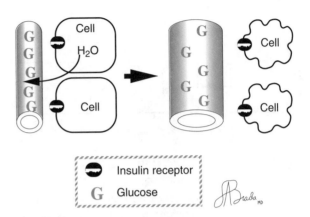

Fig. 4-15. Osmotic pressure. When the osmolarity of blood is higher than that of surrounding tissues (as in the case of diabetic hyperglycemia), water will move from the tissues into the bloodstream until both compartments have the same osmolarity. This produces a contraction of intracellular volume and an expanded intravascular volume (which is removed by the kidneys, a process known as diuresis).

CLINICAL CORRELATION *We artificially can create osmotic diuresis with agents like mannitol, a nonabsorbable sugar, to draw fluid off a swelling brain and reduce intracranial pressure.*

Three IV solutions generally are used in the field: normal saline (0.9% NaCl), lactated Ringer's, and D_5W (5% dextrose in water). Each of these solutions has been formulated to be roughly isotonic to what is normal for the body. As mentioned above, normal saline is just salt and water, the basic fluid composition of all extracellular fluid in the body. Blood, of course, is composed of more than just salt and water (see Chap. 3); it contains cells, proteins, and molecules other than NaCl. Lactated Ringer's, a solution designed to more closely approximate blood, is basically normal saline with a little bit of added potassium (K^+), calcium (Ca^{++}), and lactate (which turns into bicarbonate in the body; see below). D_5W is just sugar water. In a 5% concentration, it can't harm anyone, but remember that glucose will

pass freely into cells as long as insulin is present, leaving behind plain (hypotonic) water in the bloodstream.

CLINICAL CORRELATION *If you need IV access only to administer drugs, use D_5W. For a cardiac arrest resuscitation, use normal saline or D_5W. In any trauma patient or any patient who may have lost blood, use lactated Ringer's. In a dehydrated patient (other than blood loss), use normal saline. When in doubt use, normal saline.*

CLINICAL CORRELATION *Although lactated Ringer's is better for blood loss, you can interchange it with normal saline if you have to. Do not interchange lactated Ringer's for D_5W, however, because once the glucose enters cells, there will be no osmotic pressure to keep the water in the blood vessels. Saline does not readily enter cells, so it does a good job of keeping fluid in blood vessels where it is needed.*

Think about what happens to IV fluid when you give it to patients. Normal saline and lactated Ringer's are called **crystalloids** because they are made of salts, found in nature as crystals. Crystalloids in the intravascular space move freely throughout the extracellular space, which means a crystalloid IV will distribute evenly within the interstitial space. The interstitial space is actually larger than the intravascular space; when you give someone IV crystalloid, it travels both intravascularly and interstitially.

CLINICAL CORRELATION *For blood loss, replace lost volume with a crystalloid in a 3 to 1 ratio (e.g., if you think someone has lost 1 liter of blood, replace it with at least 3 liters of a crystalloid [lactated Ringer's or normal saline] because not all of the IV fluid is going to stay in the veins).*

CLINICAL CORRELATION *If a patient has lost a lot of blood, start large-bore (14- or 16-gauge) IVs (at least two—one on each side if possible) and infuse as much crystalloid as possible. To make fluid infuse faster, either hang the bag high or wrap the IV bag with a blood pressure cuff and inflate it, which pushes the fluid in faster.*

Protein solutions (known as **colloids**), unlike salt solutions, tend to stay mostly in the intravascular space. Colloids are not commonly used before the patient arrives at the hospital because they are very expensive, difficult to store, and of questionable value in the situations paramedics see. *Hypertonic saline* solutions are salt solutions that are much more concentrated than normal saline. Infusing hypertonic saline into the bloodstream causes the bloodstream to suck in water from the intracellular space, therefore keeping blood vessels full. Using hypertonic saline, however, hasn't been shown yet to be any more effective than using a larger volume of normal saline.

There is virtually never a contraindication to starting an IV—that is, putting the catheter in the vein and setting up a drip just to keep the vein open—but there are times when you do *not* want to give a lot of *volume* of fluid, specifically when a person is in heart failure (see Chap. 3) and has pulmonary edema. If the patient's heart is not pumping well and fluid is backing up into the lungs, the last thing you want to do is give more fluid—this can drown the patient!

CLINICAL CORRELATION *Use your stethoscope and listen to the lungs! Don't give a person with rales a lot of fluid; instead, start a small-bore IV of D_5W to keep the vein open so you have a route to give medication.*

CLINICAL CORRELATION *Isolated closed-head injuries can cause brain swelling (see Chap. 2), so don't give the patient large volumes of fluid. Isolated closed-head injuries cause an increase in blood pressure (they don't cause shock), so check blood pressure first. Although giving large amounts of fluid is contraindicated, start a large-bore IV in case the patient has sustained other trauma that eventually may cause shock.*

Don't be afraid to stick a needle in anybody, but don't start pumping in IV fluids without knowing why you're doing it.

Acid-Base Disorders

To some extent, paramedics have the ability to manipulate acid-base disorders in the body. As mentioned, most of the body is water (H_2O). Each molecule of water is made up of two atoms of hydrogen (H) and one of oxygen (O) (Fig. 4-16). It is natural for water molecules to *dissociate*, or separate, into *charged* molecules called *ions*: a hydrogen ion (H^+) and a *hydroxy* ion (OH^-). It is H^+ ion that makes something an acid.

Fig. 4-16. Dissociation of water. In solution, a small proportion of water molecules dissociate into hydrogen ions (acid) and hydroxy ions (base or alkali). The pH scale is a measure of the concentration of hydrogen ions in solution. Lower numbers on the scale indicate the presence of more hydrogen ions (more acidic), whereas higher numbers indicate the presence of less hydrogen (more alkaline).

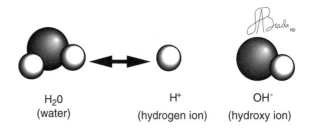

H_2O
(water)

H^+
(hydrogen ion)

OH^-
(hydroxy ion)

Acidity is measured according to the **pH scale**. (*P* stands for potens, meaning "power of," and *H* stands for hydrogen; thus, pH means the power of hydrogen, or how acidic something is.) *The lower the number on the pH scale, the more acidic something is.* The body's normal pH is 7.4, considered *neutral* for the human body. A pH lower than 7.4 is **acidic**; a pH above 7.4 is **alkalotic** (or *basic*). Stomach acid has a pH of about 1—that is, it is very acidic.

The brain needs to be kept at a neutral pH to function well. Recall that patients with diabetes can accumulate acid in their bodies that can cause a coma.

The body is very good at maintaining a neutral pH and accomplishes it in three ways: the buffer system, the respiratory system, and the kidneys. Using the *buffer system*, the quickest mechanism for the body to maintain a neutral pH, the body shifts molecules of H_2O, carbon dioxide (CO_2), and bicarbonate in the bloodstream (Fig. 4-17). A simplified way to look at this is

$$H_2O + \quad CO_2 \quad \Leftrightarrow \quad H^+ + \quad HCO_3^-$$
(water) (carbon dioxide) (acid) (bicarbonate)

The body handles CO_2 through the respiratory system and excess water and other salts/acids/bases through the kidneys; they leave the body in urine. Thus, the body's second and third mechanisms to control acid levels are the respiratory system and the kidneys, the ultimate regulators of acid.

Pouring a lot of acid into the system, as in diabetic ketoacidosis, results in the body's having a lot of extra H^+ and becoming acidotic. Draining a lot of acid out of the system, as in prolonged vomiting during which stomach acid is lost, results in the body's losing H^+ and becoming alkalotic. Holding on to a lot of CO_2 pushes the above equation to the right, resulting in the body's accumulating a lot of H^+

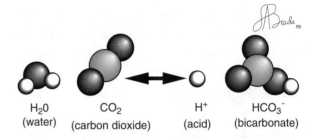

H_2O (water) CO_2 (carbon dioxide) H^+ (acid) HCO_3^- (bicarbonate)

Fig. 4-17. Bicarbonate production. One of the body's buffers against sudden swings in blood pH is bicarbonate (a base). Bicarbonate is made from carbonic acid (not shown), created by dissolving carbon dioxide in water (such as in soda and beer).

and becoming acidotic. "Blowing off," or losing a lot of CO_2, pushes the equation to the left, resulting in the body's losing H^+ and becoming alkalotic.

A person who is too acidotic has an **acidosis**; a person who is too alkalotic has an **alkalosis**. A person with too much or too little acid because of respiratory problems has either **respiratory acidosis** or **respiratory alkalosis**. A person with too much or too little acid in the system for metabolic reasons has **metabolic acidosis** or **metabolic alkalosis**.

CLINICAL CORRELATION *The biggest problem EMS people face is respiratory acidosis. A patient who is not ventilating well either because of an airway problem or some other breathing problem holds onto CO_2, causing him or her to go into respiratory acidosis. Treatment is hyperventilation. Adding oxygen is not enough; you must ventilate the patient well so air moves in and out of the lungs, allowing the body to rid itself of CO_2 and thus acid.*

CLINICAL CORRELATION *Acidosis is a cause of altered mental status, coma, and pulseless electrical activity (PEA). Therefore, anyone in PEA should be intubated and hyperventilated.*

CLINICAL CORRELATION *Anything that causes altered mental status (such as head injuries, strokes, drugs) can lead to respiratory depression, which leads to respiratory acidosis. Respiratory acidosis worsens the brain's function, so make sure that patients with mental status changes not only have enough oxygen but that they ventilate well also. A patient needs to be moving air in and out.*

The body does a great job of compensating for acid-base problems. Consider a patient in DKA. Because the body has no insulin, it cannot burn sugar for fuel and instead burns proteins, which produce acids as by-products. This acid is dumped into the system, causing metabolic acidosis. Refer to the above equation: Too much H^+ in the body drives the equation to the left, reflecting the body's effort to reduce the amount of acid by forming CO_2, which can be blown off by the respiratory system. Forming and blowing off CO_2 is the cause of Kussmaul respirations and is the body's attempt to fight metabolic acidosis.

CLINICAL CORRELATION *You can help a patient fight off metabolic acidosis by ensuring adequate ventilation. Always make sure all patients have clear airways and are breathing!*

In addition to sugar, the body needs oxygen to function normally. Without oxygen, the body switches its metabolism from *aerobic* ("with oxygen") to *anaerobic* ("without oxygen"). Lactic acid is a waste product formed from anaerobic metabolism and makes muscles cramp when the body works too hard (the muscles' oxygen demand is greater than the supply, so they have no choice but to run anaerobically). A person who is not oxygenating well (e.g., drowning) can accumulate lactic acid and develop metabolic acidosis.

Administering bicarbonate, usually in the form of sodium bicarbonate ($NaHCO_3$), is a way to treat metabolic acidosis. In water, $NaHCO_3$ quickly dissociates into Na^+, which floats off, and HCO_3^-, or bicarbonate, which neutralizes acid.

CLINICAL CORRELATION *The time to consider using sodium bicarbonate (or "bicarb") is during cardiac arrest, especially if the patient is in EMD or you suspect a long "down time" in which the patient has not been breathing. Ventilation and oxygenation generally are more important than giving bicarb, however.*

CLINICAL CORRELATION *Although it is true that diabetics in DKA are in metabolic acidosis, you should not treat them with bicarb. Their immediate problems are related to dehydration, so treat that. The metabolic needs of such patients are complex and need to be addressed in the hospital. (Too much bicarb in these patients, for example, can lower their potassium to dangerous levels.)*

Paramedics are expected to assess acid-base problems in the field. Emergency department personnel, however, fall back on a convenient lab test known as an **arterial blood gas** (ABG). Unless you work in an emergency department or do interhospital transfers, you probably will not draw an ABG, but it is useful to understand, especially when it shows up on patient follow-ups or paramedic boards.

An ABG tells you the levels of pH, CO_2, and O_2 in the blood, and oxygen saturation. CO_2 and O_2 are reported as pCO_2 and pO_2 (in this case, "p" stands for pressure because CO_2 and O_2 are actually gasses dissolved in the blood). The bicarb level is calculated from the measured pH and pCO_2 (the three levels are related in a fixed way known as the *Henderson-Hasselbalch equation*; measure any two and the third can be calculated).

On the paramedic boards, you may be given pHs and pCO_2s and asked to figure out whether someone has respiratory versus metabolic acidosis or alkalosis. First look at the pH; 7.4 is normal in the human body. A person with a pH level lower than 7.4 has an acidosis; a person with a pH level greater than 7.4 has an alkalosis.

Next, look at the pCO_2; 40 mm Hg is normal. Not breathing causes the pCO_2 to rise because the body is holding on to extra CO_2. Hyperventilating lowers the pCO_2 because the body is blowing off CO_2. Thus, a person who is acidotic and has a high pCO_2 has a respiratory acidosis from holding on to CO_2. A person who is acidotic and has a low (or normal) pCO_2 has a metabolic acidosis from trying to blow off CO_2.

Table 4-1. Acid-base disorders

Condition	pH	pCO$_2$	Serum bicarbonate
Respiratory acidosis	Down	Up*	Up
Respiratory alkalosis	Up	Down*	Down
Metabolic acidosis	Down	Down	Down*
Metabolic alkalosis	Up	Up	Up*

*Indicates that the primary event, or respiratory problems, are due to changes in pCO$_2$ with a compensation by the bicarbonate level, and that metabolic problems are due to changes in the bicarbonate level with compensation by the pCO$_2$.

A person who is alkalotic and has a low pCO$_2$ has a respiratory alkalosis (this is caused by hyperventilation). A person who is alkalotic but has a normal or high pCO$_2$ has a metabolic alkalosis (this is much more unusual) (Table 4-1). It is possible to have *mixed disorders* with a combination of problems, but those listed here are the basics you should be familiar with.

CLINICAL CORRELATION *The important thing to know in the field is that everyone needs to oxygenate and ventilate well. Also, consider giving bicarb to someone who has not been breathing for a while.*

ADRENALS

The adrenals are glands sitting on top of each kidney (Fig. 4-18) but have nothing to do with kidney function directly. They secrete a variety of hormones, the most important of which is adrenaline, and receive signals from nerve fibers of the sympathetic nervous system (see Chap. 2). When the brain sends out the "fight or flight" signal, the sympathetic nervous system is activated, and the adrenals respond to the signal by pouring adrenaline (epinephrine) into the blood. The adrenals also are responsible for producing steroid hormones such as cortisol, which help stabilize the body's stress response, and other hormones that help the kidneys regulate salt and water balance.

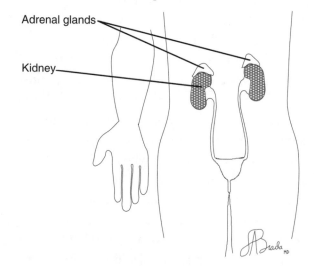

Fig. 4-18. The adrenal glands.

Adrenal glands

Kidney

VOCABULARY LIST

abdomen
: the "belly"; the region between the chest and pelvis defined by the diaphragm above and divided into four quadrants

acidic/acidotic/acidosis
: having too much acid (or H^+)

alkalotic/alkalosis
: having too much base or too little acid

appendix
: organ attached to the large intestine in the right-lower quadrant; has no function

arterial blood gas (ABG)
: a measurement of pH, O_2, and CO_2 in the blood that determines acid-base levels, ventilation, and oxygenation status

aspiration
: inhalation of fluid into the lungs, such as vomit from the stomach

bladder
: the bag in the pelvis that holds urine from the kidneys until it can be voided through the urethra

bowel
: small or large intestine

colloids
: IV protein solutions

colon
: large intestine

crystalloids
: IV salt solutions such as normal saline and lactated Ringer's

diabetes mellitus
: a disease characterized by an absence or defect in insulin function; patients untreated become hyperglycemic

diabetic ketoacidosis (DKA)
: life-threatening condition possible in some diabetics whose blood sugar levels are not well controlled (that is, they are hyperglycemic); patients have metabolic acidosis and usually dehydration; treatment is IV fluid rehydration

diuresis
: stimulated urination (e.g., from a medication or an osmotic load in the blood)

esophageal varices
: engorged veins in the esophagus; common in alcoholics; dangerous cause of GI bleeds

esophagus
: the "throat"; the soft, hollow tube connecting the mouth (oropharynx) to the stomach

extracellular
: outside of cells; a "fluid compartment" that includes interstitial and intravascular fluid; 20% of the body's weight is extracellular water

gallbladder	sac hanging below the liver that holds bile used in the small bowel for digestion; found in right-upper quadrant
gastrointestinal (GI) tract	the digestive pathway including the mouth, esophagus, stomach, and small and large intestines
GI bleed	any bleed into the GI tract; commonly caused by ulcers or esophageal varices
glucose	the form of sugar found in the blood; may be given intravenously (called dextrose or glucose)
hyperglycemia	high blood sugar; usually greater than 200 mg/dl
hypertonic	more concentrated than normal body fluid
hypoglycemia	low blood sugar; usually less than approximately 90 mg/dl
hypotonic	less concentrated than normal body fluid
insulin	hormone secreted by islet cells in the pancreas in order to control the body's blood sugar level; insulin lowers blood sugar levels by opening cells to take in sugar; diabetic patients have a defect in normal insulin function
interstitial	outside of and between cells but not in blood vessels; part of the extracellular fluid compartment
intracellular	within a cell; collectively a fluid compartment; 40% of the body's weight is intracellular water
intravascular	inside a blood vessel (artery of vein); part of the extracellular fluid compartment
isotonic	equally concentrated as normal body fluid
kidneys	paired organs in the flanks whose function is to filter blood; make urine; and regulate the body's fluid, electrolyte, and acid-base status
large intestine/bowel	part of the GI tract from the small intestine out to the rectum and anus
liver	large, solid organ in the right-upper quadrant protected partially by ribs; has numerous metabolic functions and detoxifies whatever is eaten and drunk
metabolic acidosis	acidosis for metabolic reasons such as diabetic ketoacidosis
metabolic alkalosis	alkalosis for metabolic reasons such as prolonged vomiting (loss of stomach acid)

oncotic pressure	osmotic pressure created by proteins
osmosis	the physical property in which a more concentrated fluid compartment sucks in water from a less concentrated compartment until the concentrations are equal
osmotic diuresis	urinary fluid loss due to osmotic pressure in the bloodstream (e.g., from severe hyperglycemia)
osmotic pressure	the pressure created by osmotic forces that pulls water into a concentrated compartment
pancreas	large gland below the stomach; secretes digestive juice into the small intestine; also has islets of Langerhans, which secrete the hormone insulin to control blood sugar levels
peritoneum	the membrane lining the abdominal cavity containing most of the bowels
pH scale	a measure of acidity; the lower the number, the more acid
portal vein	the common vein that drains the GI tract into the liver; backs up with blood if the liver is diseased
respiratory acidosis	acidosis for respiratory reasons; inadequate ventilation and retention of CO_2
respiratory alkalosis	alkalosis for respiratory reasons; hyperventilation (e.g., whether therapeutic or caused by a head injury)
small intestine/bowel	the long section of the GI tract filling the abdomen and connecting the stomach to the large intestine; most digestion and absorption of nutrients takes place here
spleen	solid organ in left-upper quadrant; part of the vascular and immune systems; destroys old red blood cells and fights blood infections
stomach	part of the GI tract below the heart on the left side and under the ribs; mixes food with acid and digestive enzymes
ureter	the tube that drains urine from the kidney into the bladder (one for each kidney)

SELF-ASSESSMENT QUESTIONS

1. You are called to the aid of a patient who has been stabbed in the right-upper quadrant of his abdomen. What are your initial management thoughts, and what anatomical structures are likely to be injured?

2. You are called to the aid of a patient who is vomiting blood. What is your highest priority, what are possible causes of the bloody vomit, and how would you manage this patient?

3. You are called to a community swimming pool to the aid of a teen-age boy who, after diving off of a high dive, feels week and dizzy. He tells you that he recently saw a doctor who told him that he has "mono" (mononucleosis). His vital signs are a pulse of 100; blood pressure of 110/80; respiratory rate of 18; unlabored, clear, and equal breath sounds; and an oxygen saturation of 98% on room air. What are your concerns, and what action should you take?

4. You are called to a shelter to the aid of a homeless man who has insulin-dependent diabetes. On arrival, you find a man who is sleepy, difficult to arouse, breathing very rapidly and deeply, and with markedly dry skin and poor skin turgor. What is probably wrong, and what should you do? Should you give bicarb to this patient?

5. The oral dose of verapamil can be as high as 240 mg, whereas the IV dose is only 5 mg. Why is there such a big difference, and why don't paramedics use many oral drugs?

5

Pelvis and Reproductive System

BONY STRUCTURES

Pelvis means basin in Greek. The **pelvis** in the body is a collection of bones that functionally makes a basin (or bowl) and is made up of three paired bones: the **ilium** (or iliac bones), *ischium*, and **pubic bones** (Fig. 5-1). In the back, the pelvis is joined to the sacrum, giving the pelvis a doughnut shape.

CLINICAL CORRELATION *You can't easily break a doughnut in one place. When the pelvis is broken, it almost always is broken in several places. It takes a great deal of energy to break a pelvis, and all pelvic fractures should be considered life-threatening trauma.*

The pubic bones fuse in the front and are easily palpated in the center below the abdomen. The ischium sits down low and, along with the coccyx, make up the bones we normally sit on. (If you sit on your hands you will feel the right and left ischium). The **iliac crests** can be felt on the sides and are com-

monly called the hips even though they are not the true hips at all (see Chap. 6). What we commonly call the hips are actually the crests of the iliac bones. If you slide your hands down anteriorly, you will reach a bony prominence at the end of the iliac crest, the *anterior superior iliac spine* (ASIS), an important landmark for finding the femoral artery.

CLINICAL CORRELATION *For a conscious choking patient, you easily can position your hands to perform abdominal thrusts by standing behind the patient, sliding your hands along the top of the iliac crests, and making a fist in front of the belly at that level, which should prevent you from being positioned too high and potentially damaging the xiphoid.*

CLINICAL CORRELATION *In all trauma patients, check the pelvis for stability by grasping the iliac crests (one in each hand) when the patient is supine. Press downward (posteriorly) and together (medially). Stop if you feel any instability, an indication of a fractured pelvis. Remember, pelvic fractures are serious injuries.*

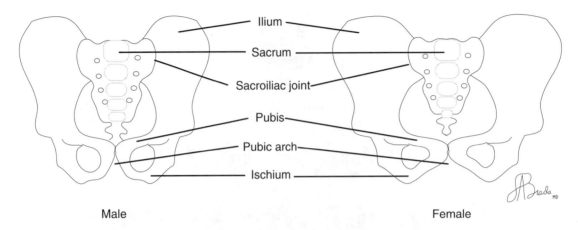

Fig. 5-1. The pelvis. Notice that the three paired bones and the sacrum join to form a ring. The inner ring of the female pelvis is somewhat wider than that of the male to allow for passage of an infant during childbirth.

CLINICAL CORRELATION *To locate the femoral pulse (see Chap. 3), feel for the ASIS (at the front tip of the iliac crest) and the pubis and then draw a line between the two. The femoral artery crosses halfway down along this line (Fig. 5-2).*

Along the lateral side of pelvis is a cup called the **acetabulum**, where the head of the femur forms the hip joint with the pelvis (see Chap. 6).

COMMON ANATOMY

Vasculature

The aorta descends into the abdomen in front of the spine. At about the level of the navel, the aorta splits into the right and left iliac arteries, which travel into the pelvis and split into the internal and external iliac arteries. The external iliac artery leaves the pelvis as the **femoral artery**. The internal iliac artery supplies the contents of the pelvis (e.g., bladder) with blood (Fig. 5-3).

Blood drains from the pelvis through a wide variety of pelvic and iliac veins. Pelvic fractures are prone to cut open pelvic veins, causing bleeding into the pelvis. The pelvis, being a large bowl or basin, can hold a lot of blood.

CLINICAL CORRELATION *A pelvic fracture can cause more than 2 liters of blood loss into the pelvis*

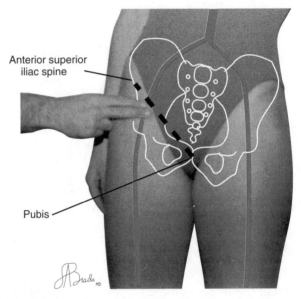

Fig. 5-2. Location of the femoral artery pulse.

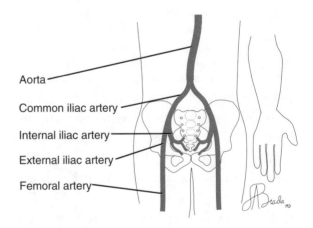

Fig. 5-3. Blood supply to the pelvis.

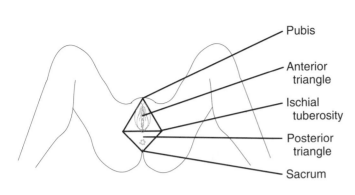
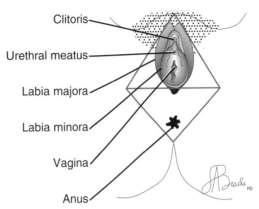

Fig. 5-4. Female external anatomy.

alone, an amount that is enough to cause shock, which is why pelvic fractures can be life-threatening. Unlike external bleeding, which you can see, or intra-abdominal bleeding, which may result in a rigid and distended belly, there is no way to see pelvic bleeding. Suspect pelvic bleeding in any patient who has suffered trauma to the pelvis, abdomen, or thighs and certainly in anyone who has an unstable pelvis.

CLINICAL CORRELATION *Military antishock trousers (MAST), or pneumatic antishock garments, are a good treatment for suspected pelvic fractures because they both stabilize the broken pelvis and may help prevent (or treat) shock.*

Urinary Tract

As previously discussed in Chap. 4, urine from filtered blood is made by the kidneys. The kidneys pass urine through the ureters (one on each side) into the **bladder,** a holding bag in the bottom of the pelvis outside of the peritoneum. It holds urine until it begins to fill up and stretch, at which time it sends a signal to the brain that you need to urinate. At the bottom of the bladder is an exit, the **urethra.** The course of the urethra varies in women and men (see below).

Full bladders and lap belts in cars can lead to bladder trauma (rupture) in automobile accidents. Fortunately, urine in the bladder is sterile, and bladder trauma is not an immediately life-threatening injury unless the person also has pelvic bone trauma and blood loss.

Kidney stones are crystals that can form in the kidneys from the urine. They often do not cause any symptoms but occasionally "pass" down the ureters, into the bladder, and out the urethra. Passing a kidney stone can be extremely painful, but nothing can be done for the patient before arriving at the hospital except transport.

FEMALE ANATOMY AND PHYSIOLOGY

External Anatomy

The **perineum** is a diamond-shaped region with its anterior tip at the pubis, its side tips at the ischia, and its posterior tip at the end of the coccyx. It has an *anterior triangle* and *posterior triangle*. The posterior triangle contains the **anus,** which leads directly to the rectum (the terminal part of the colon and gastrointestinal tract) (see Chap. 4). The anterior triangle contains the external **genitalia,** or reproductive organs. Female genitalia include the **labia major, labia minor,** clitoris, the opening of the **urethra,** and the opening of the **vagina** (Fig. 5-4).

Internal Anatomy

The **ovaries** sit high in the pelvis and low in the abdomen, one on each side. They contain *germ cells,* or *eggs,* as well as supportive cells that

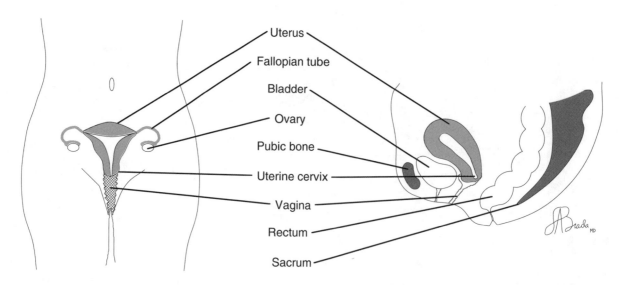

Uterus
Fallopian tube
Bladder
Ovary
Pubic bone
Uterine cervix
Vagina
Rectum
Sacrum

Fig. 5-5. Female internal anatomy.

are responsible for most of the female hormones (estrogens and progesterone). The **fallopian tubes** are hollow tubes extending from the ovaries to the **uterus**, or "womb," a hollow organ made of *smooth muscle* (different from skeletal muscles in that it is not directly under our control but does respond to the autonomic nervous system; see Chap. 2).

The uterus comes down to a "neck," called the **cervix**, which in turn opens into the **vagina**. The vagina is a soft, expandable tube, which at birth is closed partially at the end by a membrane known as the *hymen* located at the opening of the vagina in the perineum (see above). The hymen usually remains intact until a women has sexual intercourse. The part of the uterus farthest away from the opening of the uterus is called the **fundus** (Fig. 5-5).

The **bladder** sits anteriorly to the uterus. As noted, it drains via the urethra, which is very short in women. The urethral opening in the perineum is superior to the vaginal opening because the bladder is in front of the uterus.

Menses

When girls reach puberty, they begin a monthly menstrual cycle (**menses**), or "period," that lasts until they reach menopause (clinically defined as an absence of a menstrual period for at least a year, usually occurring in a woman's early 50s). Roughly every 4 weeks, an egg in one of the ovaries matures in preparation for potential fertilization by a male sperm. While an egg matures, female hormones prepare the lining of the uterus to be ready for the egg in case it is fertilized, causing the lining to become thick and vascular (full of blood).

The ovary ejects the egg when it is mature, and the fallopian tube picks up the egg and carries it to the uterus. If the egg is not fertilized, it is shed through the vagina along with the uterus lining. This monthly bloody discharge makes up a normal "period."

Gynecologic Problems

Lower abdominal and pelvic pain, common reasons for ambulance calls, usually are related to a problem with the gastrointestinal system, the urinary system, or the reproductive system (so-called "gynecologic problems"). Some conditions are life-threatening; many are not. Although pelvic pain can be severe, like abdominal pain (see Chap. 4), it is often impossible and usually unnecessary to determine its exact cause in the field, except for pregnant women (obstetric problems; see below). Again, always use vital signs as a guide.

Urinary tract infections (UTIs), technically called cystitis (inflammation of the bladder), are very common in women. Because a woman's urethra is so short, it is relatively easy for bacteria to work their way up into the bladder. Women with UTIs usually complain of pain and burning with urination. The risk for women with UTIs occurs when they don't seek medical care until after the infection spreads to their kidneys. These woman may face potentially life-threatening septic shock (see Chap. 3).

Pelvic inflammatory disease (PID) is a general term for infections of the reproductive organs: the cervix, uterus, and fallopian tubes. PID indicates sexually transmitted disease, usually *chlamydia* or *gonorrhea*, and is characterized by pelvic pain that becomes worse with motion and often associated with vaginal discharge.

CLINICAL CORRELATION *Patients with PID are at higher risk for having other sexually transmitted diseases such as hepatitis B and the human immunodeficiency virus. Follow universal precautions and protect yourself from any body fluids.*

Ovarian cysts are closed sacs in the ovary that often contain fluid. They can stretch, twist, bleed, or rupture, causing pain. *Endometriosis* is a condition in which the endometrium, the normal inner lining of the uterus, is found outside of the uterus in the pelvis or abdomen. No one knows exactly why this happens, but it can be very painful. *Fibroids* are relatively common benign tumors of the uterus that can be very painful and may cause uterine or vaginal bleeding, which usually is not life-threatening.

CLINICAL CORRELATION *There are many causes of pelvic pain that may lead women to call for help. Pelvic pain can be very intense and often is made worse by motion. Don't make a woman with PID walk any farther than absolutely necessary.*

PREGNANCY

Fertilization and Development

To fertilize the egg, a man's sperm must travel up the vagina, through the cervix, up the uterus, and into the fallopian tubes. Normal fertilization takes place in the fallopian tube. The fertilized egg (now called an *embryo*) then begins to develop as it is passed into the uterus, where it attaches to the uterine lining and sends a signal to the woman's body that she is now pregnant and stops any further menstrual periods as long as the woman remains pregnant.

CLINICAL CORRELATION *All women of child-bearing age (early teens to 50s) should be assumed to be potentially pregnant—whether they know it or not—to protect a second patient you may be treating. As a matter of course, ask any woman of child-bearing age when the start of her last menstrual period (LMP) was. If it was more than 4 weeks ago, strongly suspect that she is pregnant. Ask the patient if it is possible she could be pregnant. Birth control always can fail, and unexpected pregnancy is very common.*

The embryo usually will implant in the fundus of the uterus, where it continues to grow and develop. The time from fertilization to delivery of a baby is called the **gestation period**; in humans, the normal gestation period is 40 weeks (9 months) after which the mother is said to be "at term." Conventionally, the first day of the gestational period starts with the first day of the woman's LMP. With the aid of a nomogram, you can align the LMP with the current date to determine the **estimated gestational age** (EGA) of the baby and the mother's **estimated due date** (EDD), also known as the estimated date of confinement (EDC). Know (roughly) the due date for any pregnant patient and how far along in the pregnancy she is.

Another useful piece of information is the patient's brief obstetric history. **Gravity** (abbreviated G plus a numeral) refers to the number of times a woman has been pregnant; a gravid

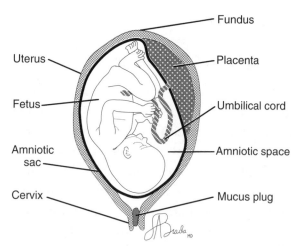

Fig. 5-6. Fetal structures. Within the uterus, the fetus obtains oxygen and nutrients from the placenta via the umbilical cord. The fluid-filled amniotic space protects the fetus from mechanical shock. Measurement of fundal height gives a good estimate of gestational age after about 20 weeks' gestation.

woman is a pregnant woman. **Parity** (abbreviated P plus a numeral) refers to the number of children a woman has delivered. For example, a woman who is pregnant for the first time is G1 P0, whereas a woman pregnant with her seventh child may be G7 P6. A woman who has lost a lot of pregnancies (see section on Abortions) may have a score like G5 P1.

CLINICAL CORRELATION *Women who are G1 P0 (that is, pregnant for the first time) tend to progress through labor very slowly (16 hours on average); multiparous women (e.g., women who have had many children) may progress through labor very quickly. Women who have lost a lot of pregnancies are more prone to having problems with future pregnancies.*

Gestations commonly are divided into three **trimesters**, namely the first, second, and third. During the first trimester, or first 3 months, the developing baby is called an embryo. After the first trimester, it is referred to as a **fetus** until it reaches term and is born.

Several new structures form inside the uterus to help support the fetus, which is contained inside a membrane called the **amniotic sac** filled with **amniotic fluid** (Fig. 5-6). Amniotic fluid is

actually the urine of the fetus (which should be sterile). The fetus is connected to the **placenta,** which sits in the top of the uterus, via the **umbilical cord,** which enters the fetus through the belly wall (after birth, it falls off, leaving the umbilicus, or navel). The placenta and fetus have their own blood separate from the mother's blood. The uterus brings mother's blood, rich with nutrients and oxygen, to the placenta, which then picks up the nutrients and oxygen and delivers them to the baby. Fresh blood is carried from the placenta to the fetus via the **umbilical vein;** old blood from the fetus is carried back to the placenta via two *umbilical arteries* (Fig. 5-7). The incoming blood vessel is called a vein because it returns blood to the fetus's heart, whereas the fetus's heart pumps blood to the placenta through arteries (see Chap. 7).

As pregnancy progresses, the fetus and uterus continue to grow. Uterine height is defined as the distance from the pubic bone over the belly to the top of the fundus and will be about 1 cm for every week of gestation. The mother's navel is approximately 20 cm above the pubic bone. A fundus at the navel represents a 20-week-old fetus, so every centimeter (about a finger's width) higher than the navel is roughly one more week.

CLINICAL CORRELATION *Women in medically underserved areas are often without any prenatal care. Feeling for the fundus to approximate fundal (uterine) height then checking it against the LMP (if known) may help establish whether a woman having pelvic pain is at term and in labor or nowhere near term and miscarrying. Believe it or not, there are women who deliver term babies not having realized they were pregnant.*

As a woman approaches term, her body undergoes numerous changes. Her average weight gain is 25–40 pounds, much of which is water. Her total blood volume increases, but since so much of it is water, she is relatively anemic. Her blood pressure may be lower, she may be prone to orthostatic hypotension (see

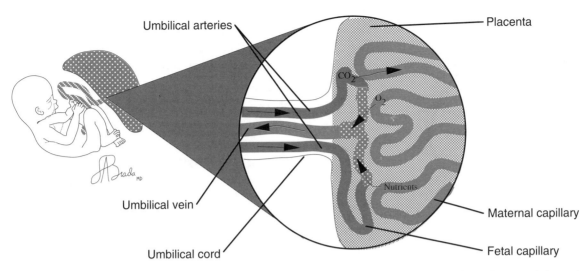

Fig. 5-7. Placental transfer. Blood from the fetal heart travels down the aorta and through one of the paired arteries to the placenta. Here, it exchanges carbon dioxide and wastes for oxygen and nutrients from the maternal bloodstream. Blood then travels back to the fetus via the single umbilical vein, which leads to the inferior vena cava and back to the heart. Remember than many drugs given to or taken by a pregnant patient also may cross the placental barrier and reach the fetus.

Chap. 3), and she may have a slightly rapid pulse. She may be short of breath because the pregnant uterus makes it mechanically difficult for her diaphragm to drop. Therefore, she may breathe more rapidly and shallowly.

CLINICAL CORRELATION *Normal vital signs of a pregnant woman are all consistent with early shock except that pregnant women should not have an altered mental status. Monitor vital signs frequently, and remember that changes in a pregnant woman's vital signs are usually more important than absolute levels.*

In addition to making breathing more difficult, a big uterus also can compress the inferior vena cava (IVC) (see Chap. 3) if the woman lies flat on her back, resulting in **supine hypotension** in which preload decreases (there is a decrease in the return of blood to the heart) and blood pressure falls.

CLINICAL CORRELATION *To keep the pregnant uterus off the IVC and avoid supine hypotension, have pregnant women lie on their left sides. Even a folded blanket under the right hip for elevation, if she cannot lie on her left side, greatly helps blood flow. (One reason cots in the backs of ambulances are on the driver's side is that when you lay patients on their left sides, they will face the crew!)*

When the fetus reaches term, it usually will lie in the uterus with its head down (Fig. 5-8). The fetus's heartbeat can be monitored using a Doppler stethoscope; it usually is very difficult to hear the heartbeat with a normal stethoscope. A normal fetal heartbeat is very rapid (120 beats per minute) and varies (the heartbeat should be irregular).

CLINICAL CORRELATION *A fetal heartbeat that is slow (less than 100 beats per minute), highly regular, or decelerating indicate possible fetal distress. Check the mother's ABCs and treat appropriately.*

CLINICAL CORRELATION *It is common to mistake the mother's heartbeat for the fetal heartbeat. Feel for the mother's pulse at the same time you check fetal pulse to make sure they are different.*

Labor and Delivery

Preparation

Labor is the process of uterine contractions leading up to the delivery of the baby. Before labor can begin, the cervix must mature, or "ripen," in preparation and undergoes two basic changes: **effacement,** in which it shortens

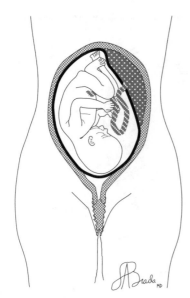

Fig. 5-8. Uterus and fetus at term. Near the end of pregnancy, the uterine fundus is about 20 cm above the navel. As it reaches up into the abdomen and displaces abdominal contents upward toward the diaphragm, it may limit the patient's ability to breathe deeply. Also, the uterus may compress the inferior vena cava if the patient lies flat or on her right side.

in length, thins, and softens, and **dilation**, in which the cervix opening begins to widen (Fig. 5-9). These processes can take place over days to weeks, but in women who have had many children, they usually take considerably less time. Effacement is measured on a relative scale from 0–100%; dilation is measured in centimeters, 10 cm being fully dilated. Effacement and dilation are determined only by an internal pelvic exam.

CLINICAL CORRELATION *It generally is considered inappropriate (and sometimes illegal) for EMS personnel to perform internal pelvic exams. Patients, however, may know how effaced or dilated they are from a recent clinic visit. If they were 100% effaced and 4 cm dilated that morning, delivery may be imminent.*

The cervix also is usually "plugged" with mucus. A woman may report a "bloody show," representing the passage of the mucus plug out the vagina and a possible sign that labor is beginning. Additionally, the amniotic

sac may rupture spontaneously, resulting in an impressive discharge of amniotic fluid, which normally looks like pale urine. This event commonly is referred to as "breaking water" or "breaking the bag of waters." Medical personnel call it a "rupture of membranes."

CLINICAL CORRELATION *Ruptured membranes (amniotic sac) is not necessarily a sign of labor. Membranes can rupture days or weeks before labor actually begins and need not rupture at all until the baby's head is coming out!*

As mentioned, amniotic fluid consists of the urine of the fetus and should be clear or nearly colorless (like clear urine), not foul-smelling, dark, or green. Stool from a fetus is called **meconium**, which is dark yellow-green to black. Fetuses usually do not pass meconium into the amniotic fluid.

CLINICAL CORRELATION *Meconium-stained amniotic fluid may be sign of fetal distress. A light yellow-green color in fluid that is almost watery is called light meconium, which may or may not be a problem. Dark, green-black, thick amniotic fluid is the result of heavy meconium staining. If you see this, support the mother's ABCs and be prepared to resuscitate the infant. Suctioning the baby's airway becomes critical. Get more help, you'll need a lot of hands.*

Stages

Labor is divided into three stages (Table 5-1). The first stage of labor begins with the onset of true labor, marked by uterine contractions, and ends with complete dilation of the cervix to 10 cm. The second stage of labor begins at this point and ends with the delivery of the baby. The third stage of labor lasts from the

Table 5-1. Stages of labor

Onset of contractions ⎫	
Complete dilation ⎬	Stage I
Delivery of the baby	Stage II
Delivery of the placenta	Stage III

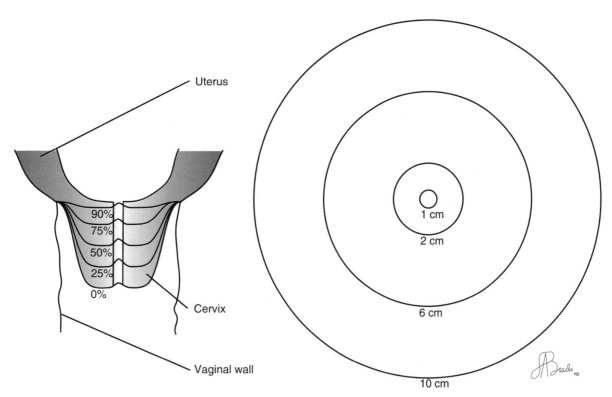

Fig. 5-9. Cervical effacement and dilatation. In order for the baby to deliver, the uterine cervix must both thin out (effacement, shown on the left) and open (dilatation, shown on the right). Here, the two processes are shown separately, though they occur simultaneously in a woman nearing delivery.

delivery of the baby to delivery of the placenta (or "afterbirth").

The first stage can last the longest, ranging from 6 to 18 hours in a first-time mother to as little as 2 hours in a multiparous woman; however, the average length of the first stage of labor is 8 hours. Remember that the uterus is a muscle and therefore has the ability to contract. When the uterus contracts, it becomes firm (something you actually can feel during an abdominal exam). When a woman is in true labor, contractions eventually settle into a pattern, occurring at regular intervals minutes apart.

CLINICAL CORRELATION *"False labor" (Braxton Hicks contractions) refers to contractions that are not associated with cervical dilation and effacement and do not lead to delivery. They are very common in the third trimester and generally not a problem. Braxton Hicks contractions, unlike true labor, do not settle into a sustained patterned. It is sometimes difficult, however, to tell them apart.*

At first, contractions may be brief in duration, mild in intensity, and far apart in frequency. As labor progresses, contractions become longer, more intense (and painful), and closer together, occurring as often as every 2–4 minutes.

Once the cervix has dilated completely to 10 cm, the second stage of labor begins and the baby begins its descent through the birth canal. The baby's trip can be likened to passing through a right-angled 4-inch stove pipe (Fig. 5-10). It is hoped the baby will travel head first, leading with its occiput, a position that allows the baby to squeeze through the smallest possible opening, usually the space between the pubis and the coccyx.

The second stage of labor is usually the most painful. In first-time mothers it may last for hours; in multiparous women, it may last for only *minutes*. As the baby descends into the vagina, its head begins to push against the

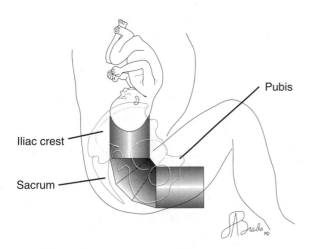

Fig. 5-10. Passage through the birth canal. To make its way from the uterus to the outside world, the infant must pass downward through the ring created by the pelvic bones, make a right-angle turn to pass beneath the pubic arch, and exit the vagina. This process is easiest when the baby descends headfirst.

labia and cause bulging. Shortly thereafter, the head becomes visible, an event called **crowning**. If you can see crowning, you, and not hospital personnel, probably will the be one to deliver the baby.

CLINICAL CORRELATION *The big decision to make when helping a women in labor is whether to stay or go—that is, you must decide whether you have time to get the woman to the hospital or whether you should instead prepare for delivery. The decision is a judgment call based on a variety of criteria: how long it takes to get to the hospital (rural EMS in the winter can be a major issue!), how many children the woman has had, how long she labored with her last child, how long she has been contracting, how far apart contractions are, whether her membranes are intact, and how she looks on exam (whether the baby is crowning).*

CLINICAL CORRELATION *If you decide to stay and deliver a baby, preparation becomes key. Have everything you need ready including extra hands to help (if possible) because you'll suddenly have two patients. Don't forget equipment for a possible resuscitation of the baby as well as equipment for the mother.*

The position of the mother during the second stage of labor is important. Lying flat on

her back, although convenient for the medic, is not a great position for delivery for several reasons: (1) gravity is not helping the mother, (2) the internal muscles of the mother's pelvic floor are in the least relaxed position (have you ever tried to move your bowels lying flat on your back? It involves many of the same muscles), and (3) the mother is more likely to develop supine hypotension. Anatomically and functionally, it is better to have the mother in a semi-sitting or semi-supine position. In parts of the world, women routinely deliver in a *squatting position*, anatomically a great idea.

CLINICAL CORRELATION *Unless women have prepared in advance to deliver in a squatting position, they are likely to think you're nuts. Try having them semi-sit. Be flexible, but avoid having women in labor lie flat on their backs if possible.*

As the baby begins to emerge from the birth canal, mothers naturally push along with the contractions. Encourage them. If the amniotic sac has not broken yet, break it yourself with a sterile, gloved finger. Avoid any sharp instruments. The important thing is to prevent a precipitous delivery—that is, you don't want the baby to deliver too quickly, which makes tearing of the mother's vagina and perineum more likely. Support the baby's head and the perineum below the head (which is the most likely part to tear). Normally, the baby presents face down (Fig. 5-11). After the head delivers, the baby's descent may pause until the next contraction, often holding the baby in place at its shoulders. Take this time to make sure the umbilical cord is not around the baby's neck.

CLINICAL CORRELATION *If the umbilical cord is around the baby's neck, simply slip the cord over its head. If you absolutely must, clamp and cut the cord. Remember, however, that the baby receives its oxygen through the cord until it starts breathing.*

As soon as possible, clear the baby's airway, even if only the head has delivered. It is impor-

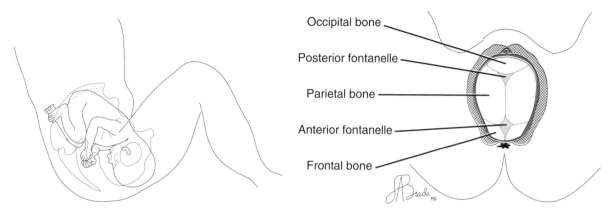

Fig. 5-11. Presentation and crowning. In a normal delivery, the infant presents with its occiput first and face turned toward the mother's back. When the baby is crowning, you can determine its orientation by observing the location of the two fontanelles ("soft spots") at the junctures of the cranial bones. Any presentation that is not occipital with the face down should alert you to the possibility of a complicated delivery.

tant to clear the airway of fluid before the baby's first breath. Use only a bulb syringe; mechanical suction is far too powerful.

CLINICAL CORRELATION *Babies breathe through their noses, not their mouths.* Suction the mouth first, then the nose. *When you suction the nose, you likely will stimulate the baby to start breathing, and if the mouth has not yet been cleared, the baby may aspirate fluid into its lungs (see Chap. 7).*

If the rest of the baby does not deliver promptly after the head, encourage the mother to push again. Don't be afraid to touch the baby! It will need guidance and support. The baby's top shoulder should deliver next, so guide the baby's head *down* to give the shoulder room. Remember that the pubis, or pubic bones, create the tightest spot for the baby to squeeze through. Once the top shoulder clears the pubis, the bottom shoulder follows, so be prepared to guide the baby *up*. Once the shoulders are out, the baby slides out easily with a gush of blood and fluid.

CLINICAL CORRELATION Babies are slippery. *It's very bad form to drop a baby. A good way to make sure you've got a firm grip on the baby is to keep your fingers laced around its ankles.*

Postpartum Management

Postpartum means after the delivery (literally, "after the parting," as in baby-from-mother) and is the third stage of labor, the time between delivery of the baby and delivery of the placenta. Before you worry about the placenta, however, tend to the baby. Remember that at this point there are now two patients.

After suctioning the baby's mouth and nose (again), clamp and cut the umbilical cord. You have some time, so don't rush. The cord is still a conduit of blood between the baby and placenta. Holding the baby too high without clamping the cord can result in the baby's losing blood due to gravity draining blood back to the placenta. Likewise, holding the baby too low can result in the baby's being overloaded with blood.

CLINICAL CORRELATION *Always clamp before you cut, leaving a couple of centimeters of cord on the baby. It can be used for venous access later if there is a problem (see Chap. 7). The cord has no nerves, so the baby will not feel pain.*

Don't be alarmed if the baby doesn't take a breath and start to cry immediately. Dry the baby, as rubbing briskly with clean, soft towels also stimulates the baby to breathe. (Spanking is no longer in vogue.) The best place to put the

Table 5-2. Apgar scoring

	0 points	1 point	2 points
Appearance	Blue, pale	Body pink, extremities blue	Completely pink
Pulse	Absent	Less than 100	Greater than 100
Grimace	None	Grimace	Strong cry
Activity	Floppy, limp	Some motion	Active motion
Respirations	Absent	Slow rate, weak cry	Good effort, strong cry

baby is on its mother's chest if possible. Skin-to-skin contact is good. After a little while, the baby even may attempt to nurse automatically, which is great for the mother because it causes an internal reflex that releases a hormone called *oxytocin*. Oxytocin causes the mother's uterus to contract and stop bleeding.

Evaluate the baby and assign **Apgar** scores that tell how well the baby is doing based on five parameters: *a*ppearance, *p*ulse, *g*rimacing, *a*ctivity, and *r*espirations (Table 5-2). The score ranges from 0 to 10 and is taken 1 minute and 5 minutes after the baby is born. A normal score is usually 7–9 at 1 minute and 9–10 at 5 minutes. Babies do not normally have pink fingers and toes, so it is unusual to get a score of 10.

CLINICAL CORRELATION   *The easiest place to feel a newborn's pulse is at the stump of the umbilical cord; even after the cord is cut, you will be able to feel a pulse there.*

Treat the ABCs for the baby as necessary; however, taking a few moments to determine the Apgar score at 1 and 5 minutes may be very helpful for later care of the baby, especially if there is a problem. Remember that you may be the only one to witness the birth, so pay attention to as much as you can.

Meanwhile, tend to the mother. After the baby is delivered, she has entered the third stage of labor. She's not finished, but the difficult part is complete. It is normal for a woman to pass blood vaginally after delivery and to continue to pass blood until after delivering her placenta. Remember that the placenta is a big, round, bloody sac attached to the inner wall of the uterus.

The uterus continues to contract in the third stage, helping to deliver the placenta and clamp down on bleeding from the inside of the uterus.

CLINICAL CORRELATION   *You can increase the contractions of the uterus by externally massaging the fundus. Nipple stimulation from a suckling baby also causes uterine contraction by increasing the release of the hormone oxytocin. Pitocin, or synthetic oxytocin, brings similar results.*

It can take as long as 30 minutes for the placenta to deliver, but normally it takes less time. You can help deliver the placenta by applying *gentle*, steady traction on the cord. Yanking or pulling hard risks ripping the cord, which makes it more difficult to retrieve the placenta.

CLINICAL CORRELATION   *When applying gentle traction to the cord, keep the pressure downward (posterior) until you see the placenta, then pull upward (anterior)—just as when delivering the baby. The placenta follows the same path. Remember to ask the mother to push hard; the placenta usually comes out easily. Keep the placenta and bring it to the hospital to be inspected for abnormalities. If the placenta is not intact (whole and complete), some of it may remain inside the mother and will have to be removed at the hospital.*

Complications of Pregnancy (Obstetric Problems)

There are a variety of complications associated with pregnancy that can occur from the time of conception until delivery of the placenta, many of which can be life-threatening often because of bleeding. It is important to able to recognize these situations quickly.

Ectopic Pregnancy

As mentioned previously, eggs are fertilized in the fallopian tubes and normally implant in the uterus. The fertilized egg, however, sometimes does not make it into the uterus and instead implants in the tube itself (a "tubal pregnancy") or floats out of the wrong end of the fallopian tube and implants in the abdomen (an "abdominal pregnancy"). The word *ectopic* means something where it doesn't belong; thus, tubal and abdominal pregnancies are known as **ectopic pregnancies**, which cannot go to term (that is, complete gestation). An ectopic pregnancy in the fallopian tube runs the risk of rupturing because the fallopian tube cannot stretch to accommodate the growing embryo.

CLINICAL CORRELATION *A ruptured ectopic pregnancy can be potentially life-threatening. A woman may not know she is pregnant but have sudden lower abdominal or pelvic pain, which can be the first symptom of a lethal event. A rupture can cause internal bleeding possibly leading to shock. Always check vital signs.*

Abortions

Many pregnancies do not make it to term. The medical term **abortion** (commonly called a **miscarriage**) refers to any pregnancy lost before the fetus has had a chance to develop far enough to survive outside the womb. There are several types of abortions: **threatened, spontaneous**, *incomplete*, and **missed**. In a threatened abortion, a woman may experience some vaginal bleeding early in the pregnancy (before 20 weeks' gestation); threatened abortions are relatively common and do not necessarily mean the woman will lose the baby.

A woman loses the pregnancy in a **spontaneous**, or **complete**, **abortion**. Along with bleeding and abdominal cramping, the *products of conception*, which often look like poorly formed bits of tissue but may also look like a small fetus, are expelled from the vagina. An incomplete abortion is an abortion in which all of the products of conception are not fully expelled; a **missed abortion** is an abortion in which the fetus dies but is retained within the uterus. Additionally, women may seek *pregnancy terminations*, also called *elective* or *therapeutic abortions*, which may be performed by a health care provider for medical or other reasons.

CLINICAL CORRELATION *When a woman has a spontaneous abortion, your first responsibility is to ensure that she is hemodynamically stable (there is the potential for significant blood loss). Additionally, recover any expelled tissue (if possible) for examination in the hospital.*

CLINICAL CORRELATION *Any fetus delivered before 22 weeks' gestation has no chance at survival. Consider the fetus as a miscarriage and do not attempt to resuscitate (see Chap. 7).*

Preterm Hemorrhage
(Vaginal Bleeding)

Normally, the fertilized egg attaches to the fundus of the uterus, so the placenta develops on top of the uterus. Occasionally, however, the placenta develops near (or over) the cervix toward the bottom of the uterus, a condition known as **placenta previa** (the placenta is a "preview" of the baby; it is closer to the exit—that is, the cervix). Placenta previas can be classified as *complete*, *partial*, or *marginal* depending on how much of the cervix the placenta covers (Fig. 5-12).

A placenta previa can cause the placenta to bleed spontaneously, which usually happens in the second or third trimester. Bleeding from a placenta previa is *painless* and starts without warning.

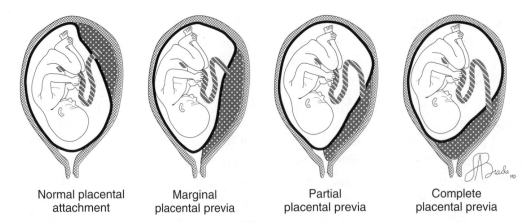

Normal placental attachment | Marginal placental previa | Partial placental previa | Complete placental previa

Fig. 5-12. Placenta previa. Sometimes the placenta attaches to the wall of the uterus too close to the cervix, growing to obstruct all or part of the opening from the uterus into the cervix. This is a common cause of second- and third-trimester bleeding and, though painless, can be quite impressive, as bright red blood is immediately apparent issuing from the vagina.

CLINICAL CORRELATION *Bleeding from a placenta previa can be fatal to both the baby and the mother. Treat for shock, keep the woman tilted toward her left, administer large volumes of IV fluids, and transport rapidly.*

The other cause of major vaginal bleeding during pregnancy is an **abruption,** or *abruptio placenta,* which occurs when the placenta prematurely separates from the uterine wall (Fig. 5-13). Abruptions occur more commonly in the third trimester and often are associated with trauma. All pregnant women who have been in significant accidents should be evaluated even if they do not report any serious injuries. Unlike placenta previas, which are painless, abruptions are usually very painful.

CLINICAL CORRELATION *In trauma, the most common cause of fetal death is death of the mother. Don't focus on the fact that a women is pregnant if she is injured—treat her injuries. In the case of abruption, give as much IV fluid as you can and transport quickly.*

Eclampsia and Preeclampsia
Preeclampsia is a condition of pregnancy characterized by *hypertension*; fluid retention and edema; and kidney, liver, and finally central nervous system abnormalities. It occurs in the second or third trimester of pregnancy,

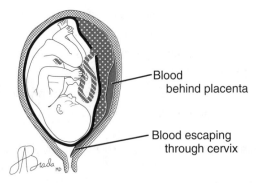

Blood behind placenta

Blood escaping through cervix

Fig. 5-13. Placental abruption. Trauma or other factors can cause part of the placenta to detach from the wall of the uterus. Though there may be significant blood lost, it is often not readily apparent, as partial detachment allows blood to be trapped between the uterine wall and the placenta. This is a common cause of bleeding in the third trimester and usually presents as pain accompanied by the passage of dark, clotted blood from the vagina.

although no one knows its cause. The final stage of preeclampsia is a seizure. Once a patient seizes, she has full-blown **eclampsia.** This condition also is known as *pregnancy-induced hypertension* or *toxemia of pregnancy,* as there may be some toxin in the body that causes it (no one knows for sure).

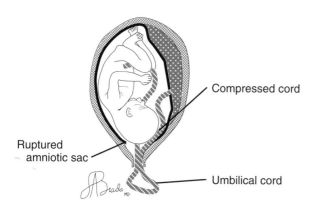

Fig. 5-14. Prolapsed umbilical cord.

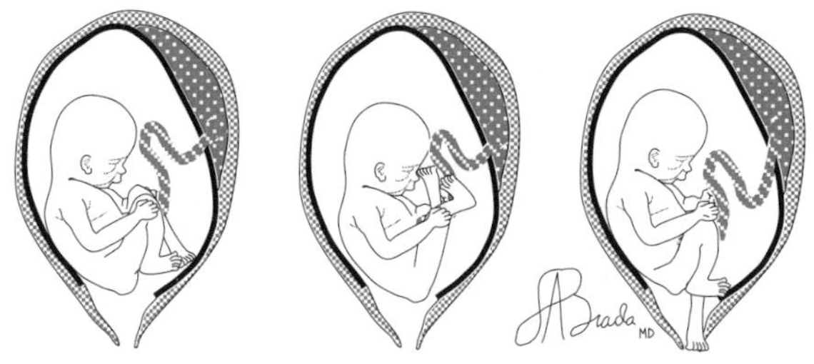

Fig. 5-15. Types of breech presentation.

CLINICAL CORRELATION *High blood pressure is not normal in pregnant women; anything greater than 140/90 should raise your suspicions that she might have preeclampsia. If the patient has mental status changes, treat her with IV magnesium sulfate to prevent a seizure. If a seizure starts, give a benzodiazepine (such as Valium) in addition to the magnesium; however, the only definitive treatment for a patient with eclampsia is delivery of the baby (usually by emergency cesarean section).*

Preterm Labor and Prematurity

At any point during the pregnancy, the mother can begin to deliver the fetus. As noted above, delivery before the fetus is *viable* (able to survive outside of the uterus) is called an abortion. The point at which a fetus becomes viable is somewhere between 23 and 28 weeks' gestation, depending on the mother, the fetus, and the availability of an experienced neonatal resuscitation team and intensive care nursery. (Remember that normal gestation is 40 weeks.) Just because a baby is delivered viable does not mean it's going to grow up and lead a normal life. Nonetheless, you need to be prepared for preterm labors and premature babies.

By 37 weeks' gestation, most fetuses are fully developed and can be delivered without much difficulty. Prior to 37 weeks, it is usually in the best interest of the fetus to delay labor if it begins.

CLINICAL CORRELATION *Terbutaline is a*

beta₂-agonist that is a smooth-muscle relaxant that stops uterine contractions (the uterus is a smooth muscle). It usually is administered subcutaneously. Magnesium sulfate also helps stop the progression of labor.

If labor cannot be stopped, be prepared to deliver a premature baby, whose immediate problem is immaturity of the lungs. Premature babies may be unable to breathe (see Chap. 7).

Complications with Delivery

As if a normal delivery weren't difficult enough, there are a variety of complications that can occur. The first you might see is a **prolapsed umbilical cord**, which comes out of the birth canal before the baby (Fig. 5-14). The problem is that the baby may compress the cord coming down the birth canal. Remember that the umbilical cord is the lifeline of the baby (like the air hose of an old-fashioned deep-sea diving suit); if the cord is pinched off, the baby "suffocates" by not getting enough oxygen.

CLINICAL CORRELATION *You normally should not see the umbilical cord before the baby's head presents. If you see the umbilical cord first, try to remove pressure from the cord by pushing back on the baby's head. Then, drive quickly to the nearest hospital capable of performing a cesarean section.*

Assuming that the baby comes out before the cord, there is still the problem with what direction the baby is lying in the uterus. Normally,

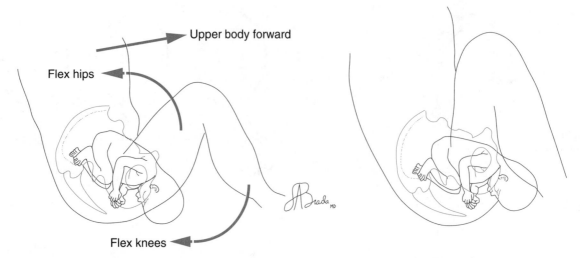

Fig. 5-16. McRobert's position. Placing the mother in McRobert's position (in which she tucks her knees up near her shoulders and basically rolls herself into a ball around her baby) is a good way to overcome shoulder dystocia.

the head presents first. If the baby's foot or bottom comes out first, the baby is **breech**, or has a breech presentation. There are three common types of breech presentations: *complete*, *frank*, and *footling* (Fig. 5-15). If a baby's bottom or foot comes out first, it is best to try to get the mother to a hospital. It is still possible to deliver the baby vaginally, but remember that the head, which is the biggest part, now is coming out last. If push comes to shove (so to speak) and you must deliver a vaginal breech, you may actively need to assist the arms and the head to deliver; they won't come out easily on their own.

CLINICAL CORRELATION *If a baby is delivering breech and the body comes out but the head is stuck, try the following: (1) have the mother push very hard repeatedly, (2) tilt and flex the baby's head and face toward the baby's chest, and (3) pull the baby with the other hand by placing your fingers over the shoulders along the neck.*

If the baby is lying sideways in the uterus, the arm or shoulder may present first.

CLINICAL CORRELATION *If a baby presents with an arm or shoulder, drive quickly to a hospital that can do a cesarean section. This baby cannot be delivered vaginally.*

Normally, the head is the widest part of the baby. Some babies, however, have overly wide shoulders, which is especially common in those with diabetic mothers. The large shoulders may become stuck under the pubis, known as a *shoulder dystocia*. A good way to help overcome shoulder dystocia is to put the mother in *McRobert's position*, with her knees bent and hips forcibly flexed back as far as they can go, to align the birth canal in the best possible position for delivery (Fig. 5-16). Fortunately, shoulder dystocia is fairly uncommon. It happens without warning, however, so you have very little time to react.

CLINICAL CORRELATION *If a baby's head starts to turn* black *because his shoulders are stuck inside, get it out by whatever means necessary. Get a finger inside the birth canal underneath a shoulder and pull. It is not unreasonable for the baby's clavicles to break; they will heal, but if the baby remains halfway in the birth canal, it will die.*

Even in an otherwise normal delivery, some trauma in the birth canal and tearing of the perineum, which can extend from the vagina all the way to the anus in extreme cases, are common.

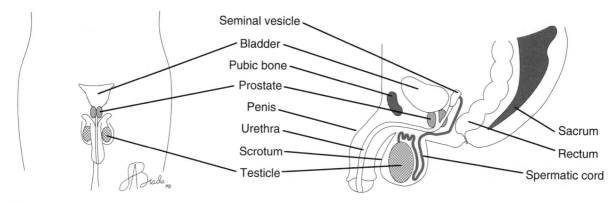

Fig. 5-17. Male external and internal anatomy.

Some physicians advocate *episiotomies* to avoid the jagged tearing, which may allow more room for the baby to come out of the perineum. Episiomoties are performed using some form of anesthesia and have no real place in the field.

CLINICAL CORRELATION *After delivery of the baby, inspect the mother for perineal tearing. In the field, it is best managed with direct pressure and, if necessary, IV fluids for blood loss.*

After the baby and placenta have been delivered, the uterus normally clamps down, contracting in a firm, hard ball, which stops the naturally occurring bleeding from the uterus. Sometimes, especially after prolonged labors, the uterus may not clamp down firmly enough, in which case the uterus continues to bleed and the patient may have a **postpartum hemorrhage.**

CLINICAL CORRELATION *Postpartum bleeding is best controlled by fundal massage, IV pitocin to help the uterus contract, and general treatment for shock, especially IV fluids.*

Another twist on pregnancy is **twins,** or *multiple gestations.* It is hoped the patient will know if she is carrying twins, but she may not. There is nothing particularly different about delivering twins except there's more work to do and more hands needed. One baby delivers, and the second follows usually a few minutes later. Keep track of which baby delivered first and save the placenta; it may be used to tell whether the twins are identical depending on how the different membranes (amniotic sac) are attached.

After delivery, an additional, potentially disastrous complication associated with pregnancy can occur: pulmonary embolism (see Chap. 3). Shortly after delivery, women are susceptible to pulmonary emboli from amniotic fluid that may get into their circulation. Unfortunately, there is nothing that can be done under these circumstances. In the days and weeks following delivery, women also are more prone to pulmonary emboli from blood clots that may form in the veins of their legs.

MALE ANATOMY

Male external genitalia include the **penis** and **testicles** (or **testes**), which are contained in the loose skin sac known as the **scrotum** (Fig. 5-17). The testicles are responsible for the production of *sperm*, which, like a woman's egg, carry genetic information. Other cells in the testicles are responsible for the production of testosterone, the male hormone responsible for muscular development, body hair, male-pattern baldness, and libido.

Sperm leave the testicles through the *spermatic cord* and travel back inside the pelvis, where they are stored in *seminal vesicles.*

underneath the pubis, into and through the body of the penis, and exits through the *meatus* at the tip, or *glans*, of the penis. The glans may be covered with a *foreskin*, but many men have had them removed (usually in infancy) by circumcision.

CLINICAL CORRELATION   *The testicles are fairly mobile. Occasionally, they* twist *within the scrotum, which can happen without warning or trauma. Such twisting is known as a* testicular torsion, *which is extremely painful. Patients with testicular torsion need surgery immediately, or they risk losing a testicle.*

CLINICAL CORRELATION   *The parasympathetic nervous system (see Chap. 2) is responsible for erection of the penis. Certain brain injuries can cause a malfunction of this system, resulting in an uncontrollable, painful erection known as* priapism. *An erection in a trauma patient may be a sign of severe head injury.*

VOCABULARY LIST

abortion	any pregnancy that terminates before the fetus is viable
abruption	separation of the placenta from the uterine wall resulting in painful vaginal bleeding
acetabulum	the cuplike groove of the pelvis where the head of the femur articulates to form the hip joint
amniotic fluid	the fluid inside the amniotic sac; formed from the urine of the fetus
amniotic sac	a fluid-filled sac within the uterus in which the fetus rests
anus	the exit of the GI tract where stool is evacuated; found in the posterior perineum
Apgar	scoring system to rate how well a baby is doing 1 minute and 5 minutes after birth
bladder	an expandable bag in the pelvis that stores urine until it is excreted from the urethra
Braxton Hicks contractions	false labor contractions; common in the third trimester
breech	when a baby descends the birth canal bottom or foot first rather than head first
cervix	the "neck" of the uterus leading into the vagina
complete abortion	a spontaneous loss of pregnancy in which the fetus is expelled from the uterus
crowning	the emergence of the baby's head from the vaginal opening during labor
dilation	the opening up of the cervix in preparation of delivery; complete dilation is 10 cm
eclampsia	the end stage of preeclampsia; seizures occurring in pregnancy
ectopic pregnancy	a pregnancy that develops outside of the uterus, commonly in the fallopian tubes
effacement	the shortening and softening of the cervix in preparation for delivery
estimated due date (EDD)	the approximate date a baby is expected to be delivered; 40 weeks after the LMP

estimated gestational age (EGA)	the approximate age of a developing fetus; the difference between the current date and the first day of the LMP
fallopian tubes	tubes that lead from the ovaries to the uterus in women
femoral artery	a continuation of the iliac artery; a branch of the aorta that supplies blood to the leg
femoral pulse	the pulse made by the femoral artery; found in the groin
fetus	a baby developing in the uterus past the first trimester
fundus	the part of the uterus farthest away from the mouth of the cervix
genitalia	internal and external organs associated with reproduction
gestation period	the time it takes for a fetus to develop from a fertilized egg to delivery; normally 40 weeks
gravity	pregnancy, or number of pregnancies; a gravid woman is a pregnant woman; a woman who is gravida 4 has been pregnant four times
iliac crests	the tips of the iliac bones of the pelvis; easily palpable on the side of the body
ilium	one of the paired bones of the pelvis that form the "waist"
labia major/minor	two skin flaps that protect the vaginal opening; part of the external female genitalia
labor	the process of uterine contractions leading to the delivery of the baby and placenta
last menstrual period (LMP)	the first day of the last menstrual period of a woman; important in determining pregnancy status or the gestational age of the fetus
meconium	the first bowel movement of the baby; if it occurs while the baby is still in the uterus, it will stain the amniotic fluid green-black and is a sign of fetal distress
menses	the monthly "period," or cycle, in women during which the lining of the uterus is shed from the vagina if the woman is not pregnant
miscarriage	common term for abortion

missed abortion	a spontaneous loss of pregnancy in which the fetus remains inside the uterus
parity	delivery of a child, or number of deliveries; a multiparous woman has delivered many children, whereas a "primipara" is on her first delivery
pelvic inflammatory disease (PID)	infection of the reproductive organs in women by sexually transmitted diseases
pelvis	the set of bones that forms a ring or basin housing the bladder and reproductive organs
penis	male external genitalia through which the urethra passes
perineum	the diamond-shaped region in the groin defined by the pubis, ischia, and coccyx; where the external genitalia and anus are located
placenta	the organ that sits on the wall of the uterus pulling oxygen and nutrients from the mother's blood supply and delivering them to the fetus via the umbilical cord
placenta previa	a condition in which the placenta implants at the bottom of the uterus near or over the cervix that results in painless vaginal bleeding; possibly life-threatening to both mother and baby
postpartum	after delivery
postpartum hemorrhage	bleeding following delivery
preeclampsia	toxemia of pregnancy that can lead to uncontrolled high blood pressure and seizures
prolapsed umbilical cord	a condition that is life-threatening to a fetus in which the umbilical cord passes into the birth canal first and therefore can be compressed by the head of the fetus
prostate gland	a gland that sits at the base of the bladder in men; responsible for the secretion of semen
pubic bones	paired bones of the pelvis that form the pubis in front
scrotum	a loose sac of skin containing the testicles in men
spontaneous abortion	spontaneous loss of a pregnancy
supine hypotension	a drop in blood pressure in pregnant women caused by the pregnant uterus compressing the IVC; occurs when pregnant women lie supine

testicles/testes	male reproductive organs contained within the scrotum; responsible for production of sperm and testosterone
threatened abortion	vaginal bleeding early in the pregnancy
trimester	a third of a pregnancy's duration (3 months)
twins	multiple birth
umbilical cord	a cord that connects the fetus with the placenta; contains one vein and two arteries; it falls off after birth, becoming the navel
umbilical vein	the major vein of the umbilical cord that carries blood into the fetus
urethra	a tube coming from the bladder that allows urine to exit the body
urinary tract infection (UTI)	a bacterial infection of the bladder; common in women; it becomes serious only if the infection spreads to the kidneys or the bloodstream
uterus	the "womb" in women; a hollow organ made of smooth muscle that houses the fetus during pregnancy
vagina	the birth canal; an expandable passageway between the uterus and the outside world

SELF-ASSESSMENT QUESTIONS

1. A loading dock worker has been caught at his hips between a truck bumper and a dock. You arrive just as he is being freed. What injuries should you anticipate, and how would you treat them?

2. You are called to the aid of a woman complaining of abdominal pain. What are some important questions you need to ask, and what are your treatment concerns as a paramedic?

3. You are called to the aid of a woman in her third trimester who has been involved in an automobile accident. What considerations should you keep in mind because she is pregnant?

4. After you assist in the delivery of a baby, you have difficulty palpating the mother's uterus and notice that she continues to bleed vaginally. What do you suspect, and what can you do?

5. You are called to the aid of a man complaining of pain and swelling in his scrotum. Could this be a life-threatening emergency?

6

The Musculoskeletal System, Extremities, and Skin

MUSCULOSKELETAL SYSTEM

Skeleton

There are 206 bones in the body, well over half of which are in the hands and feet. The skeleton is depicted in Fig. 6-1, which summarizes the major bones. Table 6-1 is a list of the major bones. The primary function of bone is to provide structure and support for the body. Bones are strong in part because they contain hardened calcium; however, they are full of living, active cells that continually renew and restore the hard bone (which is why bones can heal after they break). As we age, we tend to lose calcium from our bones, making them brittle and more easily broken, a process known as *osteoporosis*. In women, the hormone *estrogen* tends to protect bones from osteoporosis; however, some women may be at increased risk for brittle bones after menopause (when

women's ovaries stop producing estrogen, usually at about age 50) if they are not taking estrogen replacement therapy.

CLINICAL CORRELATION *Thin, older men and women who have never taken hormone replacement therapy are at very high risk for breaking bones, even from minor trauma such as a fall.*

In addition to providing structure, bones also produce blood cells. The middle of most bones contains *marrow*, a relatively soft part of the bone that is full of blood. In fact, blood is made in the marrow. A red blood cell's life begins in the bone marrow and ends in the spleen. In children, bone marrow may serve as a site for gaining access to the bloodstream (similar to starting an intravenous line [IV]; see Chap. 7).

The end of *long bones*, such as the bones of the arms and legs, is called the *epiphysis*, where growth takes place in children. The epiphysis

159

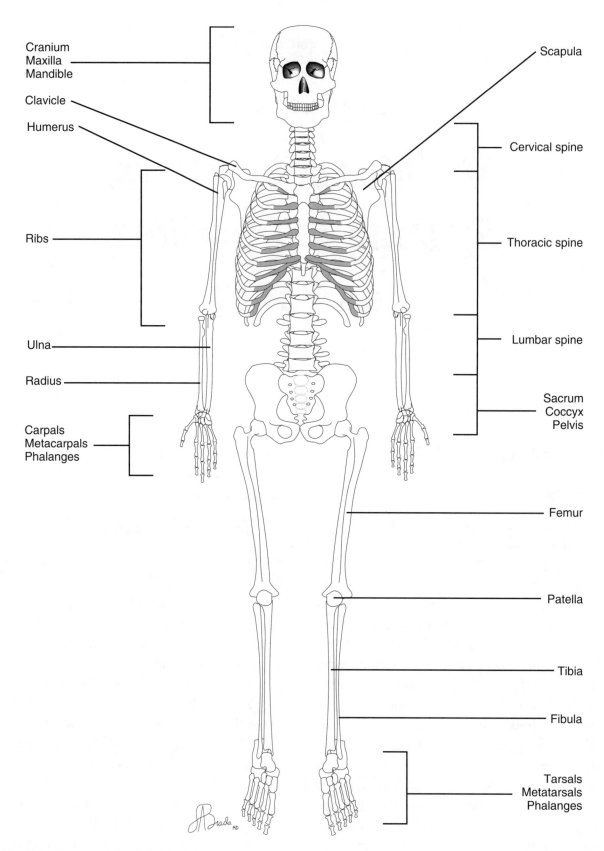

Cranium
Maxilla
Mandible

Clavicle

Humerus

Ribs

Ulna

Radius

Carpals
Metacarpals
Phalanges

Scapula

Cervical spine

Thoracic spine

Lumbar spine

Sacrum
Coccyx
Pelvis

Femur

Patella

Tibia

Fibula

Tarsals
Metatarsals
Phalanges

Fig. 6-1. The complete skeletal system.

Table 6-1. Major bones of the body

Head	Axial skeleton	Upper extremity	Lower extremity
Cranium	Vertebrae	Shoulder girdle	Pelvis
Frontal	Cervical	Scapula	Leg
Parietal	Thoracic	Clavicle	Femur
Temporal	Lumbar	Arm	Patella
Occipital	Sacral	Humerus	Tibia
Face	Coccyx	Radius	Fibula
Maxilla	Ribs	Ulna	Ankle and foot
Mandible	Sternum	Wrist/hand	Tarsals
		Carpals	Metatarsals
		Metacarpals	Phalanges
		Phalanges	

forms a *growth plate*, or epiphyseal plate, where new bone is made and lengthens the existing bone. Capping off most bones is **cartilage**, the soft "gristle" that allows for smooth contact between two bones.

The meeting of bones is called a **joint**, some of which, such as the elbow and shoulder, are designed to allow a wide range of motion (see Chap. 1). Others joints, such as between a rib and the sternum, are designed to allow only a small range of motion. In an *articulating*, or movable, joint such as the shoulder, joint space is called the *synovial cavity*, which is filled with a very slick fluid (synovial fluid) that allows bone ends to slide smoothly. Breakdown and inflammation of the joints is known as *arthritis*.

Muscles and Connective Tissue

There are three types of muscle in the body: skeletal, cardiac, and smooth muscle (Table 6-2). Cardiac and smooth muscle are not under voluntary control and often respond to stimulation by the autonomic nervous system (see Chap. 2). Skeletal muscle, also called *striated muscle* (because of its lined appearance under a microscope), is under our conscious control.

The rest of this chapter discusses skeletal muscle.

Muscles contract, or shorten; it is the only thing they can do. One end of the muscle pulls toward the other, much like a stretched rubber band. They cannot "push." You can push something with a muscle about as well as you can push something with a rubber band. Muscles are also linear—that is, they lie in lines, the ends of which are connected to a bone. Muscle crosses joints, so when the muscle shortens, it moves its two ends (or two bones) closer together, bending the joint. This is how we move about.

The brain sends signals to the muscles signals via the spinal cord, or in the case of the muscles of the head and face, through the brain stem. Every muscle is supplied by a nerve, as well as an artery and vein to supply it with blood.

CLINICAL CORRELATION *Paralysis is the inability to voluntarily move a muscle or group of muscles. Spinal cord injuries may cause paralysis below the site of the injury because the connection between the brain and muscle has been severed.*

Tendons connect muscle to bone. **Ligaments** connect bone to bone across joints. Tendons

Table 6-2. Muscle types

Type	Location	Characteristic
Skeletal	On bones	Under voluntary control
Cardiac	Heart	Contract automatically, influenced to contract harder/faster by sympathetic beta$_1$ stimulation*
Smooth	Bronchial walls Blood vessel walls Bladder, uterus	Not under voluntary control, will relax with sympathetic beta$_2$ stimulation, contract with cholinergic or sympathetic alpha stimulation*

* See discussion of autonomic nervous system in Chaps. 2 and 3.

and ligaments are structurally similar and may be referred to as connective tissue. Sacs of fluid known as *bursas* protect much of the connective tissue from irritation from the moving bones. Injuries caused by forceful or repetitive motion can lead to inflammation of tendons or bursas (tendonitis, bursitis). Joints, therefore, are fairly complex and have many components: bones, cartilage, synovial fluid, tendons, ligaments, and bursas (Fig. 6-2).

Injuries

Fractures

A **fracture** is the breaking of bone. In the field, it is important to make a distinction between suspected fractures with intact skin, called **closed** or **simple** fractures, and suspected fractures with broken skin, called **open** or **compound** fractures (Fig. 6-3). (It's possible to see bone sticking out of open wounds.) Compound fractures are worse than simple fractures for several reasons. First, it usually takes more energy to cause a compound fracture than a simple fracture; therefore, a compound fracture may represent more serious trauma, and the patient may be suffering from more extensive injuries elsewhere. Second, compound fractures are more likely to cause sig-

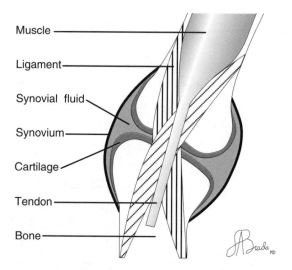

Fig. 6-2. Synovial joint. The typical mobile joint is composed of two bones with cartilage on the ends, a synovial membrane containing synovial fluid for lubrication, tendons that connect muscle to bone, and ligaments running between bones.

nificant bleeding because the broken bone causes more damage to the surrounding soft tissue. Third, broken bone ends that have moved significantly may cut nerves and blood vessels to the distal extremity, which can jeopardize the entire limb (assuming the fracture occurs in a limb). Finally, open fractures set the scene for infections that can cause tremendous complications, including loss of the limb or even death.

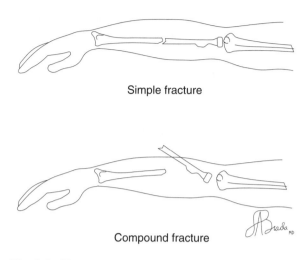

Fig. 6-3. Simple and compound fractures.

CLINICAL CORRELATION *Cover open fractures with sterile gauze moistened with sterile saline to help reduce the risk of infection later.*

A bone actually can break in a variety of ways. The classic types of fractures are *transverse*, *oblique*, *comminuted*, *impacted*, *spiral*, and *greenstick*, which are classified depending on the *mechanism of injury*—that is, how the bone was injured (Fig. 6-4). A transverse fracture occurs when bone is hit from the side—for example, a "night stick" fracture of the forearm where the patient blocked a night stick blow with the forearm, resulting in a transverse break of the ulna. Oblique fractures are similar to transverse fractures except that the fracture line is diagonal across the bone. Both oblique and transverse fractures are common in blunt trauma. A comminuted fracture occurs when a bone is shattered into multiple pieces, such as from gunshot wounds. An impacted fracture occurs when two broken bone ends are driven into each other and commonly occurs when patients fall from a height and land on their feet. (The bones of the leg break and impact.) Spiral fractures occur when twisting is involved in the injury—for example, a fracture that occurs when a skier's bindings do not release during a fall and the leg rotates

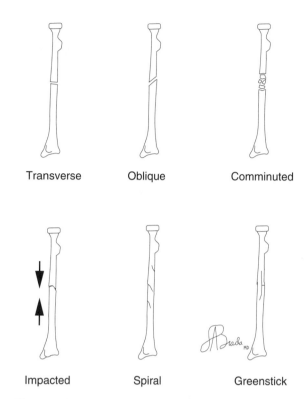

Fig. 6-4. Types of fractures.

too far (or once too many times around). Greenstick fractures occur when a bone breaks like a green tree branch—the bone does not break all the way through. Greenstick fractures occur when bones are very flexible and almost always are seen in children, as adult bones become more and more brittle with age.

CLINICAL CORRELATION *Open fractures are usually obvious, whereas closed fractures may be more subtle. Suspect a fracture whenever the mechanism of injury could cause a fracture (virtually always). A broken bone causes pain, tenderness, swelling, discoloration (from bruising and bleeding), possible deformation, loss of function, and possibly crepitus, or crepitance (the feeling of broken bone ends grating against each other).*

Whenever you suspect someone may have a fracture, your immediate concerns are the ABCs (see Chaps. 2 and 3). Assuming you have the luxury of time, there are several things you should consider with fractures. First, fractures bleed. Even if the fracture site is closed, fractures can cause considerable internal blood loss, which can be due to blood vessels being cut by a broken bone, from internal laceration of the soft tissue (muscles), or from bleeding from the marrow of the bone.

CLINICAL CORRELATION *Femur fractures can cause a loss of 1–2 liters of blood; pelvic fractures can cause a loss of 2–3 liters. The body has only 5 liters to start with, so femur or pelvic fractures can be life-threatening.*

It is possible to die from a fracture due to hypovolemic shock (see Chap. 3) as noted above. The second major complication with fractures is *loss of limb*—that is, limb fractures can lead to damage that may cause a permanent loss of the use of that limb. A fractured bone that moves may damage the nerves and blood vessels that are close to the bone (see next two sections), resulting in **neurovascular compromise**. Without an adequate blood supply, tissues in the limb *distal* to the fracture will begin to die. Moreover, a damaged nerve may prevent the limb from functioning properly.

CLINICAL CORRELATION *Check circulation, sensation, and motion (or function) at the distal end of the limb (fingers or toes) for neurovascular compromise. Check for pulses and capillary refill to determine circulation (see Chap. 3). To check motion and sensation, determine if the patient can wiggle his or her fingers and toes and feel your touch there. If circulation, sensation, and motion are normal, the patient is neurovascularly intact (he or she has no major problems with the blood vessels or nerves in that limb). In your report, say that "distal circulation, sensation, and motion were intact."*

The treatment for suspected fractures is *immobilization*, which accomplishes the desired goals of reducing the potential for bleeding, neurovascular damage, and pain. A firmly splinted fracture reduces blood loss and pain and, it is hoped, eliminates motion. (Pain may be due in part to the muscles' contracting along a broken bone that is no longer stable. As long as the muscles pull, the bone ends can grind against each other. Stabilizing the bones

Table 6-3. General guidelines for splinting

1. Treat ABCs before splinting.
2. In a life-threatening emergency, do *not* delay transport in order to splint. Use a backboard and move.
3. Use compression to help reduce bleeding and swelling.
4. Immobilize the joint above and below (distal and proximal) to a fracture.
5. Always check distal circulation, sensation, and motion, and splint in a manner that these tests can be rechecked easily after splinting. (Leave fingers and toes free.)
6. Manipulate the fracture as little as possible. (Don't move a fracture any more than necessary for safe transport.)
7. Try to immobilize the patient in a position of normal function. (Don't immobilize a limb in an unnatural position if possible.)
8. Use the patient's body as a splint (leg to leg, arm to chest, etc.).
9. Elevation of the extremity helps reduce swelling.
10. Neatness helps. ("A not neat knot is a knot needed not.")
11. Use common sense.

can help prevent the muscles from causing this type of pain.)

Immobilization is accomplished by **splinting**. There are several principles of splinting, outlined in Table 6-3. There are no hard and fast rules except do "whatever it takes."

CLINICAL CORRELATION *There are two important tips to know about immobilization: (1) Femur and pelvic fractures have the greatest risk of significant blood loss. Military antishock trousers (MAST) not only immobilize but also treat shock as well. (2) Backboards immobolize everything.*

A patient with a neurovascular compromise—that is, you can't feel a pulse distal to the fracture, capillary refill is long (>3–5 sec-

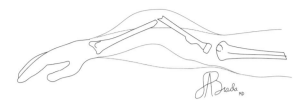

Fig. 6-5. Angulated fracture.

onds), and the patient has lost sensation or motion in the fractured limb—has a more serious problem. Rapid transport to a hospital with an orthopedic surgical service becomes imperative because the patient risks losing that limb. If the fracture is obviously *angulated*—that is, the limb is broken and now resting at an obviously unnatural angle (Fig. 6-5)—and the patient has obvious neurovascular compromise, you *might* consider *reducing* the fracture, or realigning the bone ends, in the field to help restore circulation to the limb. If transport time to a surgical facility is long, reducing the fracture may be your only chance to save the patient's limb.

CLINICAL CORRELATION *Reduce a fracture by pulling traction (until the muscles fatigue) in the direction the distal bone is lying, then moving the distal bone end to align with the proximal bone end. This, it is hoped, will restore circulation and spare the limb. Splinting then becomes crucial.*

To cut off a bone entirely (that is, to cut off the end of a limb) is an **amputation**. The major concern with amputations is controlling bleeding. Fortunately, however, clean-cut (not jagged) amputations may not bleed too badly since exposed blood vessels retract inside the stump and are clamped off partially by surrounding muscles.

CLINICAL CORRELATION *Save all amputated parts you find; a surgeon may be able to reattach them. Wrap amputated parts in (preferably sterile) gauze moistened with lactated Ringer's (or saline), put them in a plastic bag on ice, and get them to the hospital. Do not, however, overly delay transporting the patient to look for a part.*

Joint Injuries

The most common joint injury occurs when a joint is forced to move farther than it is designed to go (i.e., *hyperextension* or *hyperflexion*) or when it is moved in a direction it is not designed to go at all. When joints are moved too far or in the wrong direction, the ligaments making up the joint can become stretched or torn, known as a **sprain**. Joints, not bones or muscles, are sprained.

CLINICAL CORRELATION *The signs, symptoms, and mechanism of injury for sprains and fractures are virtually identical. It is not your job in the field to distinguish between them (one thing x-rays are good for); therefore, treat all bone and joint injuries as if they were fractures.*

The management of sprains at home is RICE: *r*est, *i*ce, *c*ompression, and *e*levation. These principles apply to acute fractures as well (see Table 6-3).

A bone end coming out of a joint is a **dislocation** of that joint; a bone coming out only partially from the joint is a partial dislocation, or **subluxation**.

CLINICAL CORRELATION *In trauma, dislocations can be associated with fractures (and have similar signs and symptoms), so treatment is the same. Some patients, however, may have chronically dislocating joints (a "trick shoulder," for example) because once dislocated, a joint is prone to future dislocations. Many of these patients can fix their own dislocations without your help.*

Soft Tissues

Soft-tissue injuries involve the skin (see Chap. 6), subcutaneous tissue, muscles, and tendons—pretty much everything but the bones and internal organs.

Incisions are clean cuts made by sharp instruments (such as scalpel blades). Knife wounds, however, are referred to as **lacerations**, which describe any other type of cut. Lacerations can be a major cause of bleeding. **Punctures**, or deep penetrating wounds, rarely cause much bleed-

Table 6-4. Soft-tissue injuries

Injury	Description
Incision	Clean cut (with a scalpel blade)
Laceration	Jagged cut (with anything else)
Puncture	Deep penetrating wound (e.g., stepping on a nail)
Abrasion	Scraping wound (e.g., a skinned knee or road burn)
Avulsion	Separation of soft tissue without amputation (no bone involvement—e.g., having an ear bitten off)

ing; ice picks (rather than knives) make typical puncture wounds. (It is important to remember that internal organs deep to the puncture site may be injured.) **Abrasions** are superficial by definition—that is, affecting primarily the skin—but can mask lacerations, especially those in motorcyclists who have been dragged along the pavement. Types of soft-tissue injuries (excluding burns) are listed in Table 6-4.

CLINICAL CORRELATION *Treatment for soft-tissue injuries is direct pressure, direct pressure, direct pressure to control bleeding. Apply direct pressure at the point of bleeding (especially a spurting artery) and use firm pressure bandages. Also, elevate the limb if possible, consider a pressure point, and resort to a tourniquet only if you are absolutely desperate and willing to sacrifice the limb to save the patient's life.*

Avulsion is the tearing away of any tissue; the only difference between an avulsion and an amputation is that an amputation involves removing a bone.

CLINICAL CORRELATION *If a piece of tissue (flesh) has been partially avulsed—that is, it is still partially connected to the rest of the body—do everything you can to preserve that connection. A tiny bridge of living tissue can help the avulsed flesh be reattached.*

Injuries to muscles from overuse (such as athletic injuries and "pulled muscles") are known as **strains**. Remember, joints are sprained; muscles are strained. It is possible to tear muscles acutely, most commonly experienced by athletes. The torn muscle no longer is attached at one end, so it will contract and form a painful, deforming lump. Apply ice, immobilize, and transport.

Blunt trauma also can cause bruises (*contusions*), or blood underneath the skin. Enough blood accumulating to form a lump is known as a *hematoma*.

UPPER EXTREMITY

Bones and Joints

The upper extremity includes the arm and shoulder, which contain the following bones: the scapula and clavicle making up the shoulder, the humerus in the upper arm, the radius and ulna in the lower arm, the carpals in the wrist, the metacarpals in the hand, and the phalanges in the fingers (Fig. 6-6).

Shoulder

There are two joints in the shoulder: the **acromioclavicular** and the **glenohumeral joints**. The acromioclavicular joint (AC joint) is formed where the clavicle meets the acromion of the scapula (Fig. 6-7). (The tip of the scapula is the *acromion*, from the Greek word "acropolis"—the highest point in the city.) Also known as the "point" of the shoulder, it normally has no motion. A hard, lateral blow to the shoulder, like that taken by a football player being tackled or a bicyclist falling, can drive the acromion (scapula) into the clavicle, separating the AC joint.

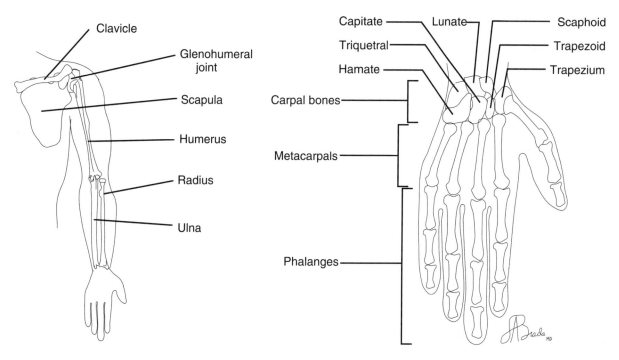

Fig. 6-6. Bones of the arm and hand.

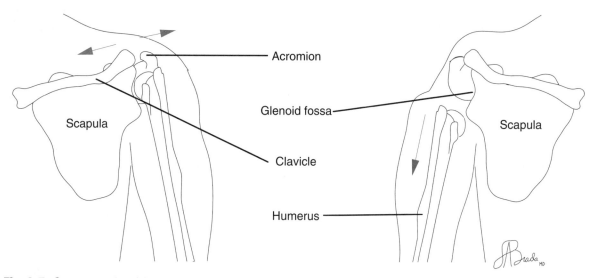

Fig. 6-7. Common shoulder injuries. A separated shoulder (left) results from a separation of the clavicle from the acromion of the scapula at the acromioclavicular joint. Shoulder dislocations occur when the head of the humerus is displaced from the glenoid fossa on the scapula. These dislocations often occur downward and anteriorly at the point of weakest support around the rotator cuff.

CLINICAL CORRELATION *A "separated shoulder," a common sports injury, is a dislocation of the acromioclavicular joint. The treatment of choice in the field is to immobilize the arm with a sling and swathe to reduce motion of the joint.*

The second joint of the shoulder is formed by the *glenoid fossa* of the scapula and the humerus. (A *glen* is a little valley; a *fossa* is an indentation. The glenoid fossa of the scapula apparently looked like a little indented valley to the ancient Greeks.) The head of the humerus is a round ball that fits into the glenoid fossa, forming the glenohumeral joint. This "ball-and-socket" joint allows for maximum mobility in almost any direction (see Chap. 1). Because it is so mobile, the glenohumeral joint is also very prone to dislocation. The joint is protected fairly well above and behind (superiorly and posteriorly) by the shape of the scapula (notice the acromion), so when the humerus is dislocated (that is, a dislocation of the glenohumeral joint) it usually goes forward and down (anteriorly and inferiorly), where the joint is not well stabilized.

CLINICAL CORRELATION *A "dislocated shoulder" is a dislocation of the glenohumeral joint where the humerus usually slides forward and down (anterior-inferior shoulder dislocation). Any motion that pries the arm over the head or jerks the arm forward can dislocate the joint. (It is possible to dislocate the shoulder posteriorly, but it is relatively unusual.) Remember that there is always a risk of a fracture when the shoulder is dislocated. Treatment in the field focuses on stabilizing the shoulder. Because the arm has been displaced forward by the injury, placing a pillow between the arm and the chest along with a sling and swathe will help stabilize the shoulder.*

The clavicle is an important bone of the shoulder whose function is to serve as a "tie rod" between the arm and the thorax (chest). The lateral end of the clavicle is anchored to the scapula as described above, and the medial end is fixed to the sternum or breastbone. Both of these joints on either end of the clavicle are actually very tight and do not give way easily. The clavicle itself, therefore, often bears the brunt of much of the trauma to the upper extremity.

CLINICAL CORRELATION *The most commonly broken bone in the body is the clavicle; any impact to the arm or shoulder may fracture it. In a way, breaking the clavicle prevents the shoulder from absorbing all of the blow. The arm of a patient with a broken clavicle droops unnaturally, and the patient has difficulty lifting it. Treatment in the field is immobilization of the upper extremity with a sling and swathe.*

Elbow

The elbow is actually a "hinge" joint between the humerus and ulna (it allows motion primarily like a hinge). The bone at the back of the elbow is the *olecranon* of the ulna. Elbow dislocations are less common in adults than in children because pulling hard enough on an adult arm usually results in a shoulder dislocation before an elbow. In toddlers and children, however, the shoulder is stronger and the elbow may dislocate first (the so-called "nursemaid's elbow"; see Chap. 7).

Wrist and Hand

The wrist is a complex joint involving the radius, ulna, and carpal bones. It rotates in a circle around the ulna whenever it is pronated or supinated (remember Oliver Twist? See Chap. 1). The wrist also can flex, extend, abduct, and adduct (pretty much move any way it wants) and is known as a "gliding joint" because the many bones glide along each other. There are eight carpal bones, but only an anatomist would expect you to know them individually by name.

CLINICAL CORRELATION *A common wrist injury is a Colles' fracture commonly resulting from a fall on an outstretched hand. When the hand snaps back, the distal radius breaks. Treatment in the field is placing a large ball of gauze (or anything) in the patient's hand and immobilizing the wrist with a simple board splint and a sling.*

The palm of the hand is made up of the metacarpal bones (numbered one through five). The fingers are each made up of three phalanges (proximal, middle, and distal), with only two in the thumb.

CLINICAL CORRELATION *Hand injuries, while not life-threatening, can have a dramatic effect on a person's life. For that reason, consider immediate transport of patients with hand injuries (especially amputations) to centers with hand specialists even if it means a helicopter flight and bypassing the nearest hospital.*

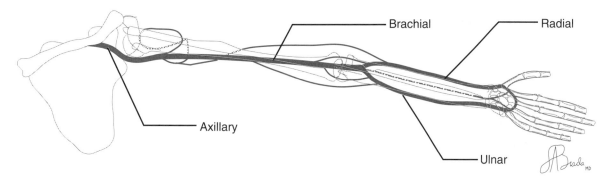

Fig. 6-8. Major arteries of the arm.

Blood Vessels and Nerves

Arteries

The purpose of arteries is to carry blood throughout the body (see Chap. 3). The *subclavian* arteries carry blood from the aorta to the arms. As the subclavian artery passes from underneath the clavicle, it becomes the *axillary* artery (in the axilla or "armpit"). As the axillary artery travels into the arm, it becomes the **brachial artery** (Fig. 6-8). The pulse of the brachial artery can be felt about halfway down the upper arm between the muscles of the biceps and triceps next to the humerus (see below).

CLINICAL CORRELATION *For arterial bleeding distally in the arm that is not well controlled by direct pressure at the bleeding site, use the brachial artery as a pressure point. Find the brachial artery pulse and squeeze it until you block the artery enough to stop bleeding. Although this sounds good in principle, it may be difficult to accomplish successfully in the field. Direct pressure and pressure bandages are usually quicker, easier, and more efficient. Do not delay transport or IV fluid resuscitation with prolonged attempts at using a pressure point.*

Branches of the brachial artery wrap behind the humerus and travel closely alongside it, which is why a humeral fracture (or any fracture) may cause blood loss.

CLINICAL CORRELATION *Remember to avoid unnecessary motion of broken bones, as most bones have arteries and nerves running closely alongside them.*

The brachial artery divides at the elbow into the **radial** and **ulnar arteries**, one following each bone of the forearm. Both arteries can be felt in the wrist, but it is usually easier to feel the radial artery, which is on the side of the thumb.

Veins

There are two basic types of veins: deep and superficial. Deep veins tend to run beside arteries. As does lacerating an artery, lacerating a vein causes bleeding, although not as immediately severe because blood in the vein is not under pressure. When cut, a vein "oozes" rather than "spurts," as does a cut artery.

CLINICAL CORRELATION *You usually can tell arterial bleeding from venous bleeding. Arterial blood is brighter red because it contains more oxygen and spurts or pulsates. Treatment for bleeding and blood loss is the same regardless of source, but keep in mind that serious arterial bleeding can lead to hypovolemic shock more quickly than simple venous bleeding.*

Superficial veins serve one purpose for EMS personnel: IV access. Superficial venous anatomy is highly variable, so go with the whatever you can find. Keep in mind, however, a few good spots to start with: the cephalic and basilic veins as shown previously in Chap. 3.

Nerves

Nerves carry instructions from the brain to the body and carry messages from the body back to the brain (see Chap. 2). When a nerve is damaged, the body part it supplies loses function (either sensation or motion). Nerve roots from C5–T1 form a complex bundle of nerves that innervate the arm. Next to control of the mouth, control of the arm and hand is one of the most complicated things the brain does. (Have you ever seen a monkey talk or knit?)

Three major nerves pass into the forearm: the *ulnar, radial,* and *median* nerves. The ulnar nerve passes behind the elbow (lateral to the ulna). When you bump your elbow and hit your "funny bone," you've actually hit the ulnar nerve, sending pain and *parasthesias* (tingling "pins and needles") down your arm to your little finger. The ulnar nerve controls most of the muscles on the posterior side of the forearm involved with wrist extension as well as some muscles in the hand.

The median nerve, as its name implies, travels down the middle of the forearm, passing through a tendinous ring in the wrist (the *carpal tunnel*) on its way to the muscles of the hand. The carpal tunnel surrounds many of the tendons that flex the fingers. People who frequently use their hands may irritate the nerve as it passes through the carpal tunnel, causing carpal tunnel syndrome.

An important branch of the median nerve, the *recurrent median nerve,* emerges along the fleshy base of the thumb and controls the muscles of the thumb (Fig. 6-9). Remember, humans are the only beings on earth with opposable thumbs, which allow us to pick up objects with control.

CLINICAL CORRELATION *Check to see if a patient with a laceration at the base of the thumb can oppose his or her thumb and little finger. Ask the patient to touch the tip of the thumb to the tip of the little finger. If he or she cannot do this normally, consider taking the patient to a hand specialty hospital, or at least point out the injury to the emergency department staff. The inability to oppose the thumb makes it difficult to perform many jobs.*

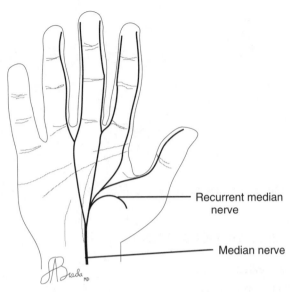

Fig. 6-9. Distribution of the median nerve to the hand. Even small lacerations to the fleshy portion of the thumb can sever the small recurrent median nerve, making it impossible for the patient to oppose his or her thumb. Be very thorough when dealing with any injury to the hand.

Muscles

The deltoid is the triangle-shaped muscle at the top of the arm on the lateral side. Its function is to raise the arm (abduct the humerus).

CLINICAL CORRELATION *The deltoid is a common site for intramuscular and subcutaneous shots.*

Some of the other muscles of the upper extremity are depicted in (Fig. 6-10).

Around the glenohumeral joint of the shoulder, a capsule known as the *rotator cuff* is formed by four muscles: the supraspinatus, infraspinatus, teres minor, and subscapularis. Rotator cuff injuries commonly occur in baseball players who have damaged this capsule.

The large chest and back muscles move the arm in various ways. Remember that muscles only shorten. Their point of attachment determines their range of motion. The pectoralis major and minor on the chest bring the arms forward; the latissimus dorsi on the back brings

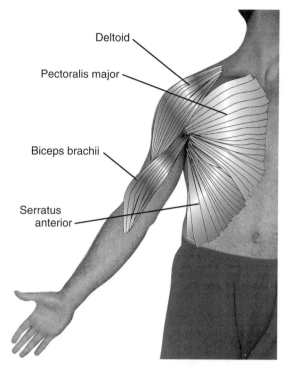
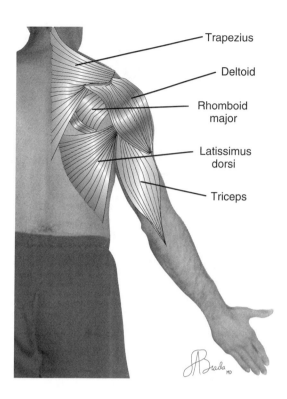

Fig. 6-10. Muscles of the upper extremity.

them down. The rhomboids in the back stabilize and rotate the scapula. The trapezius holds up the neck and helps shrug the shoulders.

In the upper arm, the biceps are anterior; when they shorten, the elbow flexes. The triceps are posterior in the upper arm; when they shorten, the elbow extends. There are a variety of wrist extensors in the forearm on the posterior side and flexors on the anterior side.

LOWER EXTREMITY

Bones and Joints

The lower extremity is made up of the legs and the "hip girdle," which contain the following bones: the pelvis, femur, patella (or kneecap), tibia (shinbone), fibula (also in the lower leg), tarsals of the ankle, metatarsals of the foot, and phalanges in the toes (Fig. 6-11).

Hip

The femur forms a ball-and-socket joint with the pelvis in the hip joint similar to the

humerus and the shoulder in the upper arm; the hip, however, is not nearly as mobile as the shoulder. The socket in the pelvic bone is known as the **acetabulum**; the head of the femur is a ball that fits snugly into the acetabulum. Notice the shape of the femur—it has a long shaft, a thin neck, and a round head. In a hip fracture, what actually breaks is the neck of the femur, not the pelvic bones.

CLINICAL CORRELATION *The neck of the femur is prone to break (a hip fracture) in elderly patients, especially women, from even minor falls. Unlike pelvic fractures, which are caused by major trauma and are life-threatening, hip fractures can be caused by minor trauma and are not immediately life-threatening. Treatment in the field is comfortable transport (supine). Use strict spinal precautions only if indicated.*

CLINICAL CORRELATION *A patient who has been in an automobile accident and caught his or her knees on the dashboard may have a femur that is jammed back into the pelvis, fracturing the acetabulum. This fracture, like any pelvic fracture, is best treated with MAST trousers.*

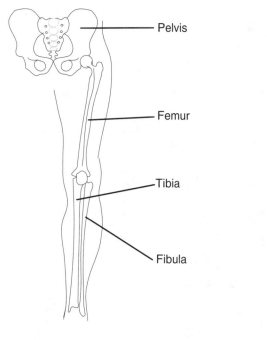

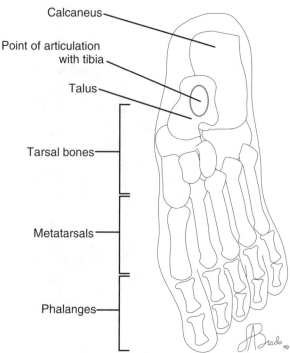

Fig. 6-11. Bones of the leg and foot.

In addition to breaking the femoral neck, the hip also is prone to dislocate, the classic mechanism being the "splits"—for example, that occurring in a person with one foot on a dock and the other on a boat that moves away from the dock before he or she can jump to one side. Pretty soon, the legs are too far apart to move, but the feet are still planted, resulting in hip dislocation. There is no specific treatment for the patient before arriving at the hospital.

The femur is the largest bone in the body. As previously noted, a midshaft femur fracture (as opposed to a femoral neck, or "hip" fracture) can be life-threatening due to associated blood loss.

CLINICAL CORRELATION *The treatment of choice for midshaft femur fractures is a traction splint, MAST trousers, or ideally both. When the leg is under traction, the fracture site is stabilized, and the big leg muscles are prevented from contracting, resulting in pain reduction and minimizing damage to muscles and blood vessels. MAST trousers aid in stabilization, treat bleeding (internal and external) in the leg, and treat for shock. The Sager style traction splint is preferable because it is fast, can be put on with MAST trousers in place, and can be used for bilateral femur fractures.*

Knee
The knee, like the elbow in the arm, is a hinge joint between the tibia and the femur. The patella, or knee cap, sits anteriorly, helping to provide mechanical advantage for the muscles of the thigh. A common sports injury is a lateral dislocation of the patella (a "trick knee") in which the patella slides to the lateral side of the leg. It is very painful and very obvious on exam.

CLINICAL CORRELATION *Laterally dislocated patellas often can be safely reduced in the field. By placing a thumb lateral to the kneecap and applying pressure to push it medially while simultaneously extending the knee, the patella usually slides back into place, resulting in considerable relief of pain. The advantage of reducing a patella sooner rather than later is that the longer it is dislocated, the more swelling and pain result, and the more difficult it is to reduce later. If there is any concern about a fracture it is best not to manipulate the knee and instead to splint in the position it is found.*

A variety of ligaments stabilize the knee, and a cartilage *meniscus*, or plate, is located on each side of the knee as well, resulting in a large number of things that can be traumatized. That is why "clipping" in football is a 15-yard

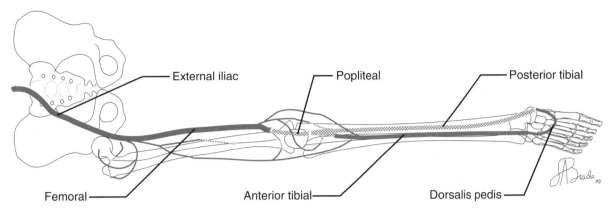

Fig. 6-12. Major arteries of the leg.

penalty because it discourages blocking from behind, which can result in knee injury.

The lower leg consists of the tibia and fibula. The tibia is the major bone of the shin; the fibula is a much smaller bone along the lateral side of the tibia. (Fibula is Latin for "safety pin." Notice that the shape of bones of the lower leg look like a safety pin.) It is difficult to break the tibia without also breaking the fibula, the so-called tib-fib fracture. This fracture will occur when a person is struck by an automobile bumper just below the knees.

Ankle and Foot

The ankle bones are known as tarsals. The foot itself is made up of metatarsals; the bones in the toes, like the bones in the fingers, are known as phalanges. (The bottom of the foot is the *plantar* surface; the top, the *dorsal* surface.)

CLINICAL CORRELATION *Isolated ankle and foot injuries are common, and it can be difficult and pointless to distinguish sprains from fractures. Large, bulky pillow splints are usually appropriate to immobilize almost any ankle or foot injury in the field.*

Blood Vessels and Nerves

Arteries

The major artery supplying the leg is the **femoral artery** (Fig. 6-12), a continuation of the iliac artery, which is a branch of the descending

aorta. The femoral pulse is best found at a point halfway along a line joining the pubis and the anterior superior iliac spine (see Chap. 5).

CLINICAL CORRELATION *The femoral artery also can be used as a pressure point to help control bleeding in the lower extremity. If MAST trousers are not available, push down on the femoral artery (using both hands, as if you were performing cardiopulmonary resuscitation).*

The femoral artery passes behind the knee as the popliteal artery and splits into several branches in the lower leg. The two common pulse points found in the lower leg are the posterior tibial and dorsalis pedis, discussed in Chap. 3.

Veins

The major vein draining the leg is the femoral vein, which runs alongside the femoral artery. There are many superficial veins of the leg as well, although they usually are not nearly as readily apparent as the superficial veins of the arm. There is no physiological reason you can't start an IV in the leg or foot, except in the case of pelvic fractures or internal abdominal injuries that might interfere with the flow of IV fluid back to the body. Starting an IV in the leg or foot, however, usually is technically more difficult and cumbersome.

CLINICAL CORRELATION *As sometimes happens with entrapments, you may be able to reach*

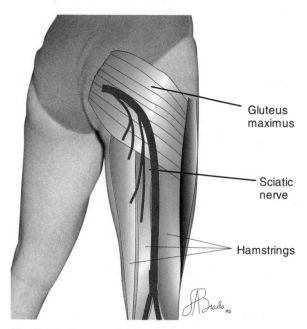

Fig. 6-13. Course of the sciatic nerve. Notice that all of the branches of the sciatic nerve exit from the inferior side as it runs beneath the gluteus maximus. All injections in this region should be placed in the upper-outer quadrant of the gluteus maximus to avoid hitting the nerve.

only the patient's foot. If necessary, start an IV there while the extrication or rescue goes on.

Nerves

Two major nerves descend into the leg: the femoral nerve in the front, which follows a course near the femoral artery and vein, and the **sciatic nerve** in the back deep in the buttocks, which leaves the sacrum and travels diagonally across the buttocks down the back of the leg (Fig. 6-13). *Sciatica* is lower back pain that may radiate down the back of the leg caused by pinching of the sciatic nerve.

CLINICAL CORRELATION   *A possible site for intramuscular injections is the buttocks; the only thing you have to avoid is the sciatic nerve. Remember to inject in the upper-outer quadrant of the buttocks to avoid hitting the sciatic nerve.*

EMS personnel often are expected to check the *Babinski reflex*, a crude means to determine whether the nerve path from the foot

through the spinal cord to the brain is intact. Rub the bottom (plantar surface) of a patient's foot with a thumbnail or car key to see how the big toe reacts. If the person jerks the foot away (the most common response in conscious people), it is meaningless—rub less briskly along the lateral side of the foot and watch the toe again. A toe that points *down* is a normal reflex. A toe that points *up* is abnormal. With an upgoing big toe, the other toes may splay apart, which also is abnormal.

CLINICAL CORRELATION   *Check the Babinski reflex in a patient with a suspected head injury, spinal injury, or stroke or who is unconscious for unclear reasons if you have time. Rub the bottom of the foot and report the response as "upgoing" or "downgoing" toes on the left, right, or bilaterally (both sides). If the toes go up, know that it is a sign of damage somewhere in the central nervous system.*

Muscles

You should know the names of the muscles in the lower extremity you may be sticking needles into, including the **gluteus maximus**, which is the major muscle of the buttocks, and the **vastus lateralis**, the lateral part of the *quadriceps* muscle group of the thigh (Fig. 6-14). The advantage of the vastus lateralis is that you can access it while the patient is supine; however, the gluteus maximus generally provides the best target.

Many muscles of the lower extremity contribute to our ability to stand and walk: the quadriceps, the biceps femoris, the soleus, and the gastrocnemius. The front of the thigh is known as the quadriceps. As the name implies, it is a set of four muscles (the vastus lateralis, intermedius, medius, and the rectus femoris). The muscle making up the back of the thigh is the biceps femoris, commonly called the "hamstring" (it flexes the knee, much like the biceps in the arm flexes the elbow). The soleus and gastrocnemius are the major muscles of the

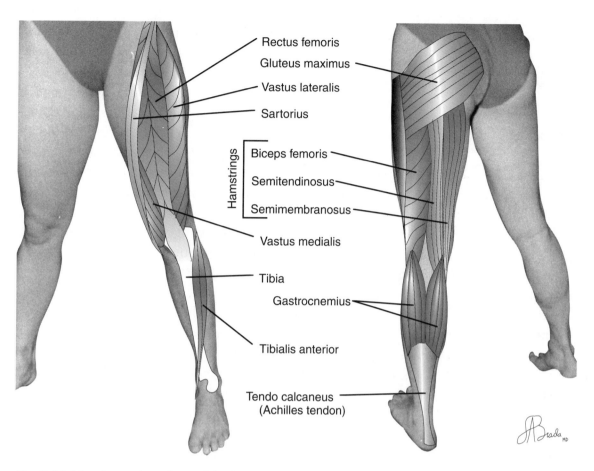

Fig. 6-14. Muscles and tendons of the lower extremity.

calf, which ends in the Achilles tendon attached to the heel bone.

THE SKIN AND ENVIRONMENTAL INJURIES

Anatomy

The skin, or *integument*, is the largest organ of the body. It is an active organ, providing the first line of defense against most infections by acting as a physical barrier. It also helps regulate body temperature.

The skin has several layers. The outermost layer is the *epidermis*; below that is the *dermis*, the thicker layer of skin full of blood vessels, hair follicles, and nerve endings. Below the dermis is the **subcutaneous** ("below the skin") connective tissue. Deep to the subcutaneous

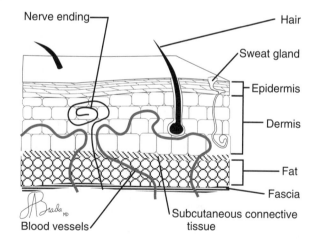

Fig. 6-15. The skin and cutaneous structures.

connective tissue is a layer of fat, which is the body's mechanism to store energy and provide insulation against the cold. Deep to the fat is *fascia*, a thin plane of connective tissue outside the underlying muscle (Fig. 6-15).

Thermoregulation

Thermoregulation is the body's ability to maintain a constant temperature. Because of its ongoing metabolism, the body internally generates heat all of the time; however, its challenge is to keep the temperature constant (not too hot or cold). The body does a very good job of maintaining a core body temperature of around 98.6°F (37°C), with the temperature control center being the brain stem. The principle organ for maintaining body temperature is the skin, which regulates how much heat the body gives off.

Heat Transfer

Heat is a form of energy that can be transferred from one thing to another. The body transfers heat according to the same laws of physics that apply to a burning building. There are four basic mechanisms of heat transfer (or in the case of humans, heat loss): **conduction, radiation, convection,** and **evaporation.**

Conduction is the transfer of heat between two touching objects. Touching a cold metal pole with a bare hand conducts a lot of heat out of the hand. Denser objects conduct heat better than less dense objects; therefore, metal conducts heat better than wood, and water conducts heat better than air. (Down jackets are so warm because they create an airspace around the body that does not conduct heat well. On the other hand, a wet cotton shirt is denser than down and thus transfers more heat from the body.)

Radiation of heat is just what the sun does. Hot objects emit heat without touching anything (we can feel the sun, but we certainly are not touching it). Human bodies have tremendous potential to radiate heat, which is why marathon runners often are given an aluminum blanket to wrap themselves in at the end of a race. Aluminum reflects the radiated heat back to the runner so he or she doesn't cool off too quickly.

Convection is the transfer of heat from a circulating current or breeze; heat is lost from the circulation. Standing in moving water feels colder than standing in still water. Likewise, breezes feel cooler than still air.

The last mechanism for heat loss is evaporation. Liquid water (such as sweat) that evaporates has been heated until it turns into a vapor; it is "boiled off," so to speak. The act of going from a liquid to a vapor consumes a tremendous amount of heat. This is why we were designed to sweat—so that we could lose heat by having sweat evaporate off our skin. As sweat evaporates, heat is drawn out of the body. (We are so miserable on humid days because sweat cannot evaporate as easily; thus, we cannot lose heat as efficiently.)

(For those of you who are not firefighters, evaporation is the same mechanism behind the "indirect attack" on a fire. By spraying water above the fire rather than directly at it, water is placed into the hottest part of the room, causing the water to evaporate quickly. The evaporating water draws off heat. Without sufficient heat, the fire extinguishes.)

Hypothermia

A body that becomes too cold is said to be **hypothermic**—that is, the patient has **hypothermia** (hypo = low, thermia = temperature). Hypothermia results when heat is lost from the body faster than the body's metabolism can produce it. Knowing the four mechanisms of heat transfer, the situations in which hypothermia takes place become clear. Cold, wet, windy days are the worst. Below-freezing temperatures are not required—just cool and damp weather.

In freezing weather, people tend to be better prepared against the "elements." Freezing weather also is usually dry (once the temperature drops enough). Dry weather, even if cold, is safer because conductive heat loss is less.

The other big risk for hypothermia is *alcohol* for two reasons: (1) Alcohol impairs judgment so patients are more likely to be stupid about protecting themselves from the elements; and (2) alcohol is a peripheral vasodilator, so it opens blood vessels in the skin (the reason why a person may become red in the face when drinking alcohol). When blood rushes to the skin, you *feel* warm because your skin suddenly is getting a lot of warm blood. The problem, however, is that sending all of this warm blood to the skin results in profuse radiation. Therefore, drinking alcohol actually causes increased heat loss.

CLINICAL CORRELATION *Alcoholics—particularly homeless ones—are at very high risk for hypothermia in inclement weather.*

When the body becomes cold, it reacts in several ways to stay warm. Goose bumps, which cause the hair to stand and form a miniature down jacket, traps a layer of air around the skin to keep it warm. Raising hair is how animals with coats retain body heat. Since most people are not as hairy as dogs, their bodies begin to shiver involuntarily. Shivering is muscle activity that generates heat. Also, blood vessels in the skin constrict to conserve heat in the body's core, which is why fingers and toes become cold first. (Fingers and toes also radiate heat well.)

Predictable signs of hypothermia occur if the cold wins out and the body's core temperature drops (Table 6-5). The organ most sensitive to cold is the brain; thus, hypothermic patients may have difficulty speaking and

Table 6-5. Signs of hypothermia

Early
  Shivering
  Slurred speech
  Blue lips
  Clumsiness
  Confusion
Middle
  Shivering stops
  Decreased mental status
  Paradoxical feeling of warmth (patient may start
    to undress)
  Bradycardia (slow heart rate)
  Bradypnea (slow respiratory rate)
  Coma
Late
  Asystole and fine ventricular fibrillation

become confused. As the temperature drops, shivering eventually stops, a bad sign indicating that the body is so cold it is saving all of its energy and not using any to shiver. At this point, patients may have impaired mental status, display bizarre behavior, and even undress, thinking they are now warm.

CLINICAL CORRELATION *Basic treatment of hypothermia is fairly straightforward. Get patients warm and dry. Get them out of their wet clothes, wrap them in a thermal or aluminum blanket, apply something warm to their trunks if possible, and transport.*

Gradually, the body in hypothermia shuts down. Metabolism nearly shuts off, the heart rate and respiratory rate slow, and the patient loses consciousness. Eventually the heart stops; however, while the patient's temperature drops, the heart is more vulnerable to going into ventricular fibrillation (V-fib).

CLINICAL CORRELATION *Avoid overstimulating profoundly hypothermic patients; they are at great risk of going into V-fib cardiac arrest. Just move them gently.*

CLINICAL CORRELATION *Hypothermic patients have slow pulses and respirations that may be difficult to detect. Check vitals carefully for up to a minute before deciding a hypothermic patient is pulseless and breathless.*

Warm the patient's core (trunk and abdomen) before warming the arms and legs if facing a long transport or if the patient is very cold (less than 86°F, 30°C). The risk of rewarming the arms and legs first is that it causes dilation of the vessels in the extremities that send excessive amounts of lactic acid back to the heart (which can cause dangerous arrhythmias).

CLINICAL CORRELATION *To treat hypothermic patients, especially those in cardiac arrest, administer warm IV fluids (preferably 109°F, 43°C). It is also important to remember to not let IV fluids become cold in the back of an ambulance out in bay at night in cold weather. Administering cold IV fluids (such as 50°) to a person with normal body temperature can induce hypothermia.*

If, after a minute, you are unable to find a pulse in a severely hypothermic patient, resuscitate following ACLS guidelines. It is useful, although difficult, to obtain a core body temperature, but it should be done, using either a tympanic (ear) or rectal probe. Oral, axillary (armpit), fingertip, or skin temperature probes are unreliable and do not accurately reflect the temperature of the patient's core (which includes vital organs, the main concern).

Resuscitation of a cold patient is not the same as resuscitation of a warm patient, especially if the core temperature is less than 86° F (30° C). Because metabolism shuts down, the hypothermic heart may not respond to defibrillation or drugs. Unmetabolized drugs can accumulate to toxic levels in a hypothermic patient.

CLINICAL CORRELATION *In the resuscitation of very cold patients (less than 86°F/30°C), limit defibrillation shocks to three and withhold IV drugs until they can be rewarmed. Once the patient is warmer than 30°C, medications should be dosed at longer intervals to avoid toxic buildups.*

CLINICAL CORRELATION *There is no such thing as a cold, dead person, only warm, dead people.*

Try to resuscitate a pulseless, cold patient, even if he or she has been "down" for a long period of time. Do not stop the resuscitation attempt until the patient has been rewarmed. The human body can show surprising resilience to cold.

Hyperthermia

Don't confuse the terms hy*po*thermia and **hy*per*thermia**, an elevation of body temperature. A fever can raise body temperature, which is a normal response to infections and a variety of illnesses and usually not a problem (except in children in whom fevers sometimes can result in seizures; see Chap. 7). The body also can be subjected to environmental extremes that may raise body temperature.

Heat exhaustion, also referred to as heat prostration, is a common problem seen in athletes or anyone working strenuously outside on a hot, humid day. Remember that when it is humid, it is difficult for the body to lose heat by evaporating sweat; the body sweats, but the sweat won't evaporate. The major problem is not heat but the combination of *heat and dehydration* that occurs when the patient has sweat a lot without drinking enough water.

The body temperature of a patient with heat exhaustion actually may be normal. The patient typically is covered in sweat (the root of the problem), and if he or she becomes dehydrated enough, the sympathetic nervous system kicks in to prevent shock (see Chap. 2). As a result, the patient's skin may be pale and clammy. The patient also is likely be tachycardic from both exercise and sympathetic tone.

CLINICAL CORRELATION *The treatment for heat exhaustion is to move the patient out of the sun into a cool environment (not too cold—avoid shivering!) and to administer oral or IV fluids (normal saline) to rehydrate.*

Heat stroke is a much more serious problem than heat exhaustion. If the patient becomes overheated so much so that his or her body can no longer cope with the heat it needs to dissipate, the brain may become overheated. An

Table 6-6. Burns

Degree	Damage	Description
First	Superficial (epidermis only)	Red, painful (e.g., sunburn)
Second	Partial-thickness (into the dermis)	Red-white, blistering, very painful
Third	Full-thickness (through the dermis into the muscle or fatty tissue) below the skin	White, black-charred, peeling blisters, no longer painful (all nerve endings in skin now burned)

overheated brain may result in thermoregulatory center dysfunction, and the body will start to lose its ability to control temperature. When this happens, the body's core temperature may start to rise dangerously (temperatures over 106°F), an urgently life-threatening event because the brain cannot tolerate such high temperatures.

Dehydration may not be an issue at all; thus, the sympathetic response seen in simple heat exhaustion may not be present. Instead, the body may attempt (with no real help from the brain) to radiate the heat by dilating all of the blood vessels in the skin, which is why heat stroke patients classically are said to have hot, red, dry skin.

CLINICAL CORRELATION *Patients do not always exactly resemble the classic textbook example of heat exhaustion (which can lead to heat stroke), so the skin may look like anything. Cool off a hot person who has altered mental status. Apply cold water or ice (if available) around the head, in the armpits, groin, and along the neck.*

CLINICAL CORRELATION *Whereas athletes outside during the summer are prone to heat exhaustion, the elderly inside during the summer are prone to heat stroke. If you walk into the house of an elderly patient during the summer, it is 95°F outside and hotter inside, and the patient still is wearing a sweater and losing consciousness, he or she is probably hyperthermic.*

Injuries

Burns

Burns are injuries to the skin and soft tissue resulting from exposure to heat, radiation, chemicals, or electricity. They commonly result from fire, direct contact with something hot, or exposure to hot liquids or steam (scalds).

CLINICAL CORRELATION *Steam burns are potentially the most serious for several reasons: (1) There is a risk of inhaling the hot gas, (2) steam more readily exposes a larger area of the patient to injury, and (3) steam holds more energy than liquid at the same temperature, making it more damaging.*

As always, your first concern with any burn injury is the ABCs. Inhalation of hot gas or steam can cause swelling in the airway or damage to the lungs (which can lead to pulmonary edema).

CLINICAL CORRELATION *Always be on the lookout for signs of inhalation injury. Look for burned nasal hair, burns around the mouth, or soot in the nose and mouth. Suspect inhalation injury in anyone who was trapped in a closed space with smoke or heat. Patients with this type of injury need oxygen and transport to a hospital even if they appear asymptomatic.*

Burns to the skin itself usually are characterized by *degree*, a measure of the extent of the damage to the skin and soft tissue caused by the burn (Table 6-6). First-degree (superficial) burns are painful but not usually a life-threatening problem. Second-degree (partial-thickness) burns are extremely painful. Third-degree (full-thickness) burns are the most serious but have the saving grace of not being painful because the nerves in the skin have been damaged. Second- and third-degree burns are both potentially disfiguring, disabling, and fatal if extensive enough. Full-thickness burns tend to be surrounded by partial-thickness areas.

In addition to the depth (or degree) of a burn, the other important factor is the *extent* of the burn. In the field, you should be able to estimate the extent of a burn by estimating the percentage of the patient's body surface area that was burned, accomplished by the **rule of nines** (Fig. 6-16). Basically, the rule divides the body into 12 parts. The groin accounts for 1% of the body's surface area and the remaining 11—head, chest, abdomen, upper back, lower back, left arm, right arm, left and right front surface of leg, and left and right back surface of leg—each account for 9%. Obviously, the more of the body covered with burn, the more severe the injury.

A more practical rule is the *1% rule*. A patient's palm represents about 1% of his or her body surface area; therefore, you can estimate the surface area of irregular burns by estimating how many of the patient's palms it would take to cover the burn.

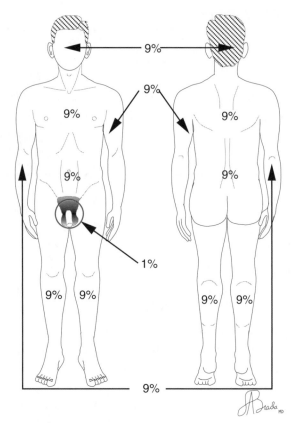

Fig. 6-16. The "rule of nines" for estimating extent of burns as a percentage of body area.

CLINICAL CORRELATION *Any burn covering greater than 30% of the body's surface area, third-degree burns greater than 10%, inhalation burns, electrical burns, deep chemical burns, burns associated with other trauma (such as fractures), and burns in patients with underlying medical problems (such as heart disease) are all critical burns that need urgent attention at a hospital equipped to handle burn patients. Additionally, burns to the hands, face, and groin, while not life-threatening, all need special attention.*

The burn itself causes two major problems: fluid loss and loss of thermoregulation. Remember that skin prevents fluid from leaking out. If enough of it is burned off, profound fluid loss from direct oozing of fluid out of the burn site and internal redistribution of fluid can result. Hypovolemia becomes an issue.

CLINICAL CORRELATION *Treat all burn patients for shock before their blood pressure drops (see Chap. 3). Quickly administer IV fluids (normal saline or lactated Ringer's).*

Without skin, the body loses its ability to regulate its temperature. In fact, patients with extensive burn injuries can become hypothermic.

CLINICAL CORRELATION *Minor first- and second-degree burns should be cooled, preferably with sterile saline, to provide pain relief and limit heat damage. If a significant percentage of a patient's body is covered with second- or third-degree burns (approximately 20% or more), do not cool the patient because he or she can lose too much heat, possibly resulting in hypothermia.*

Frostbite

The other extreme of environmental injury is frostbite, a condition in which the skin and soft tissue freeze. Typically, frostbite first affects the toes, fingers, ears, cheeks, and nose (the parts of the body most susceptible to cold). As with hypothermia, one of the biggest culprits in frostbite is wetness. When combined with freezing temperatures, wet socks are sure to result in frostbite. Another contributor to frostbite is smoking, which results in peripheral vasoconstriction. Without good circulation, it is difficult to keep toes warm.

Frostbitten extremities are fairly obvious; they are ice cold, white, stiff, and often without feeling. *Do not rub frostbitten tissue*!

Remember that frostbitten tissue is extremely damaged, so avoid traumatizing it further. The tissue needs to be gradually rewarmed, but once it is frozen, the damage has been done. Thus, there is no rush. If you are on a long transport or evacuation, do not rewarm frozen tissue unless you are positive it will not refreeze. If rewarmed tissue freezes again, it will be damaged beyond repair.

VOCABULARY LIST

abrasion	superficial "scraping" wound to the skin
acetabulum	the socket of the pelvis into which the head of the femur fits
acromioclavicular joint	the connection between the clavicle and the acromion process of the scapula; the part of the shoulder prone to "separation"
amputation	a severed bone and the surrounding flesh that are no longer connected to the rest of the body
avulsion	loss of soft tissue; similar to amputation but with no bone involvement
brachial artery	the major artery supplying the arm; a palpable pulse and pressure point in the upper arm between the biceps and triceps
cartilage	the smooth "gristle" on the ends of bones that allows them to move easily in joints
closed fracture	a simple fracture in which the surrounding skin is intact
Colles' fracture	a type of distal radius fracture commonly resulting from a fall on an outstretched hand
compound fracture	an open fracture in which the surrounding skin has been broken
conduction	a mechanism of heat transfer between two touching objects
convection	a mechanism of heat transfer in which an object loses heat in a moving breeze or current
deltoid	the triangular muscle of the upper, outer arm; a common site for intramuscular and subcutaneous needle injections
dislocation	a bone coming out of a joint
evaporation	a mechanism of heat transfer in which heat is absorbed by liquid as it vaporizes; heat is thereby lost from the body when sweat evaporates
femoral artery	the major artery supplying the leg; a palpable pulse and pressure point in the groin
fracture	a broken bone

glenohumeral joint	the joint between the humerus and the glenoid fossa of the scapula; the "ball-and-socket" joint of the shoulder; prone to dislocation
gluteus maximus	major muscle of the buttocks; site of intramuscular injections
heat exhaustion	a combination of heat and dehydration causing fatigue and possibly hypovolemia
heat stroke	a life-threatening condition in which the body loses the ability to regulate its heat loss and the patient becomes critically overheated
hyperthermia	the body's becoming too hot, as in heat exhaustion or heat stroke
hypothermia	the body's becoming too cold
joint	point at which two bones come together; an articulating joint is a joint that allows motion (e.g., "ball-and-socket" shoulder, "hinge" elbow, "gliding" wrist)
laceration	a jagged cut
ligaments	connective tissue that connects bones to bones across joints
neurovascular compromise	an interruption of the nerve fibers and blood supply to a distal extremity
open fracture	a compound fracture in which the surrounding skin has been broken
paralysis	inability to voluntarily move something; usually the result of damage to the spinal cord
puncture	a deep penetrating wound
radial artery	a major artery in the wrist found on the radial side (by the thumb)
radiation	a mechanism of heat transfer in which a hot object "shines off" heat
rule of nines	a rule to estimate body surface area to quantify the extent of a burn
sciatic nerve	a nerve that travels across the buttocks to the back of the leg; to be avoided when giving intramuscular shots in the buttocks
simple fracture	a closed fracture in which the surrounding skin is intact

splinting   stabilization of a suspected fracture or dislocation by immobilization

strains   "pulled" muscles

subcutaneous   below the skin

subluxation   a partial dislocation

tendons   connective tissues that connect muscles to bones

thermoregulation   the mechanisms by which the body is able to maintain a normal temperature

ulnar artery   a major artery in the wrist found on the ulnar side (by the little finger)

vastus lateralis   part of the quadriceps muscle group of the thigh; site of intramuscular injections

SELF-ASSESSMENT QUESTIONS

1. A patient has an isolated gunshot wound to his leg. How would you treat this person?

2. You are called to a football field to aid a player who was tackled hard and is complaining of pain in his shoulder. What injuries would you expect, and how would you treat them?

3. You are called to a ski resort to aid a skier who apparently ran off the trail and crashed into a tree. He already has been evacuated from the mountain but has received no other treatment. On your arrival, he is responsive only to painful stimuli. What are your thoughts, and how should you approach the patient's injuries?

4. It is a cold, wet, and rainy night. You are called to help a man who is apparently living underneath a highway overpass. He is lethargic, responds to verbal stimuli, but is disoriented. He smells of alcohol and urine. What are some potential problems you need to address?

5. You arrive at the scene of a house fire when firefighters bring you a patient who was apparently unconscious inside the house. She has severe second- and third-degree burns over much of her body. What are your management concerns?

7

Pediatrics

Children are not just small adults; they are very different from adults in many ways, especially in their responses to illnesses and injuries. By and large, however, most of the anatomy and physiology of children is the same as adults (only smaller!). This chapter is dedicated to the differences between adult and pediatric anatomy, function, and disease. Remember that children differ from each other too and come in all shapes and sizes (Fig. 7-1).

FETUS AND NEWBORN

Fetal Circulation

Fetus is the term for a baby still developing inside its mother's uterus (see Chap. 5). Rather than breathing air with its lungs, the fetus receives oxygen from the mother via the placenta; thus, the circulatory pathway of the fetus is different from that of adults (Fig. 7-2).

In fact, newborn babies must reroute their circulation at the moment of birth to survive outside the mother's womb.

Oxygenated blood enters the fetus from the placenta through the **umbilical vein** and then travels through the *ductus venosus*, through the liver, and into the inferior vena cava. As in adults, the inferior vena cava of a fetus drains blood into its right atrium (see Chap. 3); the difference, however, is that instead of sending blood into the right ventricle, a fetus's right atrium shunts much of the blood across to the left atrium through a hole called the *foramen ovale*. This hole allows oxygenated blood to enter the left atrium, which then sends it into the left ventricle and out the aorta to the brain and body.

Some blood goes from the right atrium into the right ventricle, which sends blood out the pulmonary artery (just as in adults); however, the pulmonary artery shunts most of its blood

187

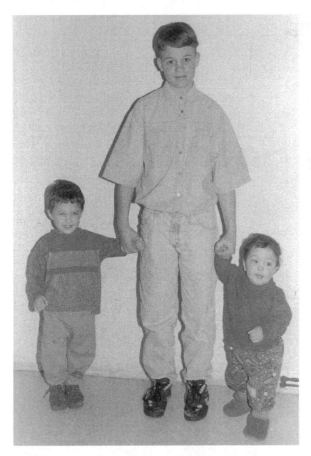

Fig. 7-1. Children come in all shapes and sizes.

through the *ductus arteriosis* into the aorta before blood has a chance to get to the lungs. The net result is that the fetus's lungs get almost no blood, which is fine because its lungs aren't used at this point.

After birth, the baby's lungs open, and the ductus venosus, foramen ovale, and ductus arteriosis start to close once the baby starts to breathe. After a few days to weeks, fetal circulatory anatomy will be the same as an adult's.

CLINICAL CORRELATION *In a newborn, the easiest way to gain intravenous (IV) access is through the umbilical vein in the umbilical cord's stump in which you can thread a 20-gauge IV catheter. Advance the catheter tip until it is just below the skin to avoid pushing it into the liver. Do not cut the umbilicus too short after the baby is born in case the baby needs IV access later.*

The arterial pathway of the fetus and newborn is virtually the same as that of adults. The only major exception is that each iliac artery gives off a branch that returns to the umbilicus to form the two umbilical arteries. These arteries return blood to the placenta and close shortly after birth.

CLINICAL CORRELATION *The easiest place to find a pulse in a newborn is the stump of the umbilical cord (even after it has been cut and clamped).*

Premature Infants

The normal gestational period for humans is 40 weeks. Any baby born before 38 weeks gestation—that is, more than 2 weeks early—is premature (see Chap. 5). With advances in neonatal medicine (medicine concerned with the care of newborns), babies born as early as 23 weeks' gestation and weighing as little as 500 g (about 1 lb) can be kept alive, although not without a lot of help.

The primary problem with premature infants is that their lungs have not developed enough to be useful. (Remember that the fetus wasn't planning to use the lungs until it was at least 38 weeks old.) The alveoli in the lungs (see Chap. 3) are all closed, unable to open. For the baby to have any hope of survival, the lungs need to be opened so that the baby can get oxygen.

Neonatal resuscitation teams use *surfactant*, which is naturally found in lungs and reduces *surface tension* on the alveoli, to open them. Each alveolus is like a small balloon. Surface tension pulls across the balloon's surface and tends to collapse it. Surfactant, on the other hand, reduces surface tension, making it easier to hold open the air sac. A premature infant's lungs, however, are like hot water bottles: tough to inflate and hold open (try to blow up a hot water bottle; it is much more difficult to inflate than a regular balloon). A

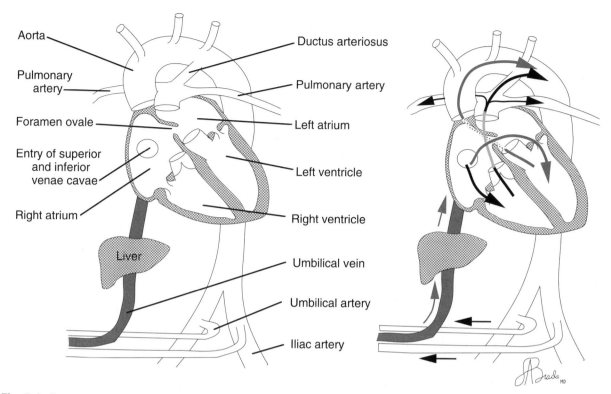

Fig. 7-2. Fetal circulation. The fetus "breathes through its liver"; oxygenated blood returning from the placenta is rerouted to the systemic circulation and away from the small pulmonary arteries via the foramen ovale and ductus arteriosus.

hot water bottle has a much higher surface tension than a balloon does. By adding surfactant, the lungs become more like balloons, which are easier to inflate.

CLINICAL CORRELATION *Surfactant is not carried routinely by most ambulances; it is used by special neonatal transport and resuscitation teams. Intubation, ventilation, and surfactant therapy keep many premature infants alive. Without surfactant, your only hope is intubation and ventilation.*

The decision of whether to resuscitate a premature infant is a difficult one. Most centers specializing in neonatal care have resuscitation guidelines based on an infant's estimated gestational age and weight at birth. This information is by and large unreliable or unavailable in the field, so, as with all resuscitations, use your local guidelines, protocols, and personal judgment to decide whether to resuscitate.

Newborn Management

Considerations for the newborn during labor and delivery are discussed in Chap. 5. Management of a newborn follows the same ABCs that govern adult care, except that in newborns, the ABCs should be thought of as: Airway, Airway, Airway, Airway, Airway, Airway, Airway, Breathing, Circulation.

With any delivery, it is important to suction out the child's airway. Recall that infants are obligate nose breathers; thus, it is important to suction the *mouth* first. If the nose is stimulated, the newborn will gasp. If the mouth has not been cleared first, the child may *aspirate*, or suck fluid into the lungs.

A major concern with newborns is aspiration of meconium (see Chap. 5). If the mother's amniotic fluid is heavily stained with dark meconium, be prepared to aggressively suction the infant's airway. Meconium in the lungs can be fatal to an infant.

CLINICAL CORRELATION *In the case of heavy meconium staining, prevent the infant from taking its first gasp by keeping it firmly wrapped in a towel immediately upon delivery. At this point, intubate the baby and apply suction to the endotracheal tube while pulling out the tube. Repeat with a new tube until you no longer see any meconium.*

As long as there is no risk of meconium aspiration, newborn care is relatively simple. The umbilical cord needs to be clamped and cut to sever the two-way blood connection with the placenta. If the baby is held high, blood can return to the placenta and the baby can effectively bleed to death. If the baby is held low, blood can flood into the baby, and he or she can "drown" from fluid overload. Avoid the risks by clamping and cutting the cord.

Babies have immature skin and cannot retain heat well; thus, it is extremely important to keep a baby warm and dry. The baby's head is disproportionately large and loses a lot of heat through it, so don't forget to place a stocking cap on the baby. The act of warming and drying a baby is usually sufficient to stimulate the baby to breathe.

If a baby has poor respiratory effort, you may need to ventilate. Babies are almost always somewhat hypoxic (have low oxygen levels) as well, so administration of supplemental oxygen is important. Babies' bodies are not habituated to high-oxygen environments, so long-term administration of 100% oxygen actually can be detrimental in the case of long interhospital transfers, especially of premature babies. In normal newborn resuscitation, however, giving excess oxygen should *not* be a concern.

CLINICAL CORRELATION *If a baby's color is poor, use "blow-by" oxygen. One easy way to do this is to take the end of oxygen tubing, cup it in your hand, and*

hold your hand near the baby's face to raise the oxygen level. Your hand also will help warm the oxygen.

Minor support with "blow-by" oxygen, brisk stimulation, and warming are usually all that is necessary for babies to spontaneously breathe adequately. It is unusual to need to intubate or ventilate a newborn. It is more unusual still to need cardiac support for a newborn. Recall (see Chap. 5) that a newborn's heart rate should be greater than 100 beats per minute. If the heart rate drops below 100, *airway* and *respiratory* support are called for. If the baby's heart rate is still below 80 after sufficient ventilation and oxygenation is established, start circulatory support (cardiopulmonary resuscitation [CPR]). If the baby's heart rate ever drops below 60, don't wait—start CPR.

CLINICAL CORRELATION *If a newborn has a clear airway and is well ventilated with extra oxygen but is still blue and floppy with a heart rate of less than 80 beats per minute, start chest compressions (CPR). If the heart rate is below 60, start CPR immediately. Do not wait until the baby is pulseless to help the heart out.*

CLINICAL CORRELATION *The last act of desperation in resuscitating a newborn is the administration of epinephrine, the preferred route being through the umbilical vein. It also can be administered through an endotracheal tube.*

HEAD, AIRWAY, AND NERVOUS SYSTEM

Bony Structure

A baby's head is proportionally much bigger than an adult's head (Fig. 7-3). As we grow, our bodies gradually catch up to our heads.

CLINICAL CORRELATION *Since a child's head is relatively big, children are more prone to head trauma than adults. Children are more likely to injure their heads rather than their necks, unlike adults. Remember: For a child or adult, treat all head injuries as if there is a neck injury as well.*

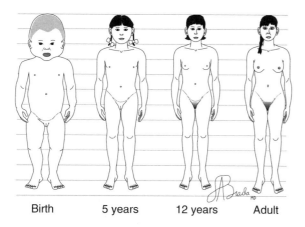

Fig. 7-3. Comparison of head size to total height at various stages of development.

Birth   5 years   12 years   Adult

Children have the same bones adults have. At birth, however, the bones of the head are not fused together, which allows the head flexibility when it descends down the birth canal (Fig. 7-4). At the junction of the frontal and parietal bones is the **anterior fontanelle**; at the junction of the parietal and occipital bones is the **posterior fontanelle**. The fontanelles gradually fill in with bone and close during the first 2 years of life. Once they close, the bones of the skull form a rigid box to protect the brain (see Chap. 2), and the brain can no longer increase in size because it has no room for expansion. While the fontanelles are still open, an increase in intracranial pressure, however, can push the fontanelles out, causing them to bulge. Likewise, too little pressure causes the fontanelles to be sucked in, or depressed.

CLINICAL CORRELATION *In infants, a bulging fontanelle is a sign of increased pressure inside the head, most likely from severe head trauma (this is bad!). A depressed fontanelle usually indicates that the baby is severely dehydrated.*

The maxilla and mandible in the skull of a child are not as large as they are in adult skulls—that is, children have relatively small faces.

Pediatric Airways

Anatomy

There are several major differences between the airway of a child and that of an adult (see Chap. 2; Table 7-1). An infant has a relatively big head, small face, big tongue, big epiglottis, high larynx, and short trachea. Also, whereas the vocal cords are the narrowest part of the airway in adults, the cricoid ring is the narrowest part of the airway in children (Fig. 7-5).

The basic principles of airway management are the same for anyone. Above all else, a patient needs a clear airway. The differences in a child's anatomy, however, leads to certain considerations (see Table 7-1), the most important being the positioning of the head to maintain an airway. Because a child's head and tongue are large and the trachea high, keep the child in a neutral, or "sniffing position," to maintain good air passage. In children, hyperextension of the head and neck may obstruct the airway.

Fig. 7-4. The neonatal skull.

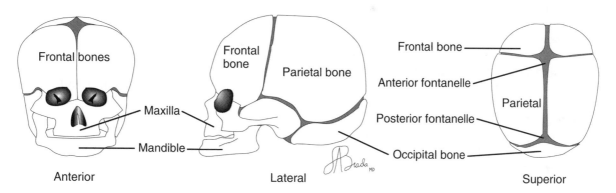

Frontal bones

Maxilla

Mandible

Anterior

Frontal bone

Parietal bone

Maxilla

Mandible

Lateral

Frontal bone

Anterior fontanelle

Posterior fontanelle

Parietal

Occipital bone

Superior

Table 7-1. Relative differences in pediatric airways

Anatomical difference	Clinical considerations
Large head	Support the shoulders and avoid hyperextending the neck to place the child in the "sniffing position."
Small face	Make sure you have the right size and shape mask for ventilations, and watch for air leaks around the face.
Big tongue Big epiglottis	Make sure you have the child in a good "sniffing position" and avoid putting any pressure on the underside of the jaw, or the airway will be blocked.
High larynx	Avoid blind finger sweeps that may lodge a foreign object in the larynx; avoid hyperextending the neck, as doing so may partially block the airway at the larynx; make sure you see the landmarks when intubating.
Short trachea	When intubating, confirm tube placement with bilateral breath sounds. Don't extend too far, and be careful of inadvertent extubation.
Narrow cricoid ring	When intubating, do not use cuffed endotracheal tubes, as the narrowest point in the airway is below the larynx.
More pliable airways	Pediatric airways are more prone to collapse than airways in adults. Children can lose an airway suddenly.
Chest wall less rigid	With a weaker chest wall, children cannot cough as effectively. Hence, they are more prone to respiratory infections that can lead to troubled breathing than are adults. Children also need less pressure and volume to ventilate than adults.

CLINICAL CORRELATION *When placing a child in the "sniffing position," support the shoulders and avoid hyperextending the neck, as doing so may partially obstruct the airway.*

The small face and large tongue are another important difference in children's anatomy. When unconscious, a child's tongue easily can cause an airway obstruction.

CLINICAL CORRELATION *When sizing a child's oropharygeal airway for tube selection (see Chap. 2), measure from the tip of the child's front teeth to the corner of the jaw. Too short an airway causes the tongue to be pushed back into the pharynx; too long an airway may cause trauma by lacerating the back of the throat.*

CLINICAL CORRELATION *Avoid pressing on the soft underside of a child's jaw because doing so may push the overly large tongue back into the airway and cause a partial obstruction.*

CLINICAL CORRELATION *Clinical rule of thumb: When sizing an endotracheal tube for a child, use the following formula:*

$$tube\ size = \frac{child's\ age + 4}{4}$$

Thus, a 4-year-old child would get a 5-mm endotracheal tube. Another guideline is to pick a tube that is the same size as the child's smallest finger.

Epiglottitis and Croup

Croup and **epiglottitis** are two problems found almost exclusively in children. Epiglottitis is inflammation of the epiglottis, usually caused by a bacterial infection. The epiglottis is relatively large in a child. When it becomes infected, it swells, which rapidly can close the airway.

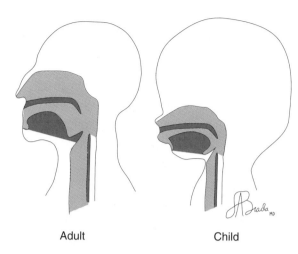

Fig. 7-5. The pediatric airway. Observe that, compared to an adult airway, a child's airway is much smaller, more anterior, and at greater risk of becoming occluded by the disproportionately large tongue.

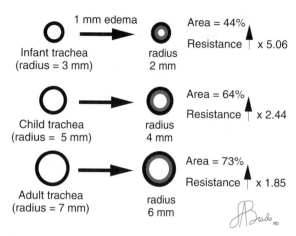

Fig. 7-6. Effects of airway edema in pediatric patients. The same degree of tissue edema (1 mm) in the airway of an infant or child affects cross sectional area (πr^2) and resistance ($1/\text{radius}^4$) more than in an adult because the proportional change is much greater. Increasing resistance greatly adds to the patient's work of breathing and easily can result in respiratory distress or failure in a small child.

Swelling in the epiglottis is problematic only in children because their airways are smaller; therefore, a little swelling causes a lot of airway obstruction (Fig. 7-6). Compare an adult airway to that of a child. The same amount of swelling in the wall of the airway causes a much greater loss of air passage in the child. (The resistance to airflow [or water flow] through a pipe is proportional to (length)/(radius)^4. This is not an important formula to memorize, but the concept is key. Firefighters who work engine pumps know that it is more difficult to pump water through small pipes. Likewise, it is more difficult to get air through small airways.) A child with epiglottitis has a very small airway made even smaller by the swelling and therefore has a difficult time moving air through it.

Epiglottitis can come on rapidly, resulting in a small change in the size of an airway that can make an extreme difference in the child's ability to move air. It usually is seen in children younger than 5 years old but can occur at any age. Children with epiglottitis naturally assume a "sniffing position" to keep their airways open. Thus, children with epiglottitis often "tripod," or sit on the edge of their seats leaning forward with their hands on their knees and their heads thrust forward. The inflammation also causes a lot of pain in the throat, so children drool because it is too painful to swallow. The narrow airway also results in inspiratory stridor (a harsh, high-pitched sound on inhalation; see Chap. 3). A swollen, inflamed epiglottis can completely shut off a child's airway.

CLINICAL CORRELATION *Epiglottitis is life-threatening to children. If you suspect it,* do not manipulate the airway in any way, *as you do not want to risk causing any spasm that might completely close the airway.* Do not upset the child, *as crying is a sure way for the child to completely lose his or her airway. Comfort the child, transport gently but quickly in a position of comfort (perhaps sitting), and give supplemental humidified oxygen. If the child goes into respiratory arrest, ventilate with 100% oxygen; you may need to "bag hard" to get air past the swollen epiglottis. Intubation is virtually impossible in such cases; the child needs a surgical airway.*

Table 7-2. Epiglottitis and croup

	Epiglottitis	Croup
Typical age of child	3–5 yrs	1–3 yrs
Infectious agent	Bacteria	Virus
Infected organ	Epiglottis	Larynx, trachea, bronchi
Time course	Rapid	Gradual
Fever	High	Minor
Stridor	Yes	Yes
Cough	Unusual	Pronounced "seal-like" bark
Drooling/tripoding	Common	Unusual
Severity	Life-threatening	Rarely serious

Croup is different from epiglottitis, but the two conditions share some similarities in that they are both upper-respiratory infections (Table 7-2). Croup is an infection of the larynx, trachea, and bronchi; hence, its medical name is *laryngotracheobronchitis*. Unlike epiglottitis, however, croup is common and rarely life-threatening. The hallmark of croup is the "barking cough."

CLINICAL   CORRELATION *Croup rarely needs specific treatment in the field. If you suspect a child has croup, consider giving supplemental humidified oxygen if warranted.*

Nervous System

Meningitis

Recall from Chap. 2 that the meninges cover the brain and spinal cord and include the dura mater, pia mater, and arachnoid. **Meningitis,** inflammation of the meninges, is potentially fatal if not treated rapidly.

Meningitis is commonly seen in infants and teen-agers. The dangerous germs that cause it usually are passed via respiratory droplets (coughing). The classic signs and symptoms are headache, stiff neck, sensitivity to light, occasionally rashes, and eventually altered mental status, seizures, and coma. These changes can come on relatively rapidly.

CLINICAL CORRELATION *Suspect meningitis in an unresponsive baby with a rash or a teen-ager with a stiff neck or who is unresponsive with a rash. Support ABCs, and protect yourself by wearing a mask and gloves.*

Seizures

Seizures are described in Chap. 2. Children can have seizures for the same reasons adults can. They are more prone, however, to two types of seizures: absence (petit mal) seizures and **febrile seizures.** Absence seizures are characterized by staring spells during which the child's brain essentially is "turned off" for a few seconds. The seizures are not alarming and do not tend to provoke 911 calls.

Febrile seizures are relatively common and *do* provoke 911 calls (*febrile* means feverish). They are caused by a rapidly increasing fever in a child, usually in the first few years of life. How hot the child finally becomes is usually not as important as how quickly the child becomes hot. Febrile seizures normally stop on their own and do not necessarily pose any immediate threat to the child. They are, however, *very* frightening to parents.

CLINICAL CORRELATION *The average ambulance response time is longer than the average duration of a febrile seizure, so it is uncommon to see a child actually seize, even though it is very common to be dispatched for it. Cool the child (but not too cold!) and support ABCs as necessary. Unlike adult patients with seizures (who routinely should get IV access and D50), advanced life support usually is not indicated in children with febrile seizures.*

CARDIORESPIRATORY SYSTEM

Respiratory Function

In early life, infants breathe strictly through their noses. Other than that, there is little difference between the mechanics of breathing for children and adults (see Chap. 3). Children are stimulated to breathe or not to breathe by the same things that stimulate adults. They also are prone to all of the same injuries. Children, however, are not prone to the same diseases as adults. The primary respiratory or lung disease seen in adults is chronic obstructive pulmonary disease (COPD), which is caused by smoking. It takes years of smoking to develop COPD, so children are too young to have it.

Alpha$_1$-antitripsin deficiency is a rare genetic (inherited) form of emphysema you may encounter in children. If you encounter it in a child in the field, treat the child as you would any patient with a COPD flare.

Asthma

Although children are too young to have COPD, they are never too young to have **asthma** (see Chap. 3), a disease in which the lower air passages—the bronchi and bronchioles—are hyperreactive. In other words, when the bronchi are stimulated, they tend to *constrict* and close. They also are prone to inflammation that causes swelling in the lower airways. Acute hyperreactive constriction that can occur in addition to swollen, irritated lower airways causes the major problem with asthma.

Children with allergies are the most likely to have asthma. The same mechanism that causes allergies (such as hay fever) also causes hyperreactivity in the airways. Allergens such as grasses, pollens, dust, dogs, cats, and molds are all common culprits that can trigger an asthma "attack," an acute episode of bronchoconstriction. During an attack, it becomes difficult for the patient to breathe and especially difficult for the patient to *exhale*. In addition to allergens, irritants such as cigarette smoke, exercise ("exercise-induced asthma"), and cold air are common triggers of asthma attacks. During exercise, patients breathe in much more deeply and quickly than normal. Outside air is usually cooler than internal body temperature and can be irritating.

CLINICAL CORRELATION *The hallmarks of an acute asthma attack are shortness of breath and expiratory wheezing. An acute attack is best treated with an inhaled (nebulized) beta$_2$-agonist such as albuterol, which causes bronchodilation.*

Another chronic illness in children that has similarities to asthma is *cystic fibrosis*, a genetic defect that makes mucus too thick. As a result, children cannot clear phlegm easily out of their lungs and are prone to constant respiratory infections and congested lungs. In a crisis, cystic fibrosis patients, like asthma patients, can be treated with oxygen and albuterol to help them breathe.

CLINICAL CORRELATION *Whatever the cause, tachypnea, or rapid respirations, is a sign of distress in a child. A breathing rate greater than 60 per minute indicates that the child is hypoxic, or not getting enough oxygen, so oxygenate.*

Sleep Apnea and Sudden Infant Death Syndrome

Two other phenomena found in children are **sleep apnea** and **sudden infant death syndrome**

Table 7-3. Ranges for pediatric vital signs

Age	Systolic blood pressure	Diastolic blood pressure	Pulse	Respirations
<30 days (newborn)	60–90	20–60	90–150	30–60
<1 yr (infant)	70–100	50–70	100–130	30–50
1–3 yrs (toddler)	80–110	50–80	100–160	20–30
4–6 yrs (preschooler)	80–110	50–80	80–110	20–25
7–12 yrs (school age)	80–120	50–80	70–100	15–20
13–18 (teen-ager)	90–140	60–80	60–100	12–16

(SIDS). Sleep apnea is a condition found in some young infants in which they stop breathing at night; their brains are not mature enough to keep them breathing all night, nor do they wake up when they are not breathing (*apnea* means not breathing). These children often are on "apnea monitors" at home that monitor the child's breathing. If the child stops breathing, the monitor goes off and awakens the parents. Once the child is stimulated, it usually breathes spontaneously again.

CLINICAL CORRELATION *If a child has sleep apnea and does not spontaneous breathe with stimulation, resuscitate it as you would any child in respiratory arrest: bag-mask ventilation with supplemental oxygen.*

SIDS, different from sleep apnea, is a horrible mystery that strikes children less than 1 year of age. By definition, SIDS is death of a child with no discernible cause. Some evidence suggests that having babies sleep on their stomachs or snugly wrapped in swaddling increases the risk of SIDS. Babies should sleep on their backs.

CLINICAL CORRELATION *SIDS babies, when found, can look horrible, as it does not take long for blood to pool on the side the baby has been lying on. (Pooling is known as* dependent lividity.*) SIDS babies look bruised and swollen—as if they were beaten, but please don't jump to any rash conclusions. Always attempt to resuscitate the infants no matter how futile it may seem, but know that your odds of success are slim to none.*

Cardiovascular Function

Vital Signs and Shock

Children do not have the same vital signs as adults. If adult standards are applied to children's vital signs, children appear as though they're in shock—that is, they have a fast pulse and respiratory rate and low blood pressure. These vital signs are normal for children, however (Table 7-3). Notice from the table that the ranges for children are large.

CLINICAL CORRELATION *Because the range of normal is so wide for children, do not "hang your hat" on any one vital sign. Instead, look at the patient as a whole and watch for changes in vital signs. Be especially worried about a change in the child's mental status.*

As in adults, the brain is the child's most sensitive organ. If the brain is hypoperfused—that is, if the child is going into shock and the brain is not getting enough blood and oxygen (see Chap. 3)—the child will begin to display changes in mental status. Unlike adults, it is useless to ask a baby, "Do you know where you are, what day is it, what's your name?" to test mental status. Instead, observe the child and talk with the parent.

CLINICAL CORRELATION *In a child, mental status changes are best determined by the parent, who can tell you that the child isn't acting the same. First, the child becomes irritable and is inconsolable by the parent. Next, the child may not recognize the parent (a bad sign). Finally, the child becomes lethargic and unresponsive.*

Children have a very dynamic circulatory system. Since children do not have heart disease the way the elderly do, their hearts and blood vessels are able to do a lot of strenuous work to meet demands placed on them; thus, children can compensate for shock extremely well (see Chap. 3) but only up to a point. When a child starts to decompensate from shock, the downhill progression can be very rapid.

CLINICAL CORRELATION *The most common cause for shock in children is hypovolemia. Unlike adults, you may not see many warning signs in a child until the he or she starts to decompensate. At this point, the child may decompensate rapidly. Be alert and prepared.*

CLINICAL CORRELATION *Early signs of shock in children are visible in the skin. Capillary refill is slow, and the child's skin color changes rapidly from pink to pale to blue or gray. The most alarming or dangerous appearance, however, is a mottled appearance with patchy areas of blue and gray skin.*

CLINICAL CORRELATION *The treatment for hypovolemic shock in children is IV fluids, 20 ml/kg—that is, a 10-kg (22-lb) baby should be given 200 ml of normal saline. You can start IVs in children, but do not let the fluid run wide open unattended, or you may rapidly overload the child with fluid. Reassess the child's status often.*

Heart Defects

Adults have heart disease from years of smoking, eating high-fat and high-cholesterol food, and not exercising enough. Children do not have this problem yet and generally do not have heart attacks, angina, or congestive heart failure as adults do. Children may, however, have congenital heart defects—that is, they may be born with hearts that don't work right.

Most children with congenital heart defects have been identified at birth. There are some, however, that may not start showing a problem until they are several months old. A common presentation is a blue baby in cardiac distress. There is no specific treatment before arriving at the hospital except to support the ABCs.

CLINICAL CORRELATION *If you have a choice of hospitals to transport patients to, it is better to transport "blue babies" to hospitals that specialize in pediatric care, such as a children's hospital. Any child in real distress should be flown, if necessary, to a children's medical center.*

CLINICAL CORRELATION *The most common cause of cardiac arrest in children is respiratory arrest. If a child appears to be having circulation problems, always check breathing first. The child's heart is probably not the cause of the circulatory problems.*

Sickle Cell Anemia

Another problem common in patients of African decent is sickle cell anemia (see Chap. 3), a genetic (inherited) disease in which the patient's red blood cells are in the shape of a sickle (a curved blade) rather than round like a doughnut. During a **sickle cell crisis,** these abnormally shaped blood cells clump up and become stuck in capillaries and small blood vessels. A sickle cell crisis usually presents as pain, often in the joints; the pain can be intense. Any blood vessels can be affected. If the lungs are affected, the patient will have the equivalent of many small pulmonary emboli (see Chap. 3) and may need extra oxygen. If blood vessels in the brain are affected, the crisis can lead to a stroke (see Chap. 2).

CLINICAL CORRELATION *Sickle cell crisis can be treated with IV hydration and O_2 if necessary.*

GASTROINTESTINAL SYSTEM, FLUIDS, AND ENDOCRINE SYSTEM

Anatomy

Children have the same organs as adults, although infants' and toddlers' livers tend to be more prominent than adults', giving them relatively large bellies.

Children have different complaints than adults. A child may not have the vocabulary or a mature enough nervous system to differentiate between feelings; therefore, a child may call almost anything a "tummy ache." Rely on your physical exam (see Chap. 4).

CLINICAL CORRELATION *Children can have acute appendicitis or a variety of other surgical emergencies. Be worried about shock if the abdomen is rigid and tender and if the child displays changes in mental status.*

Fluids

A tremendous problem seen in young children that is less common in adults is dehydration from simple illnesses. A "stomach bug," or gastroenteritis (see Chap. 4), can cause vomiting and diarrhea, problems usually dealt with easily by adults. Small children with stomach bugs, however, may not be able to drink enough to keep up with fluid loss, resulting in dehydration severe enough to cause hypovolemic shock—from simple viral infections.

CLINICAL CORRELATION *A child who looks "dry"—that is, has poor skin turgor and mottled skin, has sunken eyes and fontanelles and possibly an altered mental status, and whose parents tell you had diarrhea or had been vomiting for days—will need fluids. Oral electrolyte solutions usually are all that is necessary, but in extreme cases, give an IV bolus of normal saline or lactated Ringer's, 20 ml/kg.*

Diabetes

It is worth noting that juvenile (type I) diabetes (see Chap. 4) often shows itself for the first time when children are in their early teens. A common presentation is diabetic ketoacidosis (DKA) in a profoundly dehydrated child who is starting to go into a coma. DKA usually comes on fairly gradually, but if it has never happened before, parents will not expect it. Therefore, they may not pick up on the early signs or call for help until the child is unconscious.

CLINICAL CORRELATION *As with adults, the field treatment for DKA (hyperglycemia) is IV fluid rehydration. Start with normal saline, 10 ml/kg, and give more if necessary.*

MUSCULOSKELETAL SYSTEM

Skeleton

A child's skeleton is much more flexible than an adult's. A bone grows when the epiphyseal plate (growth plate) on the end makes new cartilage, which later fills in with hard bone (see Chap. 6).

Injuries
Because children's bones are so flexible, they are prone to "greenstick" fractures in which the bone does not break all the way through. This fracture is similar to what happens when you try to snap a "green" branch in two; because the wood is "green," it will not break all the way across.

CLINICAL CORRELATION *Fractures in children are treated in the same way as fractures in adults: ABCs first, then stabilize the extremity.*

Another injury commonly seen in toddlers is an elbow dislocation. If a child stumbles while an adult holds his or her hand, the natural response for the adult is to jerk upward to keep the child from falling. Unfortunately, while the adult pulls the hand upward and gravity pulls the child's body downward, something may give. In children, the weak point is the elbow, where the ulna dislocates from the humerus, a so-called "nursemaid's elbow."

CLINICAL CORRELATION *Splinting the arm of a child with an elbow dislocation can be difficult. Often a sling and swathe or just a swathe to keep the child immobilized is sufficient.*

Children as well as some adults (usually women) unfortunately also are subject to a form of injury not commonly seen in adult men: *nonaccidental trauma*, a polite term meaning abuse or domestic violence. By law, if you suspect a child has been the victim of abuse, you are required to report it to the appropriate authorities. Usually, clearly telling the receiving emergency room staff is sufficient.

CLINICAL CORRELATION *As an EMT, you may be able to see inside the child's home. Keep your eyes open and pay attention to what you see versus what you are told, as the mechanism of injury may not make sense. Always be suspicious of the mechanism of injury in anyone who tells you he or she "fell down the stairs." Carefully document what you see on your run sheet. Saving lives does not always involve CPR.*

Intraosseous Access

In the case of trauma, a child who has lost a significant amount of blood will go into hypovolemic shock (see Chap. 3). Although military antishock trousers (MAST) exist for children, their use is controversial because they can make it difficult for a child to breathe and may not help their circulatory status. Any patient with significant blood loss clearly needs IV fluids to avoid decompensating shock, which can lead to cardiovascular collapse and death.

Gaining IV access in children can be difficult. They are small to begin with, and if they have lost fluid, their blood vessels near the skin have vasoconstricted, making it difficult to find a vein. A quick, easy solution to administering fluids in children is to gain **intraosseous access** ("within the bone").

Recall that marrow, where blood cells are made, is found in the center of bone (see Chap. 6). Bone marrow is actually part of the body's circulatory system; therefore, there are numerous blood vessels traveling in and out of bones. Getting a needle into the bone marrow is the same as getting a needle into a vein and is most easily done in the tibia (Fig. 7-7).

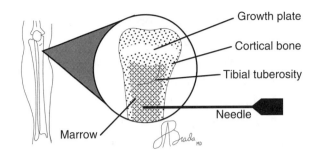

Fig. 7-7. Intraosseous access. Vascular access can be achieved in children up to 6 years of age by inserting a large-bore needle into the highly vascularized marrow space of the tibia. Proper needle positioning involves locating the tibial tuberosity and moving slightly inferiorly and medially.

CLINICAL CORRELATION *A special bone marrow needle can be inserted into the flat surface of the tibia on the anterior side (i.e., the front of the shin). The needle should be inserted one finger width (roughly 1 cm) below the tibial* tuberosity, *the bump you can feel on the front of the tibia, to avoid hitting the child's growth plate.*

The advantages to intraosseous access are that it is safe and quick. You may not be able to find a vein, but you should certainly be able to find the tibia. Any fluid or medication given intravenously can be given intraosseously.

Thermoregulation

Children regulate their body temperatures the same way that adults do (see Chap. 6), although children have relatively more surface area per body weight than adults. Since heat is transferred as a function of surface area (not as a function of volume or weight) children are more prone to the environmental extremes of hot and cold (hypothermia and hyperthermia) than are adults. The temperature control mechanism in children is also not as mature as that in an adult, so children may not realize or be able to communicate when they are too hot or cold. Remember, a sweater is something you wear when your mother is cold.

Children have one protective mechanism lost in adults: the **mammalian diving reflex,** an ancient survival reflex to keep young mammals alive if submerged in cold water that protects the brain from damage. If a child's face is submerged in cold water, the primitive reflex is triggered in the brain that tells the body to shut down. The child becomes hypothermic, heart rate slows to a near standstill, respirations stop, and most of the body's metabolism shuts down. Once rewarmed, everything may return to normal.

CLINICAL CORRELATION *Although brain damage normally occurs in adults after 3 or 4 minutes without breathing, a child submerged in cold water (for example, as a result of falling through ice on a frozen pond), may possibly be revived even if he or she has been submerged for 30 minutes or more. Never give up on a cold-water drowning, especially with a child.*

Burns

Children, like adults, are prone to burns, perhaps even more so. Toddlers reach for things they cannot see, such as coffee cups and pot handles on a stove. Spill burns on a child pose a particular problem because the hot liquids splash and may burn a large area of the child. Children also tend to look up at what they are grabbing, so their burns likely are on the face and chest.

CLINICAL CORRELATION *Facial burns should be cooled rapidly to reduce the risk of swelling around the airways.*

If a child is burned on the chest badly enough, the burned flesh may not be able to expand well. If the chest cannot expand, the child will not be able to breathe. (Recall that breathing depends on the ability to expand the chest; see Chap. 3.) A child's muscles may not be strong enough to expand the burned chest,

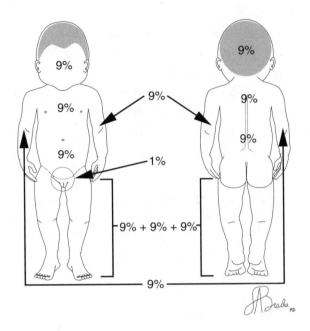

Fig. 7-8. The pediatric "rule of nines," taking into account the greater contribution of the head to body surface area.

so the child may go into respiratory arrest from the burn.

CLINICAL CORRELATION *Be prepared to assist ventilations of a child with burns to the chest, especially if they are third-degree burns.*

As with adults, the severity of a child's burn is related to the depth, or degree, of the burn, and the extent of the burn. A "rule of nines" to estimate body surface area exists for children just as one exists for adults (Fig. 7-8). According to the rule of nines for children, however, half of a nine is taken off of each leg and added to the head because babies' heads are disproportionately large. Otherwise, it follows the same rule as for adults: two nines for the head, one for the chest, one for the abdomen, one for the upper back, one for the lower back, two for the arms (one each), and three for the legs (1½ each); thus, there are 11 nines equaling 99%, plus 1% for the groin.

VOCABULARY LIST

anterior fontanelle	the "soft spot" at the junction of the frontal and parietal bones in infants
asthma	an obstructive lung disease caused by inflammation and hyperreactivity in the airways of the lungs
croup	inflammation of the larynx, trachea, and bronchi; usually caused by a virus
epiglottitis	inflammation of the epiglottis; commonly caused by a bacterial infection
febrile seizures	seizures in children caused by rapidly increasing fevers
fetus	the term for a baby developing in in the mother's uterus during the second and third trimesters
intraosseous access	placing a needle into the bone marrow to deliver fluids and medications
mammalian diving reflex	a protective reflex of young children in cold-water near-drownings
meningitis	inflammation of the meninges (membranes) that cover the brain and spinal cord
posterior fontanelle	the "soft spot" at the junction of the occipital and parietal bones in infants
sickle cell crisis	occurs in patients with abnormally sickle-shaped red blood cells that get stuck in capillaries and small blood vessels
sleep apnea	a condition in which an infant stops breathing at night while asleep
sudden infant death syndrome (SIDS)	death of an infant without any discernible cause; different from sleep apnea
umbilical vein	the blood vessel that brings oxygenated blood from the placenta into the fetus through the umbilical cord

SELF-ASSESSMENT QUESTIONS

1. While delivering a baby, you notice a lot of dark green staining of the amniotic fluid. What is the child at risk for, and what preparations do you need to make?

2. Why is it that a child with a sore throat who's drooling has a potentially life-threatening problem, while a drooling adult with a sore throat does not?

3. You are called to the house of a teen-age girl whose parents tell you she has severe asthma. Her breathing is rapid and shallow, she is straining with her neck muscles, and she has limited air movement. Expiratory wheezing is heard during a lung exam. How do you initially treat her, and what are some questions about her asthma history that might be important to you?

4. You are called to the aid of an 18-month-old boy who has been "sick" for several days. His mother tells you he has had the "flu" and a lot of vomiting and diarrhea. You find the child limp, unresponsive, warm, and dry. He has doughy skin, and his eyes appear to be sunken in. What do you need to do?

Answers to Self-Assessment Questions

CHAPTER 2

1. Your first concern is to establish and maintain an airway. Because there is significant trauma to the head, suspect cervical spine injury. Ideally, have a rescuer stabilize the patient's head while you attend to the airway. Give basic life support (BLS) first. Try to find the jaw to perform a jaw thrust, and suction with a hard catheter. The patient will need to be intubated, which is best accomplished in the field while maintaining inline stabilization of the neck. Avoid nasal intubation so that you won't intubate the brain (penetrating trauma to the head means the brain may not be well protected). If the patient is combative and you do not have drugs to sedate or paralyze him, you may have to rely on suctioning alone. A needle cricothyroidotomy is indicated if there is too much trauma to the oropharynx for intubation.

2. This woman appears to have had a stroke, or cerebral vascular accident. As always, your initial concern is managing her airway. Suction is appropriate. Consider an oral or nasal airway if she appears to have great difficulty managing secretions. Although intubation is the ultimate airway intervention, she seems to be awake and alert, meaning (1) she may not need such an invasive airway, and (2) she may not tolerate your attempt at it. Remember that just because she cannot speak doesn't mean she doesn't understand everything being said. Inability to speak is known as *aphasia*, of which there are a variety of forms. Some involve understanding language while others involve the motor skills necessary to speak. The form of aphasia depends on the part of the brain affected by the stroke. In general, however, assume that all patients can hear and understand you even if they cannot speak. Other than maintaining an airway, there is no specific treatment. Monitor her electrocardiogram (ECG) and vital signs closely and gain prophylactic intravenous (IV) access in case something else goes wrong.

3. This man is starting to have a grand mal, or generalized motor, seizure. Remember that the patient can have tonic (rigid) contractions, clonic (rapid moving contractions), or both. It is unusual but not unheard of to actually catch a seizure in progress, although it is much more common to arrive after the seizure has stopped. Your job is to stop the seizure; there are a variety of causes you can treat. The fact that he is young, slender, pale, diaphoretic (perspiring profusely), and acting strangely all point to hypoglycemia (low blood sugar), which you can treat quickly and easily (see Chap. 4). Hold his arm still and start an IV while he is convulsing and administer a rapid bolus of dextrose, which alone may stop the seizure completely. If not, try lorazepam or diazepam. Don't be too aggressive about opening an airway while he is seizing, however. Also, ECGs and blood pressure readings are profoundly unreliable (due to artifact) during a seizure. Other measures include giving oxygen and administering naloxone and thiamine.

4. The fact that the bicyclist is up, walking, and talking ("ambulatory at the scene") is reassuring. Amnesia, or loss of memory, however, is never normal and should be taken very seriously. By definition, he has at least a concussion (that is, a head injury with alteration of consciousness). He may have suffered a much worse head injury, however—namely, an epidural hematoma. Furthermore, neither you nor the patient knows how long he was unconscious; lucid periods are typical in such injuries. He needs to be convinced to be taken to the hospital for a thorough neurological examination, as he may have a neurosurgical emergency requiring immediate surgery to save his life despite his reports of feeling fine.

5. Your greatest concern is personal safety. It is likely that your patient was exposed to a toxic agent such as an insecticide that contains organophosphates. Assuming that your exposure risk is minimal, your next concern is the patient's airway (when in doubt, the answer is always either "safety" or "airway"). Organophosphate poisoning prevents the body from turning off the parasympathetic nervous system; therefore, patients with this type of poisoning have an abnormally increased parasympathetic tone. Massive salivation (drooling) is common, as is a decreased level of consciousness, so it is imperative that you suction his airway. Increased parasympathetic tone also will dangerously slow the heart, but a more immediate concern is respiratory difficulty. Parasympathetic tone causes constriction of bronchial smooth muscles—that is, the muscles constrict lower airways, as in an asthma attack. This patient needs airway maintenance, oxygen, and IV atropine (a parasympathetic blocker) to help reverse the effects of the poison on the lungs and heart.

CHAPTER 3

1. This patient was shot just to the right of the middle of the chest. Your first concern is the airway. It is possible that he injured the esophagus and may have regurgitated blood into the pharynx. This is unlikely, but nonetheless, always evaluate the patient's airway. It is more likely that the bullet hit the right lung. If the parietal pleura is punctured, the patient will have an open pneumothorax (sucking chest wound). Whether he appears to be sucking air into his wound or not, place an occlusive dressing over the hole. Additionally, he may develop a tension pneumothorax, so examine the chest closely. Look and feel for an asymmetric chest rise or tracheal deviation in the sternal notch. Listen with your stethoscope for equal lung sounds and be prepared to perform a needle chest decompression. Finally, even though the bullet entered the right side, you have no idea what path it traveled once inside the patient's body; thus, the heart or major blood vessels could be injured. Anticipate internal bleeding, start large-bore IV lines, and treat for shock.

2. When a person has a heart attack (myocardial infarction), part of the heart muscle is deprived of blood and is starting to die. If the heart attack involves damaged muscles in the left ventricle (which is common), the left ventricle may not work well, which can lead to acute (sudden) heart failure. During acute heart failure, blood backs up behind the poorly functioning left ventricle, causing fluid to accumulate in the lungs. Recall that the lungs drain fluid into the left side of the heart. Fluid build-up in the lungs leads to pulmonary edema, which can cause great difficulty in breathing. Some patients, especially the elderly, may have heart attacks without any chest pain at all.

3. Morphine benefits a person having either angina or a myocardial infarction with associated pulmonary edema. It causes venodilation, in which the major veins such as the inferior vena cava dilate and pool blood, which helps reduce the amount of fluid in the lungs. Venodilation, in turn, reduces preload, which reduces the amount of work the left ventricle needs to do. Reducing the left ventricle's workload decreases myocardial oxygen demand, which helps protect the heart from overworking, thus helping reduce damage to the heart and improving cardiac performance. Morphine also works directly to reduce the patient's perception of pain. (Decreasing the heart's workload can reduce chest pain indirectly if the pain is caused by oxygen starvation to the heart muscle.) By reducing the pain, you can poten-

tially reduce stress levels and sympathetic tone, which also reduces the heart's workload.

4. If you suspect the patient is having a heart attack (myocardial infarction), excessive PVCs are worrisome (see Fig. 3-21). PVCs may be caused by ischemic (oxygen-deprived) areas of the heart. The concern is that patients with both myocardial infarctions and excessive PVCs may go into ventricular tachycardia (V-tach) or ventricular fibrillation (V-fib) cardiac arrest.

5. By definition, the patient is symptomatically bradycardic, given that she is hypotensive and has an altered mental status. The wide-complex bradycardia is likely to be an advanced heart block (second-degree type II or third-degree) or a ventricular escape rhythm. By no means is it V-tach; thus, giving lidocaine to this woman would be a lethal error on your part. The exact type of bradycardia is not important for now. It is sufficient that she is symptomatic and needs to be treated. Give BLS first: Administer oxygen and put the patient in the Trendelenburg position. Start an IV and administer atropine. Recall, however, that atropine blocks only the vagal tone on the AV node. If she has a block in the conduction path distal to the AV node (in the His-Purkinje system) or if the AV node is permanently damaged (as from scarring from previous heart attacks), atropine probably will not work. The ventricle is innervated by the sympathetic nerves but not by the vagus nerve. So, to speed it up, she will either need to be paced, or you may have to use a beta-agonist such as epinephrine. Pacing is preferable to epinephrine because it does not cause the positive inotropic effect epinephrine causes, thus sparing the heart from any extra work.

6. This woman is having an anaphylactic reaction, which can be caused by a wide variety of foods. She needs an immediate subcutaneous shot of epinephrine, which has a mix of alpha and beta effects that work in just the right balance to counteract anaphylaxis. The alpha effect causes vasoconstriction, which reduces swelling in the airway (laryngoedema); the beta$_2$ effect relaxes the smooth muscles along the bronchi, dilating them and allowing her to breathe. The vasoconstrictive effects also help the developing hypotension caused by the swelling and hiving (angioedema).

7. This man has chronic obstructive pulmonary disease (COPD) (the home oxygen is a dead giveaway) and is having an acute exacerbation, most likely caused by a pneumonia (witnessed by the green sputum). This is an extremely common scenario. At a minimum, he needs oxygen. He may stop breathing but seems to be a candidate for intubation regardless. Next, he needs a nebulized beta-agonist such as albuterol. With his failing mental status, however, he may not have the coordination to breathe in the nebulizer. Again, be prepared to intubate and ventilate. When listening to his lung sounds, you will hear wheezes, rhonchi, and rales. Just because you hear rales, however, don't be too quick to give furosemide. In addition to CHF, pneumonia and COPD cause rales too.

CHAPTER 4

1. Always determine safety, then treat the ABCs. If the stab was the result of an upward thrust, there is a good chance the knife may have punctured the diaphragm and the pleural lining of the lungs. Watch for a pneumothorax or breathing difficulty and consider an occlusive dressing. The main organ likely to be injured is the liver, which bleeds profusely if stabbed, so watch for shock.

2. Treat the ABCs. People who vomit blood (the medical term is hematemesis) are at high risk of aspiration—that is, getting vomit into

their lungs. Suction the airway, keep patients on their sides or sitting up so vomit can drain, or intubate. The blood is most likely from a bleeding ulcer in the stomach or possibly due to ruptured (bleeding) esophageal varices. Either way, once the airway is secured, IV access and fluid replacement are your next priorities.

3. Patients with "mono" (infectious mononucleosis) develop *splenomegaly* (an enlarged spleen). Minor trauma can easily rupture an enlarged spleen. Although he may not be in much initial distress, he can rapidly bleed to death internally if he has a splenic rupture. His tachycardia (heart rate of 100) and light-headedness are early warning signs. Start two large-bore IVs and begin fluid replacement.

4. This is a typical presentation of hyperglycemic coma or possibly diabetic ketoacidosis. Diabetes is a common disease homeless people are certainly not immune to, so don't confuse his symptoms with alcohol intoxication (although both may happen at the same time). This patient's major immediate problem is dehydration from osmotic diuresis caused by hyperglycemia; therefore, he needs IV fluid rehydration. The heavy breathing is probably Kussmaul respirations, a sign of respiratory compensation for metabolic acidosis that comes about from burning proteins instead of sugar. Avoid giving bicarbonate, however, because without a formal blood gas analysis, managing acid-base disorders is hazardous to the patient.

5. A drug taken orally is absorbed by the gastrointestinal (GI) tract into the bloodstream. Recall that the blood draining the GI tract collects in the portal vein, which goes into the liver. The liver then metabolizes blood contents before blood is returned to the heart and circulated throughout the rest of the body, a process known as the "first pass effect." Anything we swallow, including oral drugs, first passes through the liver, where it often may be metabolized into something completely different before it is circulated throughout the rest of the body. When a drug is administered intravenously, it immediately enters systemic circulation, avoiding the liver completely. Paramedics generally do not give oral drugs because (1) oral drugs take too long to be absorbed, (2) the oral drug's effect is more difficult to predict because of the metabolic effects the liver has on it, and (3) the oral drug often stays in the body too long (again, because it is held up in the liver). In the case of oral verapamil, the 240-mg preparation is designed to be slowly released from the GI tract, so the pill needs to be taken only once a day for a sustained effect. It is of no use in an emergency.

CHAPTER 5

1. Crush injuries to the hips, waist, and pelvis are a common mechanism for pelvic fractures. Bleeding—internally or externally—is more likely when the external pressure that has trapped a person is removed. The external pressure, the truck in this case, acted like military antishock trousers (MAST) by applying pressure to the entire region. Treat the ABCs, take full spinal precautions, and presumptively treat for a pelvic fracture with bilateral large-bore IVs, backboard, and MAST trousers.

2. Initially, you cannot make a distinction between an abdominal problem and a pelvic problem based solely on the complaint of "pain," especially in women. Before the patient arrives at the hospital, your concerns are the ABCs. Abdominal or pelvic problems can lead to circulation problems (shock) if the patient has sustained a lot of fluid or blood loss. Ask the patient if he or she has been vomiting, vomiting blood, or had diarrhea or bloody or tarry stools. If the patient is a woman, ask also if she has had vaginal dis-

charge or vaginal bleeding and when her last menstrual period was. If you have the slightest doubt about whether a patient could go into shock, establish IV access in case the patient becomes hemodynamically unstable.

3. It is important to remember that in cases of trauma, the leading cause of death of a fetus is death of the mother. Save the mother's life first and foremost. Remember that when women are pregnant, they have vital signs that appear "shock-like"—that is, they are prone to being tachycardic and hypotensive at baseline. Don't be fooled by vital signs. Always presume pregnant women in trauma potentially are going into shock and don't dismiss their vital signs as being solely determined by pregnancy. Remember to avoid transporting pregnant women flat on their backs, as the gravid uterus will compress the inferior vena cava (the baby will push down on the blood vessels returning to the heart), causing the mother to become hypotensive (from the loss of preload). Also, the abdominal section of MAST trousers should be avoided. You can deliver a baby through MAST trousers if you have to.

4. Following delivery of the baby, the mother's uterus should continue to contract, forming an easily palpable, tight ball that can be felt above the pubic bones. If the woman's uterus is not contracting, it may be *atonic* (without tone) and continue to bleed. Increase uterine contraction by massaging the fundus, by allowing the baby to rest on the mother's chest and attempt to nurse (which stimulates natural oxytocin release), or by administering IV Pitocin, a synthetic version of oxytocin. Additionally, establish IV access and replace lost volume with lactated Ringer's.

5. Men are prone to a variety of problems affecting their groins, the most common being hernias. A hernia is protrusion of visceral contents (usually the small intestine) where they do not belong and usually happens because of defects or weak areas in the abdomen's muscular walls. Common hernia sites include into the scrotum, in the groin lateral to the penis, down into the thigh, or out the navel (umbilicus). Hernias themselves are not necessarily dangerous unless they become *incarcerated*. An incarcerated hernia is a protrusion of tissue that becomes pinched off and cannot go back where it belongs—for example, the bowel may become pinched off and not able to go back into the abdomen. The pinched bowel then starts to die and leak, or perforate, spilling bowel contents into the peritoneum, which can cause fatal peritonitis. So, if a man has a painful mass (lump) in his groin or a big bulge in his testicle, consider it a surgical emergency and get him to an appropriate hospital promptly. Testicular torsions also can present this way as a painful mass in the testicle. and are surgical emergencies. The only treatment for incarcerated hernias or torsions before arriving at the hospital is prompt recognition, IV access, and transport.

CHAPTER 6

1. Treat ABCs first (as always) and immediately control the hemorrhage. Anyone with a gunshot wound deserves bilateral large-bore IVs and rapid transport. Assuming that the patient's ABCs are otherwise stable, a gunshot wound to an extremity should be treated as a compound fracture; it is highly likely that the bone is injured, and a gunshot wound is certainly an open wound. Use a pressure bandage and splint as appropriate.

2. This was a trick question. If the player was hurt badly enough to call an ambulance, you are practically obligated to put him in a cervical collar and on a backboard, regardless of the exact mechanism of injury. It is not your job to rule out cervical spine injuries in the field. As far as his shoulder is concerned, the most likely injury is a clavicle fracture, broken rib, or shoulder separation. A backboard is sufficient treatment for any of them. Don't forget ABCs. Football field trauma also can cause a pneumothorax.

3. Almost anything could be wrong with this skier. Remember the ABCs. Establish an airway, intubate if necessary while maintaining cervical spine control, and get vital signs. Once he is stable enough, examine him. (You've got to remove all of his clothes, so make sure you're in a warm place.) Possible causes of his unconsciousness are head trauma, hypovolemia and hemorrhagic shock from internal injuries, fractures of large bones such as the femurs and pelvis, or hypothermia. Apply basics: airway, ventilation, oxygen, cervical collar and backboard, clothes off in a warm ambulance, bilateral IVs, high-flow fluids if hypovolemia or fractures are suspected, MAST trousers, and/or traction splinting as appropriate.

4. Such patients are both a frustration and a challenge for paramedics because there are a variety of things that may be going on, including hypothermia, acute intoxication, withdrawal, seizures, hypoglycemia, hyperglycemia, acute trauma, or chronic trauma (subdural hematomas). The patient described in this question is at high risk for all of these. For the sake of discussion, consider the risk of hypothermia and why this man is vulnerable. The weather conditions are perfect for hypothermia; cold, wet, and windy conditions are conducive to conductive, radiative, and convective heat loss. He is also someone who likely has impaired judgment and few options (that is, no dry clothes or warm place to go). Alcohol, in addition to impairing his judgment, causes vasodilation and increased radiative and conductive heat loss. Always consider hypothermia in such patients.

5. Treat the ABCs. He is at high risk for an inhalation injury caused by the heat and hot gasses in the fire. He likely will need to be intubated and given oxygen. His airway may swell shut from being burned by hot gasses, and it may be difficult for him to expand his ribcage with burns in this area. (Burned flesh, also known as *eschar*, is very stiff and will not move easily.) Thus, if the patient has a lot of eschar across his chest, he will not be able to expand his ribs well and will not be able to ventilate on his own. He will need to be intubated and ventilated with positive pressure. You also should be concerned about his circulatory status. Second- and third-degree burns are associated with fluid loss because the skin no longer can hold in fluid effectively; therefore, start large-bore IVs and begin fluid resuscitation as you would with any trauma patient. Also, without intact skin, the body cannot regulate heat loss, so be prepared to treat the patient for hypothermia.

CHAPTER 7

1. The dark green staining is meconium, the baby's first bowel movement. Seeing it in the amniotic fluid means that the baby was likely in some form of distress during labor. Be prepared to clear the baby's airway by getting four or more endotracheal tubes out and setting up low-powered suction. Once the baby comes out of the birth canal, rather than encouraging it to breathe, have someone rapidly wrap a towel around the baby's chest to pre-vent it from gasping and breathing in the meconium. Repeatedly intubate and suction until you get all of the meconium out of the baby's lungs.

2. A small, drooling child with a sore throat is a classic presentation for epiglottitis. (Adults do not get epiglottitis nearly as often as children.) Even slight swelling in a child's airway can cause a major airway compromise because the child has such a small airway to begin with (see Fig. 7-6), and small reductions in an airway size can lead to big increases in airway resistance.

3. You initially should treat her with a nebulized beta-agonist such as albuterol. The worst thing that could happen is that she could go into respiratory failure and no longer be able to breathe well enough for herself. Ask her or her family if she has ever been intubated before. If she has, there is the chance she may have to be intubated again by you. It is hoped that the beta-agonists will work. Remember that beta stimulation causes relaxation of bronchial smooth muscle. When bronchial smooth muscle relaxes, the bronchi become larger and the airways open more.

4. This baby is terribly dehydrated. Even without knowing any vital signs, know that any child who has lost enough fluid to become unresponsive is now in deep trouble. Start an IV and give a bolus of fluid (normal saline) at 20 mg/kg. Look in the antecubital fossa or scalp for veins. Then, get the child to a hospital with a pediatric service.

Bibliography and Recommended Reading

GENERAL EMERGENCY MEDICINE

Caroline NL. *Emergency Care in the Streets* (5th ed). Boston: Little, Brown, 1995.*

Caroline NL. *Emergency Medical Treatment: A Text for EMT-As and EMT-Intermediates* (3rd ed). Boston: Little, Brown, 1991.

U.S. Dept. of Transportation. *Emergency Medical Care.* Washington, DC: US Government Printing Office, 1983.†

Campbell JE. *Basic Trauma Life Support* (2nd ed). Englewood Cliffs, NJ: Prentice-Hall, 1988.*

Demarest JH (ed). *Pre-Hospital Trauma Life Support.* Akron, OH: Educational Direction, 1986.

GENERAL ANATOMY

Netter FH. *Human Anatomy.* Summit, NJ: Ciba-Geigy, 1989.†

Scanlon VC, Sanders T. *Essentials of Anatomy and Physiology.* Philadelphia: FA Davis, 1991.

*The best books to get, "must reading" for an active paramedic.
†Definitive books, excellent resources but more difficult to use as primary textbooks.

Philo R et al. *Guide to Human Anatomy.* Philadelphia: Saunders, 1985.

Snell RS, Smith MS. *Clinical Anatomy for Emergency Medicine.* St. Louis: Mosby, 1993.

Snell RS. *Clinical Anatomy for Medical Students* (3rd ed). Boston: Little, Brown, 1986.

GENERAL PHYSIOLOGY

Scanlon VC, Sanders T. *Essentials of Anatomy and Physiology.* Philadelphia: FA Davis, 1991.

GENERAL PHARMACOLOGY

Katzung BG (ed). *Basic and Clinical Pharmacology* (4th ed). Norwalk, CT: Appleton & Lange, 1989.

Katzung BG, Trevor AJ. *Pharmacology: Examination and Board Review.* Norwalk, CT: Appleton & Lange, 1990.

Melmon KL, Morrelli HF, Hoffman BB et al. *Clinical Pharmacology.* New York: McGraw-Hill, 1992.

HEAD AND NECK AND NEUROLOGY

Netter FH. *The Ciba Collection of Medical Illustrations. Vol. 1. Nervous System.* West Caldwell, NJ: Ciba Pharmaceutical, 1986.
Katzung BG (ed). *Basic and Clinical Pharmacology* (4th ed). Norwalk, CT: Appleton & Lange, 1989. Pp 59–69.
Reeves AG. *Disorders of the Nervous System* (2nd ed). West Lebanon, NH: Imperial, 1989.

HEART AND LUNG AND CARDIOLOGY

Netter FH. *The Ciba Collection of Medical Illustrations. Vol. 5. Heart.* West Caldwell, NJ: Ciba Pharmaceutical, 1991.
Netter FH. *The Ciba Collection of Medical Illustrations. Vol. 7. Respiratory System.* West Caldwell, NJ: Ciba Pharmaceutical, 1980.
American Heart Association. Guidelines for cardiopulmonary resuscitation and emergency cardiac care. *JAMA* 268:2135, 1992.†
American Heart Association. *Textbook of Advanced Cardiac Life Support.* Dallas: American Heart Association, 1994.
Dubin D. *Rapid Interpretation of EKG's* (4th ed). Tampa, FL: Cover Publishing, 1990.*

GASTROINTESTINAL SYSTEM, KIDNEYS, AND FLUIDS

Netter FH. *The Ciba Collection of Medical Illustrations. Vol. 3. Digestive System, Parts 1–3.* West Caldwell, NJ: Ciba Pharmaceutical, 1989.
Netter FH. *The Ciba Collection of Medical Illustrations. Vol. 6. Kidneys, Ureters, and Urinary Bladder.* West Caldwell, NJ: Ciba Pharmaceutical, 1979.
Valtin H. *Renal Function* (2nd ed). Boston: Little, Brown, 1983.
Valtin H, Gennari FJ. *Acid-Base Disorders.* Boston: Little, Brown, 1987.
Lawrence PF. *Essentials of Surgery.* Baltimore: Williams & Wilkins, 1988.

PELVIS, OBSTETRICS, AND GYNECOLOGY

Netter FH. *The Ciba Collection of Medical Illustrations. Vol. 2. Reproductive System.* West Caldwell, NJ: Ciba Pharmaceutical, 1988.
Hacker NF, Moore JG. *Essentials of Obstetrics and Gynecology* (2nd ed). Philadelphia: Saunders, 1992.

MUSCULOSKELETAL SYSTEM

Netter FH. *The Ciba Collection of Medical Illustrations. Vol. 8. Musculoskeletal System, Parts 1–2.* West Caldwell, NJ: Ciba Pharmaceutical, 1987.

PEDIATRICS

American Heart Association and American Academy of Pediatrics. *Textbook of Pediatric Advanced Life Support.* Dallas: American Heart Association, 1990.*
Silverman BK. *APLS: The Pediatric Emergency Medicine Course* (2nd ed). American Academy of Pediatrics and American College of Emergency Physicians, 1993.†
Eichelberger MR, Stossel-Pratsch G, (eds). *Pediatric Emergencies Manual.* Rockville, MD: Aspen, 1984.
Allen MC, Donohue PK, Dusman AE. The limit of viability—neonatal outcome of infants born at 22 to 25 weeks' gestation. *N Engl J Med* 329:1597, 1993.
Ponsonby AL et al. Factors potentiating the risk of sudden infant death syndrome associated with the prone position. *N Engl J Med* 329:377, 1993.

*The best books to get, "must reading" for an active paramedic.
†Definitive books, excellent resources but more difficult to use as primary textbooks.

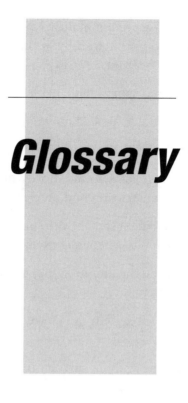

Glossary

abdomen   the "belly"; the region between the chest and pelvis defined by the diaphragm above and divided into four quadrants

abortion   any pregnancy that terminates before the fetus is viable

abrasion   superficial "scraping" wound to the skin

abruption   separation of the placenta from the uterine wall resulting in painful vaginal bleeding

absence seizure   Petit mal seizures, staring spells common in children

absolute refractory   part of the refractory period during which the cardiac

accessory muscles of respiration   muscles other than the diaphragm that can assist with breathing, including intercostal muscles, abdominal muscles, and muscles of the neck and back

acetabulum   the cuplike groove of the pelvis where the head of the femur articulates to form the hip joint

acidic/acidotic/acidosis   having too much acid (or H^+)

acromioclavicular joint   the connection between the clavicle and the acromion process of the scapula; the part of the shoulder prone to "separation"

213

adrenaline (epinephrine) a predominantly beta-sympathetic stimulant produced both naturally in the body and synthetically as a medication

adrenergic referring to the sympathetic nervous system

afterload the pressure the heart has on its outflowing side

alkalotic/alkalosis having too much base or too little acid

alpha-receptor sympathetic receptor found mostly on blood vessels; causes vasoconstriction and increases blood pressure

alveoli small, grapelike clusters at the ends of the bronchial airways in the lungs where gas exchange occurs

amniotic fluid the fluid inside the amniotic sac; formed from the urine of the fetus

amniotic sac a fluid-filled sac within the uterus in which the fetus rests

amputation a severed bone and the surrounding flesh that are no longer connected to the rest of the body

anaphylactic shock compromise, bronchoconstriction, and vasogenic shock

anaphylaxis/ a widespread allergic reaction that can cause airway
anatomical position the common reference point in describing anatomy: standing upright, with the palms facing forward

aneurysms bulging weak spots in blood vessels, especially the aorta

angina chest pain usually brought on by exercise caused by insufficient blood supply to the heart muscle

angle of the mandible the corner of the jaw

antecubital veins veins found in the antecubital fossa, or the arm in front of the elbow

anterior fontanelle the "soft spot" at the junction of the frontal and parietal bones in infants

anterior the front, or toward the front with respect to a frontal plane

anticholinergic anything that blocks the effects of the parasympathetic nervous system

anus the exit of the GI tract where stool is evacuated; found in the posterior perineum

aorta the great blood vessel that carries blood out of the left ventricle to the body

aortic dissection	a condition in which blood flows between the layers of the aortic wall rather than inside the lumen of the aorta
aortic valve	the valve on the outflow tract of the left ventricle leading to the aorta
apex	the point of a cone, top of the lungs
Apgar	scoring system to rate how well a baby is doing 1 minute and 5 minutes after birth
apnea	not breathing at all
appendix	organ attached to the large intestine in the right-lower quadrant; has no function
arterial blood	blood pumped away from the heart; when not in the lungs, arterial blood has a lot of O_2 and little CO_2
arterial blood gas (ABG)	a measurement of pH, O_2, and CO_2 in the blood that determines acid-base levels, ventilation, and oxygenation status
artery	any blood vessel carrying blood away from the heart
arytenoid cartilage	a visual landmark for intubation posterior to the vocal cords
aspiration	inhalation of fluid into the lungs, such as vomit from the stomach
asthma	an obstructive lung disease caused by inflammation and hyperreactivity in the airways of the lungs
asystole	absence of any heart contraction or electrical activity; "flatline"
atrial fibrillation (A-fib)	an abnormal tachyarrhythmia in which the atria have lost all electrical coordination; characteristically "irregularly irregular"
atrial flutter (A-flutter)	an abnormal tachyarrhythmia in which the atria rapidly contract in a "fluttering" pattern; characterized by the "sawtooth" pattern on the ECG
atrial tachycardia	an abnormal tachyarrhythmia arising from a site in the atria
atrioventricular node/ junction (AV node/) junction	the secondary pacemaker of the heart and the "gatekeeper" of electrical impulses to the ventricles
atropine	the prototype anticholinergic drug; a parasympathetic blocker

aura	a vague feeling some patients have preceding a seizure or migraine
automaticity	a characteristic of cardiac cells that allows them each to act as pacemakers
autonomic nervous system	the part of the nervous system that controls involuntary functions
avulsion	loss of soft tissue; similar to amputation but with no bone involvement
base (of the lungs)	the bottom, or inferior-most part, of the lungs
basilar skull fracture	a fracture of the bottom of the cranium
Battle's sign	ecchymosis about the mastoid; a sign of a basilar skull fracture
beta-blocker	any drug that blocks the beta responses of the sympathetic nervous system; propranolol is the prototype
beta$_1$-receptor	a sympathetic receptor found mostly in the heart; causes an increase in heart rate and force of contraction
beta$_2$-receptor	a sympathetic receptor found mostly in the lungs and bronchi; causes bronchodilation, which makes breathing easier
bigeminy	a cardiac rhythm in which every other beat is a PVC
bladder	an expandable bag in the pelvis that stores urine until it is excreted from the urethra
block	anything that prevents or slows normal cardiac conduction
bowel	small or large intestine
brachial artery	the major artery supplying the arm; a palpable pulse and pressure point in the upper arm between the biceps and triceps
bradyarrhythmia	any slow cardiac rhythm
bradycardia	slow heart rate
brain	part of the central nervous system; controls all higher functions in humans
brain stem	found at the base of the brain; connects the brain to the spinal cord; responsible for primitive body functions such as breathing and autonomic responses

Braxton Hicks contractions	false labor contractions; common in the third trimester
breech	when a baby descends the birth canal bottom or foot first rather than head first
bundle branch (left/right)	the major divisions of the bundle of His as it leads into the Purkinje fibers
bundle of His	the conduction path leading from the AV node into the Purkinje fibers
capillaries	the smallest blood vessels that connect arteries to veins; where cells exchange molecules such as O_2 and CO_2
capillary refill	the time it takes for capillaries to refill with blood after it has been squeezed out (e.g., by pressing on a finger-nail bed)
carbon dioxide (CO_2)	the gas that is the normal waste product of the body's metabolism
cardiac output	how much the heart is able to pump; stroke volume × heart rate
cardiogenic shock	shock due to failure of the heart
cardiovascular system	the circulatory system; includes the heart and blood vessels
carina	the point at which the trachea forks; the desired point for the end of an endotracheal tube
carotid arteries	the major arteries arising from the aorta that supply blood to the head and brain
carotid body/ carotid sinus	found just below the angle of the mandible; can be stimulated to produce a vagal response
carotid sinus massage	a vagal maneuver performed by briskly massaging the carotid body to slow the heart
cartilage	the smooth "gristle" on the ends of bones that allows them to move easily in joints
central nervous system (CNS)	the brain and the spinal cord
central neurogenic hyperventilation	a breathing pattern of deep, rapid breaths associated with head injuries
cerebellum	part of the brain responsible for coordination
cerebrospinal fluid (CSF)	the clear, colorless fluid that bathes the central nervous system and acts as a shock absorber

cerebrovascular accident (CVA)	a stroke; a neurological deficit caused by an area of the brain becoming ischemic
cerebrum	part of the brain responsible for higher function
cervical spine	seven vertebrae immediately below the head
cervix	the "neck" of the uterus leading into the vagina
chamber	one of the four compartments of the heart; the right and left atria and ventricles
chest wall	includes the rib cage and muscles between the ribs
Cheyne-Stokes respirations	abnormal breathing pattern in which respiratory rate speeds up, slows down, stops, starts again, and so forth.
cholinergic	referring to the parasympathetic nervous system
chordae tendinae	fibrous chords anchoring the flaps of the tricuspid and mitral valves to the papillary muscles
chronic bronchitis	an element of COPD characterized by chronic inflammation and mucus secretion in the bronchi that causes airway obstruction
chronic obstructive pulmonary disease (COPD)	chronic lung disease with elements of emphysema and chronic bronchitis; a disease that obstructs the flow of air in the lungs
chronotropy/ chronotropic	referring to the heart rate
circulatory system	the cardiovascular system; the heart and blood vessels
clavicle	the collarbone; extends from the sternum to the scapula
closed fracture	a simple fracture in which the surrounding skin is intact
coccyx	fused tailbone; the end of the spine
collateral circulation	blood vessels that develop over time to help the coronary arteries feed the heart muscle
Colles' fracture	a type of distal radius fracture commonly resulting from a fall on an outstretched hand
colloids	IV protein solutions
colon	large intestine
complete abortion	a spontaneous loss of pregnancy in which the fetus is expelled from the uterus

complex partial seizure   a seizure that starts in a focused area of the brain and causes an alteration in level of consciousness without necessarily becoming a grand mal seizure

compound fracture   an open fracture in which the surrounding skin has been broken

conduction   a mechanism of heat transfer between two touching objects

congestive heart failure   a condition in which the heart cannot effectively pump and fluid backs up behind the failing ventricle

conjunctiva   the highly vascular membrane covering the inside of the eyelid and the surface of the eye; the inside of the eyelid is normally pink

contract   the shortening of a muscle (e.g., the lowering of the diaphragm or the beating of the heart)

convection   a mechanism of heat transfer in which an object loses heat in a moving breeze or current

cor pulmonale   right-sided heart failure secondary to chronic lung disease

coronary arteries   the arteries feeding the heart muscle

crackles   sounds heard when fluid is in the lungs; rales

cranium   the bones of the head that form a rigid protective shell around the brain

cricoid cartilage   cartilage that sits anterior in the neck; lower border of cricothyroid membrane

cricothyroid membrane   a membrane stretching between the cricoid cartilage and thyroid cartilage; a good site for emergency airway access

croup   inflammation of the larynx, trachea, and bronchi; usually caused by a virus

crowning   the emergence of the baby's head from the vaginal opening during labor

crystalloids   IV salt solutions such as normal saline and lactated Ringer's

cyanosis   blue extremities (fingers, lips); a sign that an inadequate O_2 supply is being circulated

deltoid   the triangular muscle of the upper, outer arm; a common site for intramuscular and subcutaneous needle injections

depolarize	occurs when a cardiac muscle or conduction cell gets an electrical signal and then "fires" or contracts
diabetes mellitus	a disease characterized by an absence or defect in insulin function; patients untreated become hyperglycemic
diabetic ketoacidosis (DKA)	life-threatening condition possible in some diabetics whose blood sugar levels are not well controlled (that is, they are hyperglycemic); patients have metabolic acidosis and usually dehydration; treatment is IV fluid rehydration
diaphragm	the flat, dome-shaped muscle separating the thorax from the abdomen; the principle muscle of respiration
diastole	the relaxation of the heart
diastolic	during diastole
dilate/dilated/dilator	referring to the opening up, or relaxing, of a tube such as a blood vessel or a bronchus
dilation	the opening up of the cervix in preparation of delivery; complete dilation is 10 cm
dislocation	a bone coming out of a joint
distal	away from the trunk (along an extremity)
diuresis	stimulated urination (e.g., from a medication or an osmotic load in the blood)
dorsal	posterior
dorsalis pedis	artery found on the back of the foot
dura mater	"tough mother," the outermost meninge covering the central nervous system
ecchymosis	pooling of blood beneath the skin; bruising
eclampsia	the end stage of preeclampsia; seizures occurring in pregnancy
ectopic beats	any heartbeat that does not originate from the SA node
ectopic pregnancy	a pregnancy that develops outside of the uterus, commonly in the fallopian tubes
ectopy	having a lot of ectopic beats
effacement	the shortening and softening of the cervix in preparation for delivery

electrical mechanical dissociation (EMD)	a type of pulseless electrical activity of the heart (PEA)
embolus	any free-floating particle in the blood stream such as a blood clot
emphysema	an element of COPD characterized by irreversible destruction of lung/alveolar tissue
endocardium	the inside layer of the heart muscle
epicardium	the outermost layer of the heart muscle located inside the pericardial sac
epidural hematoma	collecting of blood in the epidural space secondary to trauma
epidural space	the space between the dura and the skull
epiglottis	the "flapper valve" protecting the top of the trachea
epiglottitis	inflammation of the epiglottis; commonly caused by a bacterial infection
epilepsy	a diagnosis of seizures with no other known cause
epinephrine	adrenaline, the prototype sympathetic stimulator
escape beats	abnormal beats arising from the junction or ventricles after a long pause
esophageal varices	engorged veins in the esophagus; common in alcoholics; dangerous cause of GI bleeds
esophagus	the "throat"; the soft, hollow tube connecting the mouth (oropharynx) to the stomach
estimated due date (EDD)	the approximate date a baby is expected to be delivered; 40 weeks after the LMP
estimated gestational age (EGA)	the approximate age of a developing fetus; the difference between the current date and the first day of the LMP
evaporation	a mechanism of heat transfer in which heat is absorbed by liquid as it vaporizes; heat is thereby lost from the body when sweat evaporates
expiration	exhaling, normally a passive process
extend/extension	straightening out a joint
external jugular vein	vein that runs across the sternocleidomastoid muscle; a good site for emergency peripheral intravenous line access

extracellular   outside of cells; a "fluid compartment" that includes interstitial and intravascular fluid; 20% of the body's weight is extracellular water

fallopian tubes   tubes that lead from the ovaries to the uterus in women

febrile seizures   seizures in children caused by rapidly increasing fevers

femoral artery   major artery feeding the leg; can be felt in the groin; a palpable pulse and pressure point in the groin

femoral pulse   the pulse made by the femoral artery; found in the groin

fetus   the term for a baby developing in in the mother's uterus during the second and third trimesters

first-degree atrioventricular block   mild delay through the AV node; P-R interval lengthened longer than 0.2 seconds

flail chest   two or more ribs broken in two or more places

flex/flexion   bending a joint

focus   point of origin. An ectopic focus is an abnormal point of origin for a beat within the heart

fracture   a broken bone

frontal plane   a vertical plane separating the front from the back

frontal   the bone of the forehead; part of the cranium

fundus   the part of the uterus farthest away from the mouth of the cervix

gallbladder   sac hanging below the liver that holds bile used in the small bowel for digestion; found in right-upper quadrant

gastrointestinal (GI) tract   the digestive pathway including the mouth, esophagus, stomach, and small and large intestines

genitalia   internal and external organs associated with reproduction

gestation period   the time it takes for a fetus to develop from a fertilized egg to delivery; normally 40 weeks

GI bleed   any bleed into the GI tract; commonly caused by ulcers or esophageal varices

glenohumeral joint   the joint between the humerus and the glenoid fossa of the scapula; the "ball-and-socket" joint of the shoulder; prone to dislocation

glottis	the space between the vocal cords that needs to be visualized during intubation in order to pass an endo-tracheal tube into the trachea
glucose	the form of sugar found in the blood; may be given intravenously (called dextrose or glucose)
gluteus maximus	major muscle of the buttocks; site of intramuscular injections
grand mal seizure	a primary generalized seizure characterized by periods of muscle tension and spastic movements
gravity	pregnancy, or number of pregnancies; a gravid woman is a pregnant woman; a woman who is gravida 4 has been pregnant four times
heart failure	any condition in which the heart cannot pump an adequate supply of blood, causing a backup of blood behind the side of the heart that is failing
heat exhaustion	a combination of heat and dehydration causing fatigue and possibly hypovolemia
heat stroke	a life-threatening condition in which the body loses the ability to regulate its heat loss and the patient becomes critically overheated
hemothorax	blood in the pleural space
hyperglycemia	high blood sugar; usually greater than 200 mg/dl
hypertension	high blood pressure
hypertensive	having high blood pressure
hyperthermia	the body's becoming too hot, as in heat exhaustion or heat stroke
hyperthyroid	an excess of thyroid hormone; causes an overactive metabolic state
hypertonic	more concentrated than normal body fluid
hyperventilation	too much ventilation; breathing too much, too rapidly and deeply, thereby reducing the amount of CO_2 in the blood
hypoglycemia	low blood sugar; usually less than approximately 90 mg/dl
hypotension	low blood pressure
hypotensive	having low blood pressure

hypothermia	the body's becoming too cold
hypothyroid	a deficiency of thyroid hormone; causes an underactive metabolic state
hypotonic	less concentrated than normal body fluid
hypovolemia	too little fluid in the body
hypovolemic shock	shock caused by having too little fluid in the body
hypoxia	low O_2 level
hypoxic drive	a condition found in COPD patients in which they breath only in response to low O_2 levels
iliac crests	the tips of the iliac bones of the pelvis; easily palpable on the side of the body
ilium	one of the paired bones of the pelvis that form the "waist"
inferior	toward the feet, referring to the transverse plane
inferior vena cava (IVC)	the great vein that collects blood from the lower body (except from the gastrointestinal tract)
inotropy/inotropic	how hard the heart is able to beat
inspiration	breathing in; normally accomplished by contraction of the diaphragm
insulin	hormone secreted by islet cells in the pancreas in order to control the body's blood sugar level; insulin lowers blood sugar levels by opening cells to take in sugar; diabetic patients have a defect in normal insulin function
intercostal arteries	arteries found on the bottom of each rib
intercostal retraction	contraction of the muscles of the intercostal space that aids failing respirations
intercostal space	the space between one rib and the rib above or below it; intercostal spaces are numbered by the rib above it (e.g., the second intercostal space is below the second rib)
internal jugular vein	great vein that drains the brain; best found just superior to the sternum and clavicle
internodal pathways	conduction pathways between the SA and AV nodes going through the atria
interstitial	outside of and between cells but not in blood vessels; part of the extracellular fluid compartment

intracellular	within a cell; collectively a fluid compartment; 40% of the body's weight is intracellular water
intracranial pressure (ICP)	the pressure inside the head; is elevated by any bleeding inside the cranium
intraosseous access	placing a needle into the bone marrow to deliver fluids and medications
intravascular	inside a blood vessel (artery of vein); part of the extra-cellular fluid compartment
ischemia	inadequate blood flow getting to where it's needed
ischemic	deprived of blood
isotonic	equally concentrated as normal body fluid
joint	point at which two bones come together; an articulating joint is a joint that allows motion (e.g., "ball-and-socket" shoulder, "hinge" elbow, "gliding" wrist)
jugular venous distention (JVD)	engorgement of the jugular veins, especially the internal jugular; a sign of right-sided heart failure
junctional tachycardia	an abnormal tachyarrhythmia arising from the AV junction
kidneys	paired organs in the flanks whose function is to filter blood; make urine; and regulate the body's fluid, electrolyte, and acid-base status
Kussmaul respirations	"air hunger"; deep, rapid breathing pattern
labia major/minor	two skin flaps that protect the vaginal opening; part of the external female genitalia
labor	the process of uterine contractions leading to the delivery of the baby and placenta
laceration	a jagged cut
large intestine/bowel	part of the GI tract from the small intestine out to the rectum and anus
larynx	the voice box, protected in front by the thyroid cartilage; contains the vocal cords
last menstrual period (LMP)	the first day of the last menstrual period of a woman; important in determining pregnancy status or the gestational age of the fetus
lateral	away from the midline, toward the side
left atrium	the chamber of the heart that receives blood from the lungs and passes it onto the left ventricle

left   the patient's left

left ventricle   the largest chamber of the heart; pumps blood to the body

ligaments   connective tissue that connects bones to bones across joints

liver   large, solid organ in the right-upper quadrant protected partially by ribs; has numerous metabolic functions and detoxifies whatever is eaten and drunk

lucid interval   a period of normal consciousness between an initial loss of consciousness and a coma; characteristic of epidural hematomas

lumbar spine   the large spine of the lower back

lung sounds   the sound of breathing heard when listening to lungs with a stethoscope

lungs   the organs of respiration consisting of airways (bronchi, bronchioles) and alveoli

mainstem bronchi   the two principle airways leading to each lung and arising just proximal to the carina

mammalian diving reflex   a protective reflex of young children in cold-water near-drownings

mandible   the jaw

mastoid process   the bony prominence at the base of the skull behind the ear

maxilla   the facial bones below the nose

meconium   the first bowel movement of the baby; if it occurs while the baby is still in the uterus, it will stain the amniotic fluid green-black and is a sign of fetal distress

medial   toward the midline

median   in the midline

mediastinum   the space in the chest between the lungs and the contents therein

meninges   the coverings of the brain and spinal cord

menngitis   inflammation of the meninges (membranes) that cover the brain and spinal cord; may be caused by an infectious agent

menses	the monthly "period," or cycle, in women during which the lining of the uterus is shed from the vagina if the woman is not pregnant
metabolic acidosis	acidosis for metabolic reasons such as diabetic ketoacidosis
metabolic alkalosis	alkalosis for metabolic reasons such as prolonged vomiting (loss of stomach acid)
midline	the centerline of the body, defined by the midsagittal plane, separating the body's left from right
midsagittal plane	a sagittal plane down the center of the body, separating the body's left from right
miscarriage	common term for abortion
missed abortion	a spontaneous loss of pregnancy in which the fetus remains inside the uterus
mitral valve	the valve connecting the left atrium and ventricle
myocardial infarction	"heart attack," death of heart muscle
myocardium	the heart muscle
myxedema coma	loss of consciousness accompanied by facial swelling; caused by hypothyroidism
nares	nostrils, the openings of the nose
narrow complex tachycardia	any tachycardia with a narrow QRS complex, required to classify an SVT in the field
nasal septum	the internal divider between the left and right side of the nose made mostly of cartilage
nasopharynx	the airway passage through the nose
negative chronotropic effect	anything that makes the heart beat slower
negative inotropic	anything that makes the heart beat less strong**effect**
neurogenic shock	a shock state caused by widespread vasodilation due to loss of sympathetic tone, secondary to spinal trauma
neurovascular compromise	an interruption of the nerve fibers and blood supply to a distal extremity
neutral position	neither flexed nor extended (with regard to the neck and back, hips, and wrist)

occipital	the bone on the back of the cranium
oncotic pressure	osmotic pressure created by proteins
open fracture	a compound fracture in which the surrounding skin has been broken
open pneumothorax	"sucking chest wound"; air in the pleural space caused by a penetrating (open) wound
orbits	eye sockets
organophosphate poisoning	poisoning characterized by overactive parasympathetic tone and treated with atropine
organophosphates	common poisons found in most insecticides
oropharynx	the airway passage through the mouth
orthostatic hypotension	low blood pressure when standing or sitting up
osmosis	the physical property in which a more concentrated fluid compartment sucks in water from a less concentrated compartment until the concentrations are equal
osmotic diuresis	urinary fluid loss due to osmotic pressure in the bloodstream (e.g., from severe hyperglycemia)
osmotic pressure	the pressure created by osmotic forces that pulls water into a concentrated compartment
oxygen (O_2)	the gas vital for life; 21% of the atmosphere
oxygen saturation	the percentage of red blood cells carrying O_2; a measure of oxygenation
oxygenated blood	blood with a lot of O_2 in it
oxygenation	getting O_2 into the blood; the measure of how much O_2 is in the blood
P wave	the first part of the ECG that corresponds to atrial contraction
pancreas	large gland below the stomach; secretes digestive juice into the small intestine; also has islets of Langerhans, which secrete the hormone insulin to control blood sugar levels
papillary muscles	the muscles inside the heart that keep the tricuspid and mitral valves closed during systole
paradoxical movement of the abdomen	"see-sawing" motion of the chest and abdomen accompanying respirations that occur when abdominal muscles attempt to help with failing respirations

paralysis	inability to voluntarily move something; usually the result of damage to the spinal cord
parasympathetic blocker	any drug that blocks the effects of the parasympathetic system; atropine is the prototype
parasympathetic nervous system	the part of the autonomic nervous system that tends to slow the body down, decrease heart rate, bronchoconstrict, and vasodilate
parietal pleura	the outside lining of the lung closer to the chest wall
parietal	the bones on the top of the cranium on each side
parity	delivery of a child, or number of deliveries; a multiparous woman has delivered many children, whereas a "primipara" is on her first delivery
paroxysmal	sudden onset, as in paroxysmal junctional tachycardia
pedal edema	fluid retained in the feet causing swelling
pelvic inflammatory disease (PID)	infection of the reproductive organs in women by sexually transmitted diseases
pelvis	the set of bones that forms a ring or basin housing the bladder and reproductive organs
penis	male external genitalia through which the urethra passes
pericardial tamponade	a life-threatening condition in which the pericardial sac fills with blood and compresses the myocardium
pericardium/ pericardial sac	the fibrous sac surrounding the heart
perineum	the diamond-shaped region in the groin defined by the pubis, ischia, and coccyx; where the external genitalia and anus are located
period	cells are repolarizing and heart cells are absolutely unready to depolarize (fire) again
peritoneum	the membrane lining the abdominal cavity containing most of the bowels
pH scale	a measure of acidity; the lower the number, the more acid
pharynx	the upper "throat"; the airway passage connecting the mouth and nose to the larynx
phrenic nerve	the major nerve of respiration coming off of the spinal cord at C3-4-5; innervates the diaphragm

pitting edema	any swelling (e.g., pedal edema) that leaves behind an impression, or "pit," when a finger is pressed into it
placenta previa	a condition in which the placenta implants at the bottom of the uterus near or over the cervix that results in painless vaginal bleeding; possibly life-threatening to both mother and baby
placenta	the organ that sits on the wall of the uterus pulling oxygen and nutrients from the mother's blood supply and delivering them to the fetus via the umbilical cord
pleurae	the outside linings of the lungs consisting of the visceral and parietal pleurae
pleural space	the potential space between the two pleural layers that can fill with air (pneumothorax) or blood (hemothorax)
pneumothorax	air in the pleural space
portal vein	the common vein that drains the GI tract into the liver; backs up with blood if the liver is diseased
positive chronotropic effect	anything that makes the heart beat faster
positive inotropic effect	anything that makes the heart beat harder
posterior fontanelle	the "soft spot" at the junction of the occipital and parietal bones in infants
posterior	the back, or toward the back with respect to a frontal plane
posterior tibial	artery found behind the tibia on the medial side of the ankle
postictal	a period of confusion or decreased level of consciousness immediately following grand mal seizures
postpartum	after delivery
postpartum hemorrhage	bleeding following delivery
preeclampsia	toxemia of pregnancy that can lead to uncontrolled high blood pressure and seizures
preload	the volume that fills the heart before contraction
premature atrial complex (PAC)	premature beats arising from the atria
premature beats	ectopic beats that occur earlier than expected

premature junctional complex (PJC)	premature beats arising from the AV junction
premature ventricular complex (PVC)	premature beats arising from the ventricles
prolapsed umbilical cord	a condition that is life-threatening to a fetus in which the umbilical cord passes into the birth canal first and therefore can be compressed by the head of the fetus
prone	facedown or pronated (palm down)
prostate gland	a gland that sits at the base of the bladder in men; responsible for the secretion of semen
proximal	toward the trunk (along an extremity)
pubic bones	paired bones of the pelvis that form the pubis in front
pulmonary artery	the artery carrying blood from the heart to the lungs
pulmonary edema	fluid in the lungs; usually caused by heart failure
pulmonary embolus	any embolus, such as a blood clot, that was free-floating and becomes lodged in the pulmonary artery system, preventing blood flow to that part of the lung
pulmonary veins	a set of veins that drain the lungs and return oxygenated blood to the left atrium
pulmonic valve	the valve on the outflow of the right ventricle leading to the pulmonary artery
pulse pressure	the difference between the systolic and diastolic blood pressures; may widen with increased intracranial pressure
pulseless electrical activity	heart activity that produces some form of electrical signal but not a pulse or effective circulation
puncture	a deep penetrating wound
pupil	the normally round, dark circle in the center of the eye; both pupils should become smaller when light is shined into either eye
Purkinje fibers	fibers carrying electrical impulses out into the ventricular heart muscle; the last part of the cardiac conduction system
QRS complex	the part of the ECG that corresponds to the ventricles contracting
R-on-T pattern	a pattern in which a PVC falls on the preceding beat's T wave

raccoon eyes	ecchymosis about the orbits; a sign of basilar skull fracture
radial artery	a major artery in the wrist found on the radial side (by the thumb)
radiation	a mechanism of heat transfer in which a hot object "shines off" heat
rales	sounds from the lungs heard when fluid is present in the lungs; crackles
refractory phase/period	period during which a cardiac cell repolarizes
relative refractory period	the part of the refractory period during which heart cells are normally repolarizing/relaxing; during this period heart cells are susceptible to impulses that may cause them to depolarize (fire) prematurely
repolarization	a cell's "recharging" after it has depolarized
respiratory acidosis	acidosis for respiratory reasons; inadequate ventilation and retention of CO_2
respiratory alkalosis	alkalosis for respiratory reasons; hyperventilation (e.g., whether therapeutic or caused by a head injury)
respiratory arrest	not breathing at all; failure to ventilate or oxygenate; apnea
respiratory depression	inadequate breathing; failing breathing
respiratory system	everything in the body having to do with breathing, delivering O_2 to the blood, and exhaling wastes such as CO_2
rhonchi	coarse, raspy breathing sounds due to congestion in the bronchi
ribs	bones of the chest; one pair is attached to each thoracic vertebra
right atrium	the chamber of the heart into which venous blood returns and is passed on to the right ventricle
right	the patient's right
right ventricle	the chamber of the heart that receives blood from the right atrium and pumps it into the lungs
rule of nines	a rule to estimate body surface area to quantify the extent of a burn
sacrum	the "butt bone," a fused bone of the spine between the lumbar spine and the coccyx

sagittal plane · a vertical plane separating left from right

scalp · the layers of skin stretched across the head; tends to bleed profusely if cut

scapula · the shoulder blade

sciatic nerve · a nerve that travels across the buttocks to the back of the leg; to be avoided when giving intramuscular shots in the buttocks

scrotum · a loose sac of skin containing the testicles in men

second intercostal space · below the second rib; the normal point where a needle is placed to decompress a tension pneumothorax

second-degree atrioventricular block (types I and II) · advanced blocks through the AV node where some impulses are not conducted

shock · cardiovascular failure; hypoperfusion; a condition in which not enough blood is delivered to vital tissues

sickle cell crisis · occurs in patients with abnormally sickle-shaped red blood cells that get stuck in capillaries and small blood vessels

simple fracture · a closed fracture in which the surrounding skin is intact

sinoatrial node (SA node) · the body's natural pacemaker; sinus node

sinus bradycardia · a rhythm originating from the sinus node at a rate of less than 60 beats per minute

sinus tachycardia · normal variant of sinus rhythm with a rate more than 100 beats per minute

sleep apnea · a condition in which an infant stops breathing at night while asleep

small intestine/bowel · the long section of the GI tract filling the abdomen and connecting the stomach to the large intestine; most digestion and absorption of nutrients takes place here

spinal cord · the major nervous pathway connecting the brain and the body; is protected by the spine

spine · the backbone or spinal column; a long series of vertebrae

spleen · solid organ in left-upper quadrant; part of the vascular and immune systems; destroys old red blood cells and fights blood infections

splinting	stabilization of a suspected fracture or dislocation by immobilization
spontaneous pneumothorax	a pneumothorax that forms without warning or obvious injury
spontaneous abortion	spontaneous loss of a pregnancy
status asthmaticus	an unstoppable, life-threatening asthma attack (bronco-constriction)
status epilepticus	seizures that will not stop or seizures that recur before the patient can regain consciousness
sternal angle	a palpable ridge on the sternum marking the spot where the second rib attaches to the sternum
sternal notch	the notch at the top, or superior-most part, of the sternum
sternocleidomastoid muscle	the large strap-like muscle of the neck; a landmark for the carotid artery and the internal jugular vein
sternum	breastbone; bone in the front of the chest
stomach	part of the GI tract below the heart on the left side and under the ribs; mixes food with acid and digestive enzymes
strains	"pulled" muscles
stridor	high-pitched inspiratory wheezing from upper airway obstruction
stroke volume	the volume pumped out of the heart in each beat
subclavian artery	a major artery arising from the aorta found below the clavicle that feeds the arm
subcutaneous mphysema	air underneath the skin that can indicate ae pneumothorax
subcutaneous	below the skin
subdural hematoma	bleeding into the subdural space that is usually caused by even minor trauma
subdural space	the space below the dura mater outside the brain
subluxation	a partial dislocation
sucking chest wound	open pneumothorax
sudden infant death syndrome (SIDS)	death of an infant without any discernible cause; different from sleep apnea

superior   toward the head, referring to the transverse plane

superior vena cava (SVC)   the great vein that collects blood from the arms and upper body

supine   face up (on your back), or supinated (palm up)

supine hypotension   a drop in blood pressure in pregnant women caused by the pregnant uterus compressing the IVC; occurs when pregnant women lie supine

suprasternal retraction   contraction of the neck muscles above the sternum to aid with failing respirations

supraventricular tachycardia (SVT)   an abnormally fast rhythm arising from somewhere above the ventricles (usually a narrow complex tachycardia)

sympathetic nervous system   the part of the autonomic nervous system representing the body's "fight or flight" response; its general effect is to speed the body up, increase heart rate, bronchodilate, vasoconstrict, and raise blood pressure

sympathetic tone   activation of the sympathetic nervous system, a baseline that can be increased or blocked (decreased)

sympathomimetic   any drug that mimics the sympathetic nervous system

syncope   fainting; psychogenic shock; vasovagal response

systole   the contraction of the heart

systolic   during systole

T wave   the part of the ECG that corresponds to relaxation of the ventricles

tachyarrhythmia   any abnormally fast cardiac rhythm

tachycardia   a rapid heart rate

tachypnea   rapid respiratory rate (not necessarily hyperventilating)

temporal lobe epilepsy   a common type of epilepsy that results in complex partial seizures characterized by bizarre behavior and activity not necessarily accompanied by grand mal seizures

temporal   the bones on the side of the head; the temples

tendons   connective tissues that connect muscles to bones

tension pneumothorax   a life-threatening emergency in which air fills the pleural space and collapses a lung, causing a mediastinal shift

testicles/testes	male reproductive organs contained within the scrotum; responsible for production of sperm and testosterone
thermoregulation	the mechanisms by which the body is able to maintain a normal temperature
third-degree AV block	complete block in the AV node; no electrical communication between the atria and ventricles
thoracic spine	the spine of the chest and rib cage between the cervical spine and the lumbar spine
thoracic vertebrae	the 12 bones of the spine that make up the chest
thorax	the chest, defined externally by the rib cage and internally by the organs above the diaphragm
threatened abortion	vaginal bleeding early in the pregnancy
thrombus	a blood clot
thyroid cartilage	the "Adam's apple"; cartilage in the neck that protects the larynx
thyroid gland	butterfly-shaped gland to the side of the thyroid cartilage that maintains the body's metabolic rate
thyrotoxic storm	resulting in life-threatening tachyarrhythmias
thyrotoxicosis/ trachea	an emergency caused by hyperthyroidism usually the windpipe; airway passage leading from the larynx to the mainstem bronchi
transient ischemic attack (TIA)	a "mini-stroke" similar to a cerebrovascular accident but lasting only minutes to hours and producing no permanent deficit
transverse plane	any horizontal plane across the body
triangle of auscultation	a point just medial and inferior to the bottom tip of the scapula; the best place to hear the bases of the lungs
tricuspid valve	the valve that connects the right atrium and ventricle
trimester	a third of a pregnancy's duration (3 months)
turbinates	plates on the lateral side of the nose that warm and filter air
twins	multiple birth
ulnar artery	a major artery in the wrist found on the ulnar side (by the little finger)

umbilical cord	a cord that connects the fetus with the placenta; contains one vein and two arteries; it falls off after birth, becoming the navel
umbilical vein	the blood vessel that brings oxygenated blood from the placenta into the fetus through the umbilical cord
ureter	the tube that drains urine from the kidney into the bladder (one for each kidney)
urethra	a tube coming from the bladder that allows urine to exit the body
urinary tract infection (UTI)	a bacterial infection of the bladder; common in women; it becomes serious only if the infection spreads to the kidneys or the bloodstream
uterus	the "womb" in women; a hollow organ made of smooth muscle that houses the fetus during pregnancy
vagal maneuvers	procedures that increase the body's vagal tone, or level of parasympathetic stimulus
vagal response	a response that stimulates the parasympathetic nervous system
vagina	the birth canal; an expandable passageway between the uterus and the outside world
vagus nerve	the major nerve of the parasympathetic nervous system
vallecula	the soft tissue anterior to the epiglottis that must be displaced forward during endotracheal intubation
Valsalva maneuver	a vagal maneuver performed by bearing down as if having a bowel movement
vasogenic shock	shock caused by problems with the vasculature; distributive shock
vasovagal	a response occurring after parasympathetic stimulation that causes vasodilation and usually results in a sudden drop of blood pressure and syncope (fainting)
vastus lateralis	part of the quadriceps muscle group of the thigh; site of intramuscular injections
vein	a blood vessel that carries blood back to the heart
venous blood	blood returning to the heart; blood from the body (not the lungs) has very little O_2 and a lot of CO_2
ventilation	moving air in and out of the lungs; required to "blow-off" the body's CO_2

ventral	anterior
ventricular fibrillation (V-fib)	a potentially terminal rhythm in which the heart has lost all electrical coordination
ventricular tachycardia (V-tach)	life-threatening tachyarrhythmia arising from the ventricles
vertebra	one of the bones of the spine; plural: vertebrae
visceral pleura	the outside lining of the lung that is closer to the lung itself
vocal cords	cords within the larynx that allow us to speak, appear to be a white inverted V during endotracheal intubation
Wenkebach's block	second-degree AV block type I
wheezes	expiratory lung sounds made from lower airway constriction
wide complex tachycardia	any tachycardia with a wide QRS complex; to be considered V-tach until proven otherwise
Wolff-Parkinson-White syndrome (WPW)	a syndrome caused by a bypass conduction pathway around the AV node; tends to cause tachyarrhythmias
xiphoid	the lower, or inferior-most tip, of the sternum, made of cartilage

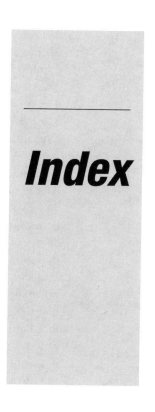

Index